POTENCY RANKING OF COMMON TOPICAL STEROIDS*

Group	Brand name	Generic name
1	Diprolene Creme	Betamethasone dipropionate
	Diprolene Ointment	Betamethasone dipropionate in optimized vehicle
	Psorcon Ointment	Diflorasone diacetate
	Temovate Cream/Ointment	Clobetasol propionate
	Ultravate Cream/Ointment	Halobetasol propionate
2	Cyclocort Ointment	Amcinonide
	Diprolene AF Cream	Betamethasone dipropionate
	Diprolene Ointment	Betamethasone dipropionate
	Elocon Ointment	Mometasone furoate
	Florone Ointment	Diflorasone diacetate
	Halog Cream	Halcinonide
	Lidex Cream/Gel/Ointment	Fluocinonide
	Maxiflor Ointment	Diflorasone diacetate
	Maxivate Ointment	Betamethasone dipropionate
	Topicort Cream/Ointment	Desoximethasone
3	Aristocort Cream	Triamcinolone acetonide
	Diprosone Cream	Betamethasone dipropionate
	Florone Cream	Diflorasone diacetate
	Halog Ointment/Solution	Halcinonide
	Lidex-E Cream	Fluocinonide
	Maxiflor Cream	Diflorasone diacetate
	Maxivate Cream	Betamethasone dipropionate
4	Aristocort Ointment	Triamcinolone acetonide
	Cordran Ointment	Flurandrenolide
	Elocon Cream	Mometasone furoate
	Kenalog Ointment	Triamcinolone acetonide
	Synalar Cream (HP)/Ointment	Fluocinolone acetonide
	Topicort LP Cream	Desoximethasone
5	Cordran Cream	Flurandrenolide
	Diprosone Lotion	Betamethasone dipropionate
	Elocon Lotion	Mometasone furoate
	Kenalog Cream/Lotion	Triamcinolone acetonide
	Locoid Cream/Ointment	Hydrocortisone butyrate
	Maxivate Lotion	Betamethasone dipropionate
	Synalar Cream	Fluocinolone acetonide
	Westcort Cream	Hydrocortisone valerate
6	DesOwen Cream/Lotion/Ointment	Desonide
	Aclovate Cream/Ointment	Aclometasone dipropionate
	Synalar Solution	Fluocinolone acetonide
	Tridesilon Cream	Desonide
7	Nutracort Cream/Lotion	Hydrocortisone

Other topicals with hydrocortisone, dexamethasone, flumethalone, prednisolone, and methylprednisolone

*Group 1 is most potent, with Group 7 being the least potent.

SKIN DISORDERS

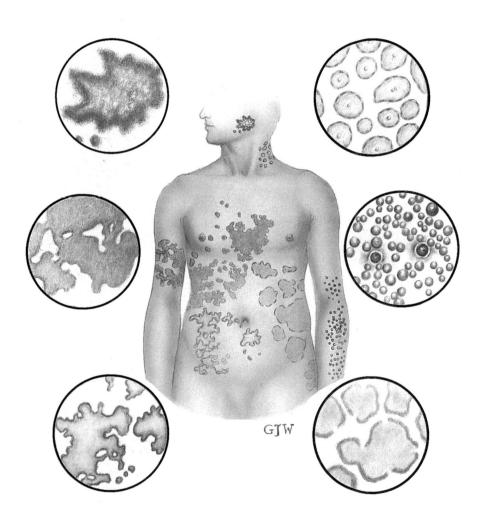

GJW

Mosby's Clinical Nursing Series

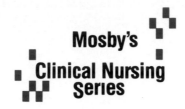

Mosby's Clinical Nursing Series

Cardiovascular Disorders
by Mary Canobbio

Respiratory Disorders
by Susan Wilson and June Thompson

Infectious Diseases
by Deanna Grimes

Orthopedic Disorders
by Leona Mourad

Renal Disorders
by Dorothy Brundage

Neurologic Disorders
by Esther Chipps, Norma Clanin, and Victor Campbell

Cancer Nursing
by Anne Belcher

Genitourinary Disorders
by Mikel Gray

Immunologic Disorders
by Christine Mudge-Grout

Gastrointestinal Disorders
by Dorothy Doughty and Debra Broadwell Jackson

Blood Disorders
by Anne Belcher

Ear, Nose, and Throat Disorders
by Barbara Sigler and Linda Schuring

Women's Health Care
by Valerie Edge and Mindi Miller

AIDS and HIV Infection
by Deanna Grimes and Richard Grimes

Skin Disorders
by Marcia Hill

SKIN DISORDERS

MARCIA JO HILL, M.S.N., R.N.

Manager, Dermatology Therapeutics,
The Methodist Hospital;
Assistant Clinical Professor, Dermatology,
Baylor College of Medicine,
Houston, Texas

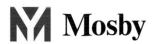 Mosby

St. Louis Baltimore Berlin Boston Carlsbad Chicago London Madrid
Naples New York Philadelphia Sydney Tokyo Toronto

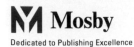

Publisher: *Alison Miller*
Editor: *Sally Schrefer*
Developmental Editor: *Penny Rudolph*
Project Manager: *Mark Spann*
Production Editor: *Stephen C. Hetager*
Manuscript Editor: *Christine O'Neil*
Layout: *Doris Hallas*
Design: *David Zielinski*
Manufacturing Supervisor: *Betty Richmond*

Composition by The Clarinda Company
Printed by Von Hoffmann Press

Printed in the United States of America

Mosby–Year Book, Inc.
11830 Westline Industrial Drive
St. Louis, Missouri 63146

ISBN 0-8016-8055-7

94 95 96 97 98   9 8 7 6 5 4 3 2 1

Contributors

Chapter 3 Diseases of epidermal origin

Noreen Heer Nicol, M.S., R.N., F.N.C.
Dermatology Clinical Specialist/Nurse Practitioner,
National Jewish Center for Immunology and Respiratory Medicine;
Clinical Senior Instructor,
University of Colorado Health Sciences Center,
Denver, Colorado

Chapter 7 Bites, stings, and infestations

Gwendolyn W. Roof, R.N., B.S.N.
Unit Manager, Medicine/Dermatology,
Parkland Memorial Hospital,
Dallas, Texas

Chapter 8 Tumors of the skin

Anne E. Belcher, Ph.D., R.N.
Professor of Oncology Nursing,
American Cancer Society;
Associate Professor,
University of Maryland School of Nursing,
University of Maryland at Baltimore,
Baltimore, Maryland

Chapter 10 Acne and rosacea

Lynda Hiatt, B.S., M.S., R.N.
Dermatology Nurse,
Dallas, Texas

Chapter 13 Drug therapy for skin disorders

Gregory D. Mudd, R.Ph.
St. Louis, Missouri

Original illustrations by

George J. Wassilchenko
Tulsa, Oklahoma
and
Donald P. O'Connor
St. Peters, Missouri

Original photography by

Patrick Watson
St. Louis, Missouri

Preface

Skin Disorders is the fifteenth volume in *Mosby's Clinical Nursing Series*, a new kind of resource for practicing nurses.

The *Series* is the result of the most elaborate market research ever undertaken by Mosby. We first surveyed hundreds of working nurses to determine what kinds of resources practicing nurses require to meet their advanced information needs. We then approached hundreds of clinical specialists—proven authors and experts—and asked them to develop a consistent format that would meet the needs of nurses in practice. This format was presented to nine focus groups composed of working nurses and refined between each group. In the later stages we published a 32-page full-color sample so that detailed changes could be made to improve physical layout and appearance, page by page.

Skin Disorders presents an overview of disorders that mainly affect the skin, accompanied by guidelines for intervention, prevention, and health promotion. The content focuses on common disorders that may be seen at any age. Rare disorders are sometimes discussed as deemed necessary for continuity. The five-step nursing process is used to outline nursing care for both specific and general skin disorders.

In response to requests from scores of nurses participating in our research, a distinctive feature of this book is its usefulness for patient teaching. Background material increases the nurse's ability to answer common patient questions with authority. The illustrations in the book, particularly those in the assessment chapter, are specifically designed to support patient teaching. Chapter 12 is a compilation of patient teaching guides that supplement the patient teaching sections of each care plan. The patient teaching guides are ideal for reproduction and distribution to patients.

Skin Disorders was written in the hope that it would give nurses in any specialty a basic reference to dermatologic nursing, assist them in providing comprehensive, scientifically based, holistic care, and stimulate them to strive for quality in nursing practice.

ACKNOWLEDGMENTS

I would like to acknowledge and thank Sally Schrefer and Penny Rudolph for their guidance during the development of this book. I want to thank Lynda Hiatt, Noreen Nicol, and Gwen Roof for their contributions.

To the most important role models in my life, my parents, I thank you. I also thank my family, Carl, Carrie, and Corbin, for their encouragement and patience during the long hours of manuscript preparation. All these individuals continually keep me striving to do my very best.

Marcia Jo Hill

Contents

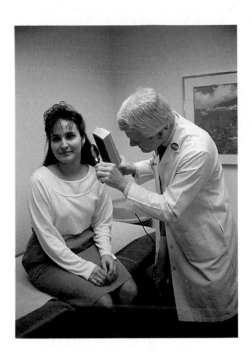

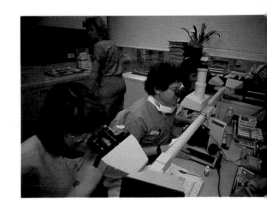

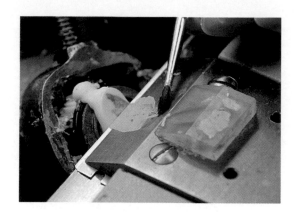

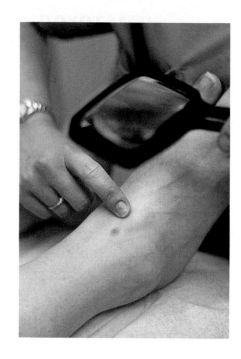

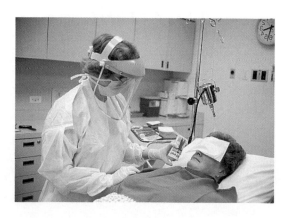

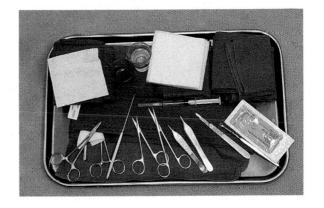

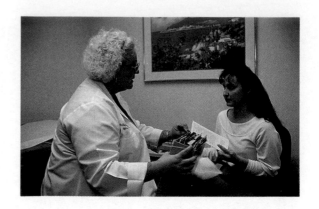

COLOR PLATES

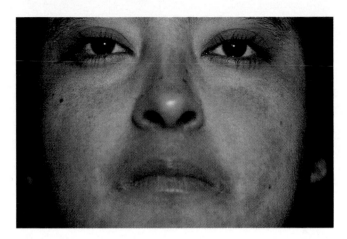

PLATE 1 Eczema of the face.

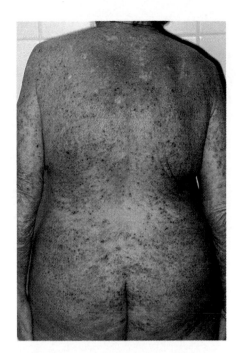

PLATE 2 Eczema of entire body.

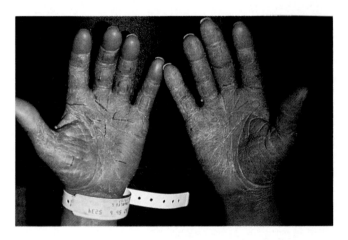

PLATE 3 Severe eczema of the hand.

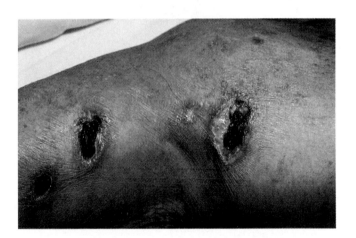

PLATE 4 Dermatomyositis.

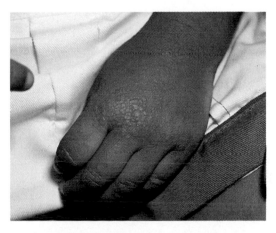

PLATE 5 Gottron's papules of dermatomyositis.

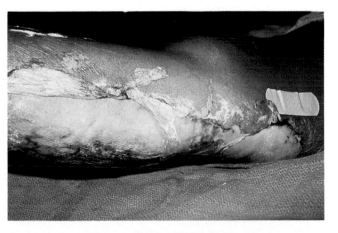

PLATE 6 *Staphylococcus* cellulitis with full thickness loss.

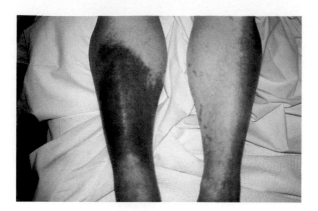

PLATE 7 Cellulitis with capillaritis.

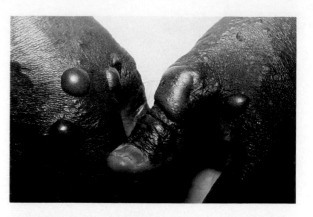

PLATE 8 Bullous pemphigoid.

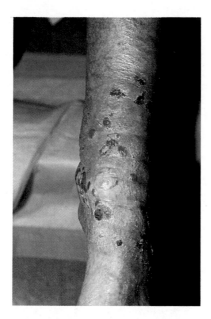

PLATE 9 Bullous pemphigoid, localized.

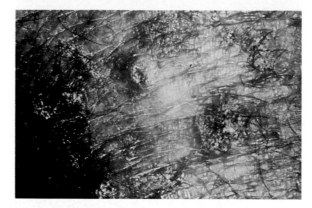

PLATE 10 Actinic keratosis.

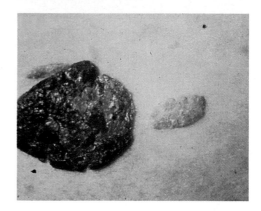

PLATE 11 Seborrheic keratosis.

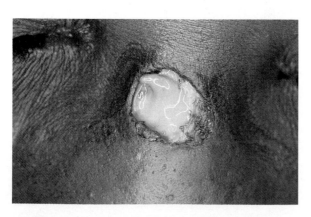

PLATE 12 Discoid lupus (neglected) with full thickness loss.

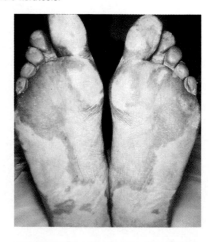

PLATE 13 Discoid lupus erythematosus.

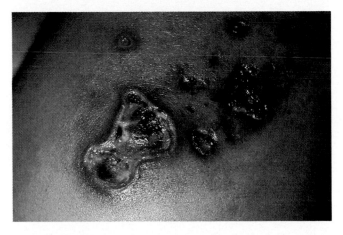

PLATE 14 Discoid lupus erythematosus.

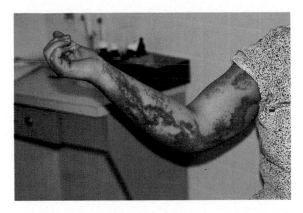

PLATE 15 Discoid lupus erythematosus with dermatomyositis.

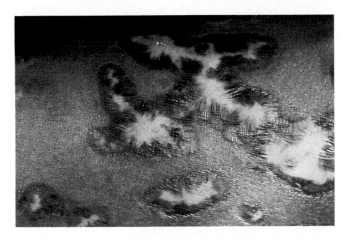

PLATE 16 Discoid lupus erythematosus on the extremity.

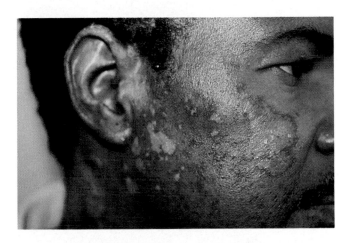

PLATE 17 Discoid lupus erythematosus on the face.

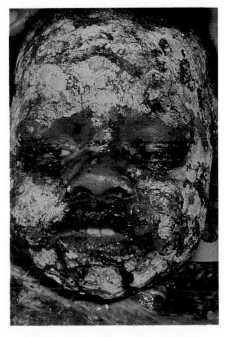

PLATE 18 Toxic epidermal necrolysis (TEN).

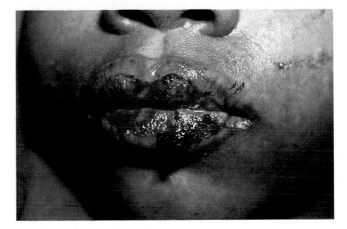

PLATE 19 Toxic epidermal necrolysis (mucous membrane involvement).

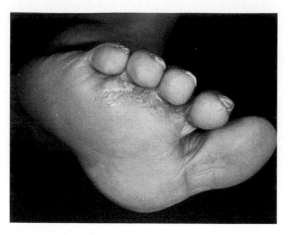

PLATE 20 Tinea pedis.

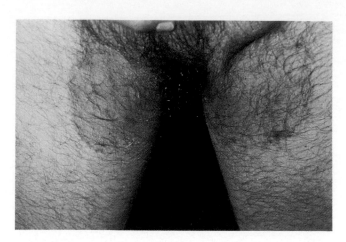

PLATE 21 Tinea cruris.

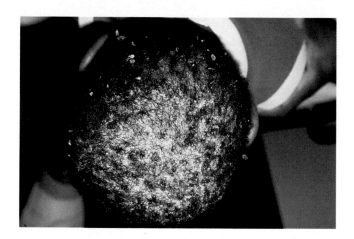

PLATE 22 Tinea capitis.

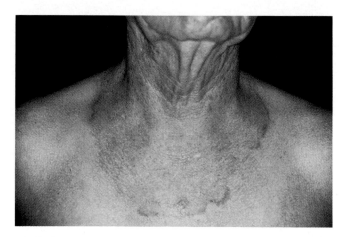

PLATE 23 Tinea corporis on the neck.

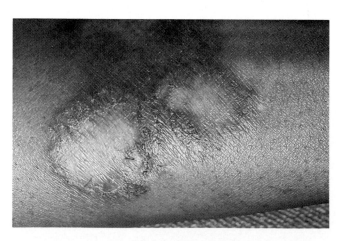

PLATE 24 Tinea corporis, classical presentation with central clearing.

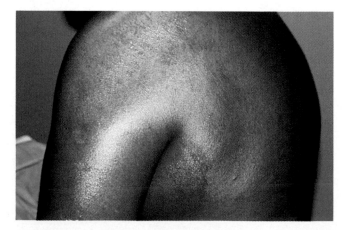

PLATE 25 Erythroderma.

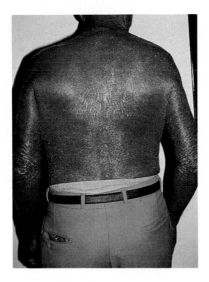

PLATE 26 Psoriatic erythroderma.

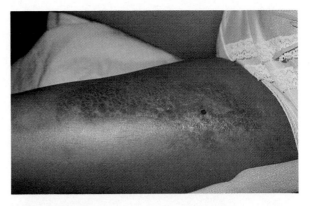

PLATE 27 Morphea.

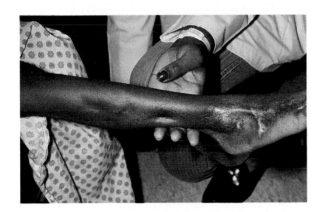

PLATE 28 Linear morphea.

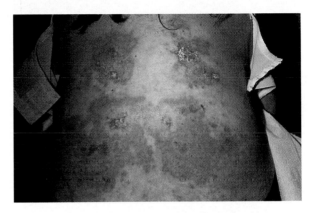

PLATE 29 Systemic lupus erythematosus on the back.

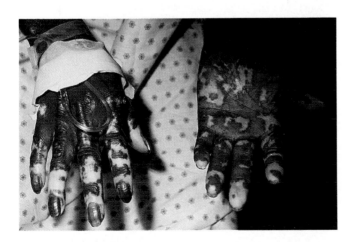

PLATE 30 Systemic lupus erythematosus in black skin.

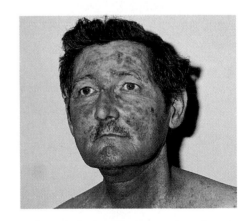

PLATE 31 Systemic lupus erythematosus, butterfly rash.

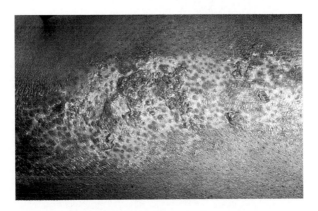

PLATE 32 Systemic lupus erythematosus, resolving ulceration.

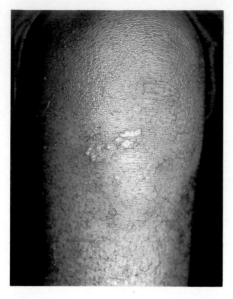

PLATE 33 Herpes simplex virus.

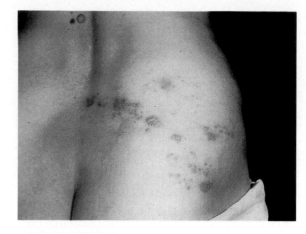

PLATE 34 Herpes zoster (shingles).

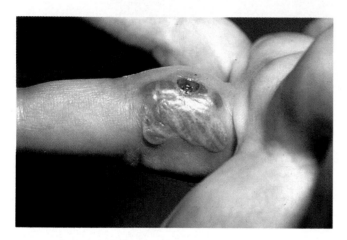

PLATE 35 Herpetic whitlow.

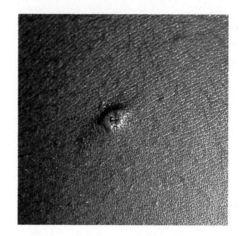

PLATE 36 Chickenpox (varicella).

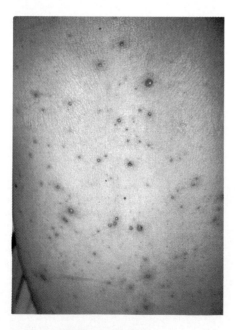

PLATE 37 Chickenpox (varicella).

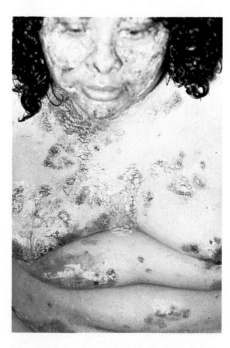

PLATE 38 Pemphigus foliaceus, generalized.

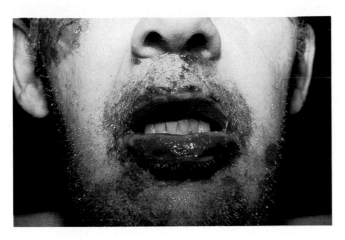

PLATE 39 Pemphigus foliaceus, mucous membrane involvement.

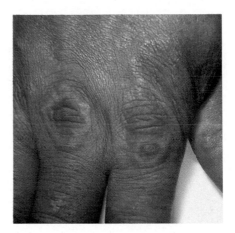

PLATE 40 Erythema multiforme in black skin.

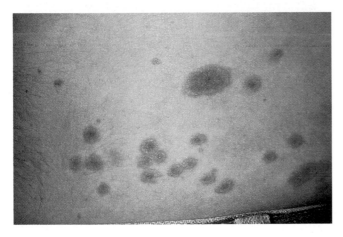

PLATE 41 Erythema multiforme in white skin.

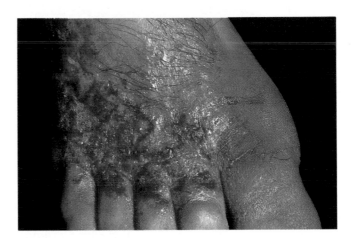

PLATE 42 Scleroderma (secondary ulceration).

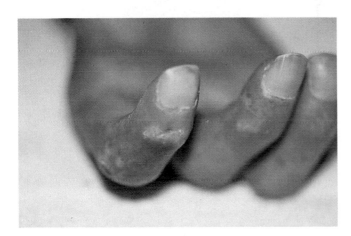

PLATE 43 CREST syndrome of scleroderma.

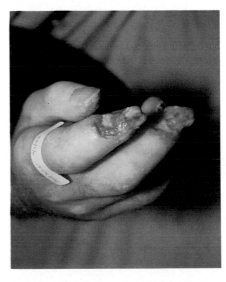

PLATE 44 Scleroderma—calcinosis cutis.

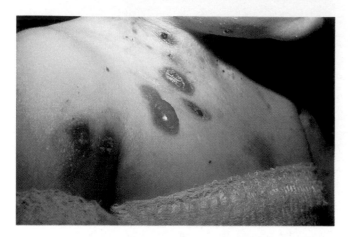

PLATE 45 Epidermolysis bullosa dystrophica on the upper trunk.

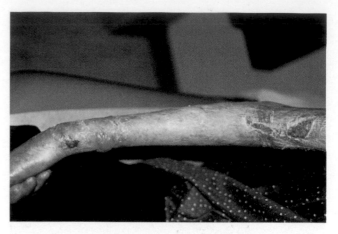

PLATE 46 Epidermolysis bullosa dystrophica, recessive.

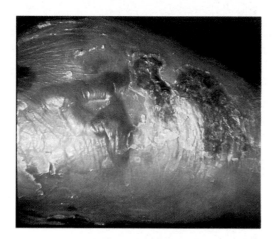

PLATE 47 Epidermolysis bullosa dystrophica, advanced involvement with scarring.

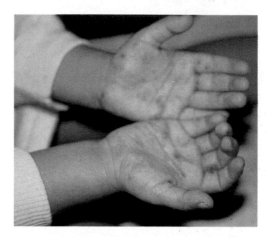

PLATE 48 Scabies, palmar involvement.

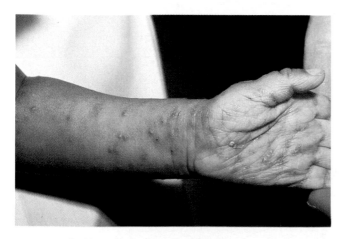

PLATE 49 Scabies with involvement of the arm.

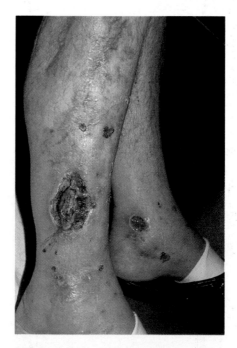

PLATE 50 Pyoderma gangrenosum.

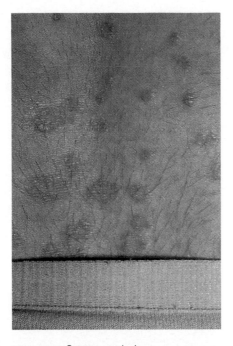

PLATE 51 Guttate psoriasis.

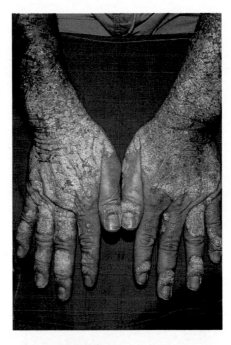

PLATE 52 Psoriasis.

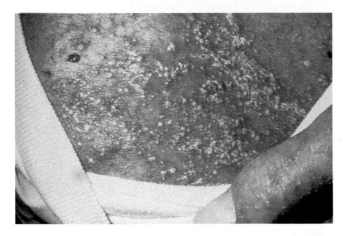

PLATE 53 Pustular psoriasis (sterile pustules).

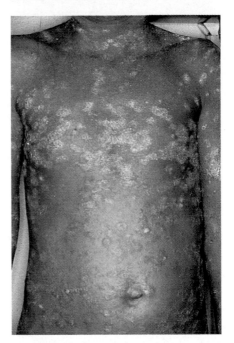

PLATE 54 Pustular psoriasis induced by systemic steroids (sterile pustules).

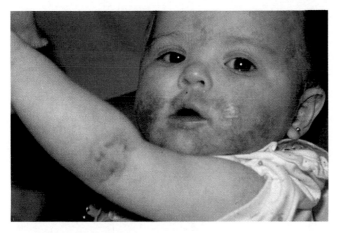

PLATE 55 Atopic dermatitis.

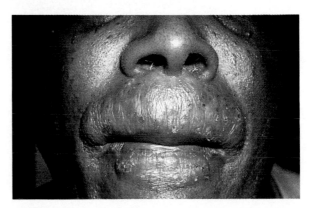

PLATE 56 Severe atopic dermatitis.

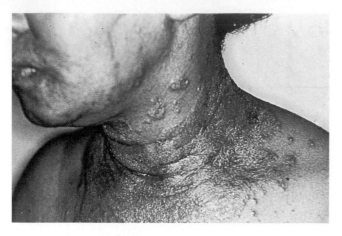

PLATE 57 Contact dermatitis.

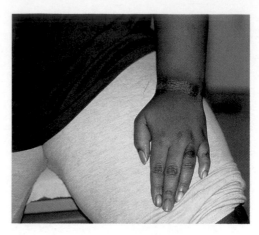

PLATE 58 Contact dermatitis—nickel.

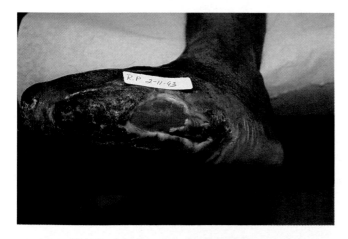

PLATE 59 Contact dermatitis—rubber.

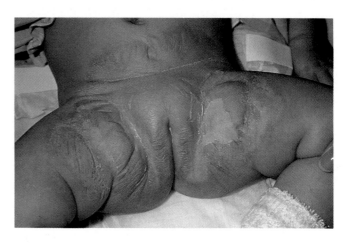

PLATE 60 Contact dermatitis, resolving.

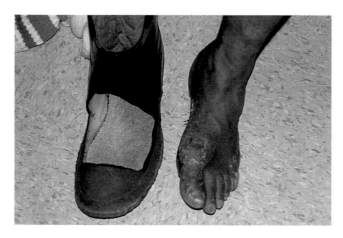

PLATE 61 Diabetic ulcer, lateral aspect of the foot.

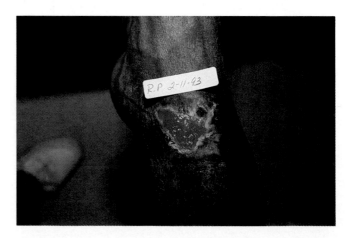

PLATE 62 Diabetic ulcer, dorsal aspect of the foot.

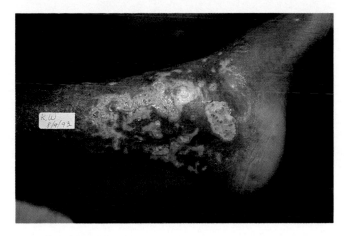

PLATE 63 Sickle cell anemia ulcer.

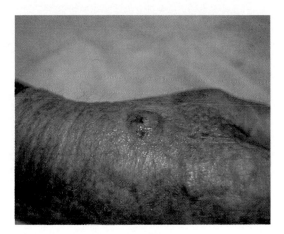

PLATE 64 Basal cell epithelioma.

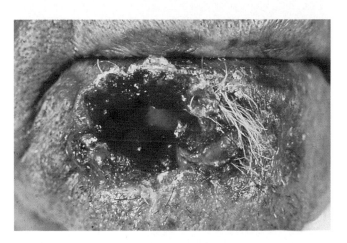

PLATE 65 Basal cell epithelioma—untreated.

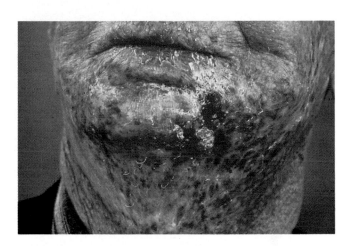

PLATE 66 Squamous cell carcinoma with extensive solar damage.

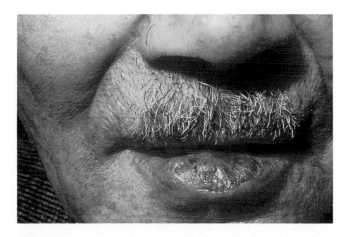

PLATE 67 Squamous cell carcinoma.

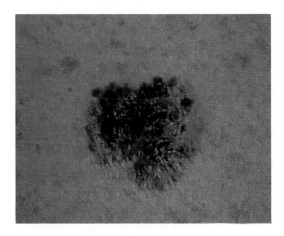

PLATE 68 Malignant melanoma.

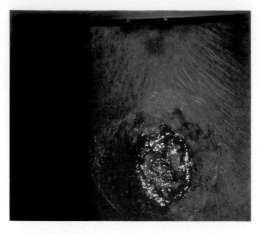

PLATE 69 Brown recluse spider bite after 48 hours of treatment. (Courtesy Dr. William N. New, Dallas, Texas.)

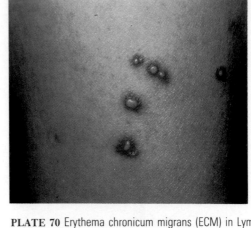

PLATE 70 Erythema chronicum migrans (ECM) in Lyme disease. (Courtesy Dermatology Department, University of Texas Southwestern Medical School, Dallas, Texas.)

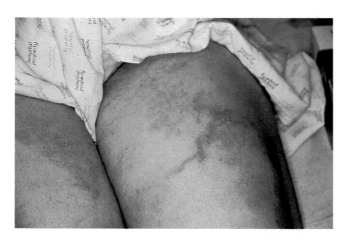

PLATE 71 Multiple bites of the imported fire ant. (Courtesy Dermatology Department, University of Texas Southwestern Medical School, Dallas, Texas.)

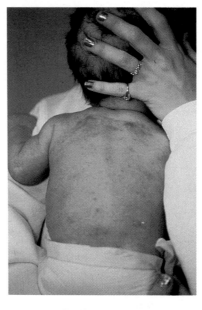

PLATE 72 Erythematous papules and burrows of scabies mite in an infant. (Courtesy Dermatology Department, University of Texas Southwestern Medical School, Dallas, Texas.)

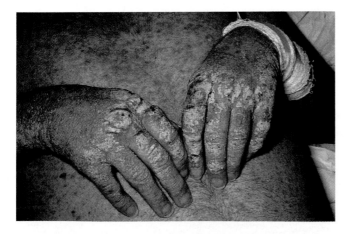

PLATE 73 Disseminated papular eruption with hyperkeratotic lesions with fissures on the hands of a patient with AIDS. (Courtesy Joseph Knipper, Parkland Memorial Hospital, Dallas, Texas.)

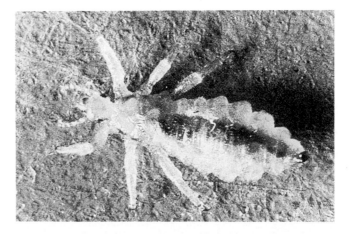

PLATE 74 *Pediculus corporis*, or body louse. (Courtesy Dermatology Department, University of Texas Southwestern Medical School, Dallas, Texas.)

CHAPTER 1

Color Atlas of the Skin

The skin (integument) and its appendages (nails, hair, and certain glands) form the largest single organ of the body. The skin ranges in thickness from less than 0.1 mm at its thinnest part to more than 1 mm at its thickest part. It is a dynamic organ composed of many types of cells whose functions are crucial to health and survival. The functions of the skin include protection, maintaining homeostasis, thermoregulation, vitamin synthesis, sensory perception, excretion, processing of antigenic substances, and cosmetic adornment. Each function correlates to specific structures and properties in the epidermis and dermis.

FUNCTIONS OF THE SKIN

Protection
Maintenance of homeostasis
Thermoregulation
Vitamin synthesis
Sensory perception
Excretion
Processing of antigenic substances
Cosmetic adornment

EPIDERMIS

The epidermis, the dermis, and the subcutaneous tissue make up the three distinct layers of the skin (Figure 1-1). The epidermis, the outermost layer of the skin, has two major regions: the inner region of viable, moist cells *(malpighian layer)* and the outer region composed of anucleated, flattened, nonviable, desiccated cells *(stratum corneum,* or *horny layer).* The basal layer *(stratum basale),* the spinous layer *(stratum spinosum),* and the granular layer *(stratum granulosum)* are the regions in which the living cells are recognized (Figure 1-2).

Keratinocytes originate in the lowermost cell layer of the epidermis (the stratum basale) and are called basal cells. Basal cells go through three stages of development—germinative, differentiation, and protective—before becoming the anucleated, flattened cells of the horny layer, or stratum corneum. Columnar basal cells in the stratum basale (germinative layer) continually divide and migrate upward, changing as they move to the skin's surface.

The process of keratinization begins in the stratum spinosum. The basal cells become polyhedral and are connected by desmosomes. Keratin filaments form in the cytoplasm, along with keratohyaline and lamellar

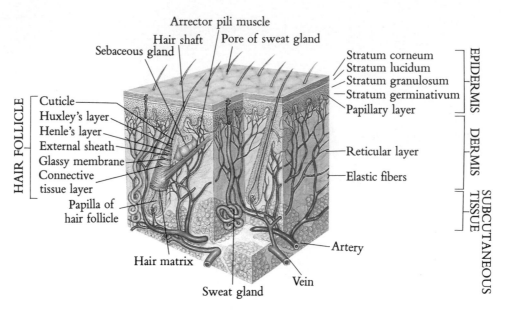

FIGURE 1-1
Anatomic structures of skin. (From Seidel et al.[59])

granules. As the cells migrate from the stratum spinosum to the stratum granulosum, they go through the final stage of keratinization. This process involves flattening and the loss of water as the intracellular substances move into the intercellular space. The nucleus is destroyed by enzymes that are released during this process. The enzymes also convert the remaining cellular contents into tough, insoluble keratin. A thickened cellular envelope of stratum corneum cells forms, with the property of extreme resistance to degradation by various chemicals.

Keratinocytes, the cells of the stratum corneum, are continually shed from the surface of the skin at a rate of 0.5 to 1 g daily, which is imperceptible. The normal cell turnover time from the stratum basale to the stratum corneum and shedding is approximately 28 days. In diseases of epidermal proliferation, such as psoriasis, this turnover time is greatly accelerated.

Of all the skin's functions, protection is the most vital. For people to survive, they must be protected from their environment. The stratum corneum provides this protection through its barrier function. Its low permeability to water retards water loss, slowing or preventing dehydration. Breaks in the stratum corneum may allow potentially dangerous substances or organisms to enter the body, setting up infection, or they may allow transepidermal water loss, which may

lead to compromised homeostasis. The efficient barrier function of the stratum corneum regulates the percutaneous absorption of topical medications. When treating extremely inflamed skin with topical steroids, it is important to remember that the barrier function of the skin is compromised, leading to increased absorption. Increased absorption can lead to the same side effects seen with systemic steroids.

SPECIALIZED CELLS OF THE EPIDERMIS

Melanocytes are found in the stratum basale (germinative layer). They synthesize yellow, red, and brown biochromes (melanin) and are the major determinants of skin color. Melanocytes also help absorb harmful solar ultraviolet radiation. Melanin is produced at a steady rate. All individuals have approximately the same number of melanocytes, and the number is not affected by either race or sex. Normal differences in skin color are determined by the intensity of pigmentation, or melanin production. Pigmentation may be influenced by ultraviolet light (tanning) or hormones (Addison's disease).

Langerhans' cells are found between the keratinized cells in the stratum spinosum. They participate in immunologic responses by reactivating lymphocytes in the epidermis in response to an antigen.

The structures found at the dermal-epidermal junc-

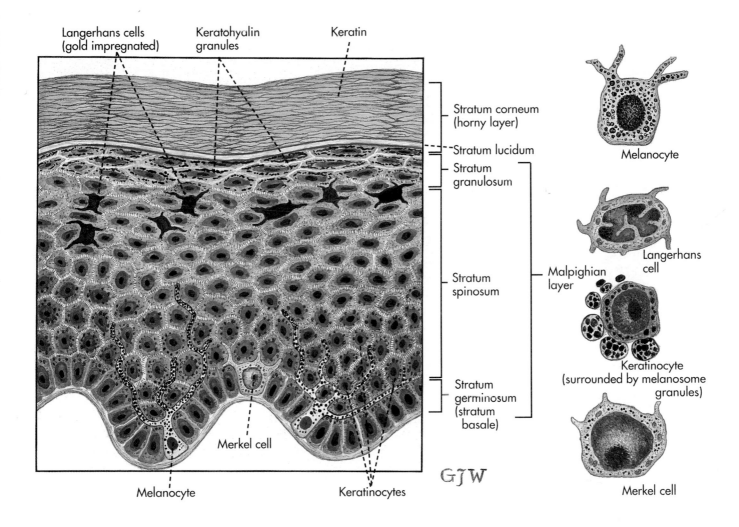

FIGURE 1-2
Structures of the epidermis.

tion cement the epidermis to the underlying dermis. These structures also act as a barrier to the movement of inflammatory and neoplastic cells between the dermis and epidermis. The upward projections seen at the dermal-epidermal junction are called *dermal papillae,* and the downward projections are called *rete ridges.* Collagen is found at the dermal-epidermal junction and helps secure the epidermis to the dermis.

Epidermal cells differentiate and specialize, some early in fetal life, to form the appendages or structures of the epidermis. These specialized cells, which are set apart from regular keratinocytes, form such things as the hair, nails, and sebaceous glands. The sweat glands, the arrectores pilorum muscles, and the sebaceous glands are also appendages of the epidermis.[48]

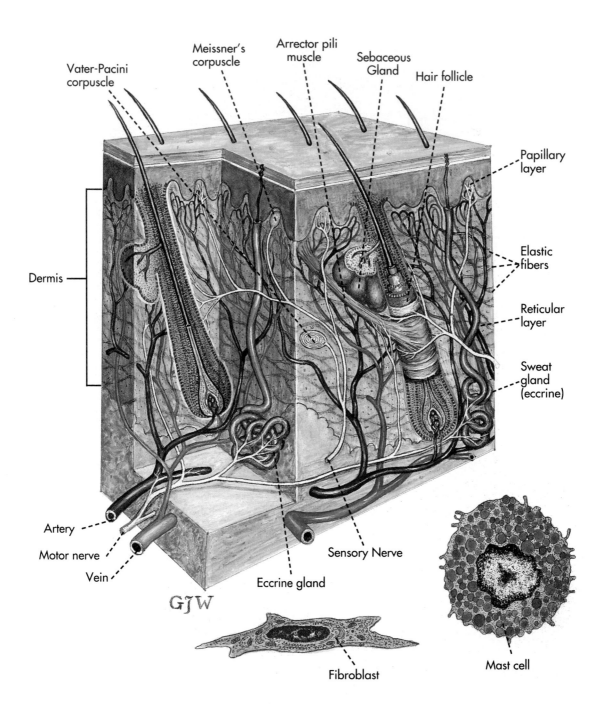

Vater-Pacini corpuscle

Meissner's corpuscle

Arrector pili muscle

Sebaceous Gland

Hair follicle

Papillary layer

Dermis

Elastic fibers

Reticular layer

Sweat gland (eccrine)

Artery

Motor nerve

Vein

Eccrine gland

Sensory Nerve

GJW

Fibroblast

Mast cell

FIGURE 1-3
Structures of the dermis.

DERMIS

The thicker layer beneath the epidermis, the dermis, gives the skin its substance, or feel. It also plays a role in the protective function of the skin by cushioning deeper structures from mechanical injury. The dermis provides nourishment to the epidermis and is important in wound healing and remodeling. It is composed of collagen and elastin fibers, which give the skin its strength and elasticity. Sweat glands and pilosebaceous units are found in the dermis, where they are provided support and protection (Figure 1-3).

The primary functional component of the dermis is the cutaneous vasculature. This vasculature consists of reticulum and elastin fibers, with the bulk of the fibers being collagen. Blood vessels, nerves, and lymphatics course through the dermis. Fibroblasts, which are also found in the dermis, have a number of functions. They help maintain the integrity of the dermis, participate in the wound healing cascade and the removal of foreign bodies, combat infections, and help mediate certain reactions of the skin that occur in the dermis.

The dermis is the structural support for the epidermis. Its makeup, especially the mucopolysaccharides, enables it to resist compression and to absorb and reduce environmental stress and strain on the body. The dermis is heavily innervated with sensory nerve fibers. Many postganglionic sympathetic fibers supply the blood vessels, sweat glands, and arrectores pilorum muscles.

SPECIALIZED CELLS OF THE DERMIS

Mast cells and *fibroblasts* are found in the dermis, with fibroblasts being the predominant cell. Fibroblasts are involved in the synthesis of collagen and elastic fibers and the ground substance. Mast cells are important in the inflammatory reaction seen in the skin. Granules within the mast cells contain heparin, histamine, and protease. Histamine increases capillary permeability and initiates vasodilation, evoking redness and edema. Granules within mast cells also synthesize leukotrienes and prostaglandins, evoking severe inflammatory reactions characterized by redness, edema, and pruritus.

Cutaneous circulation serves two distinct functions, nutritive and thermoregulatory. Nutritive arteries, capillaries, and veins, in conjunction with extensive subcutaneous venous plexus and arteriovenous anastomoses, accomplish these two important functions. Temperature is regulated through four mechanisms: (1) sweating, (2) insulation, (3) vasodilation, and (4) temperature receptors.

SUBCUTANEOUS TISSUE

The deepest layer of the skin is the subcutaneous tissue. It consists mainly of adipose tissue and sometimes is called the *adipose layer*, or *panniculus adiposus*. It varies in thickness in all areas of the body and is completely absent in the eyelids, penis and scrotum, nipples and areolae, and skin over the tibias. The distribution of subcutaneous tissue depends on secondary sex characteristics and also is influenced by age, heredity, and caloric intake. Subcutaneous tissue insulates the underlying tissues from extreme heat or cold and acts as a mechanical shock absorber.

APPENDAGES OF THE SKIN

GLANDS

Three types of glands are found in the skin: the *eccrine sweat glands*, the *apocrine sweat glands*, and the *sebaceous glands*. (Figure 1-4). Eccrine glands are part of the body's thermoregulatory system. These coiled glands are widely distributed throughout the dermis and open directly onto the skin's surface. The eccrine glands produce a hypotonic solution, which is delivered to the skin's surface and provides evaporate cooling. Production of this solution is stimulated by the hypothalamus. Increases in the body's core temperature stimulate sensors in the hypothalamus, which in turn stimulate the eccrine sweat glands. Thermoregulation is one of the skin's most important functions. If the skin is severely compromised, it becomes extremely difficult, as well as dangerous, to maintain a stable body temperature.

Apocrine glands are found in the axillae, anogenital area, mammary areolae, and external auditory canal. They produce a viscous material that causes body odor when acted upon by surface bacteria. The production of the secretory substance of the apocrine glands is controlled by both sympathetic and parasympathetic nerve fibers. The apocrine gland empties into the upper part of the hair follicle, which communicates to the skin's surface. Apocrine glands begin functioning at puberty and have no known biologic function.

Sebaceous glands are found in all areas of the skin's surface except for the palms and soles. These glands secrete a lipid substance called sebum. The size and number of sebaceous glands vary; they are most prominent on the scalp, face, and upper torso and in the anogenital region. Sebum can be delivered to the skin's surface through the hair follicle or directly by

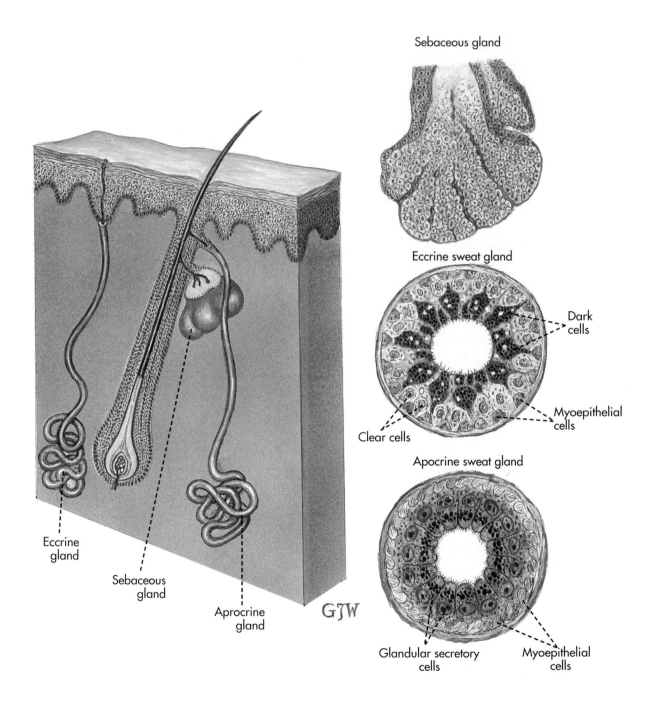

FIGURE 1-4
Structures of the glands.

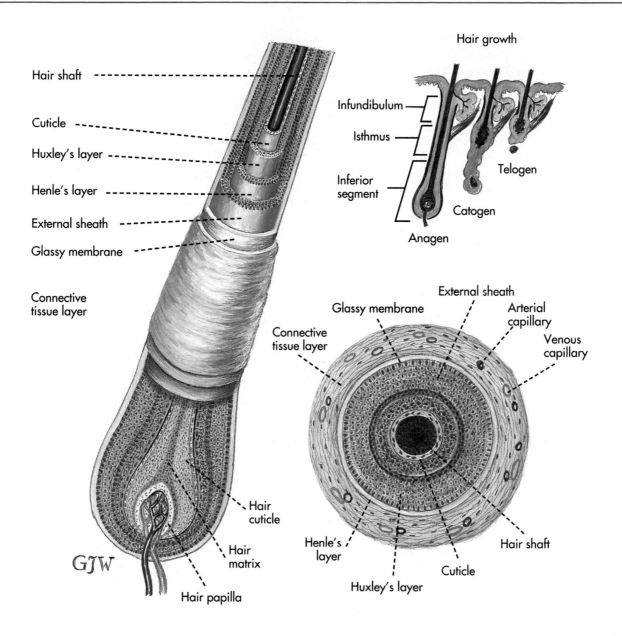

FIGURE 1-5
Structures of the hair follicle.

the sebaceous duct. Sebum may help lubricate the skin, waterproof the hair and skin, and promote the absorption of fat-soluble substances into the dermis. Sebum production is controlled by androgen, and the sebaceous glands become very active during puberty. Sebum plays a role in the production of vitamin D, and it may have some antibacterial function.

HAIR

Hair is a keratin structure of the epidermis. It is found on all parts of the body except for the palms, soles, and mucocutaneous junctions.

Hair follicles are formed in the embryo by a downward growth of epidermal cells. The epidermal cells invaginate into the dermis, forming the papilla of the hair follicle (Figure 1-5). The papilla contains capillaries that provide nourishment for mitosis, which causes the hair to grow. Stress, nutritional problems, drugs, or disease can severely alter mitotic activity and thus hair growth. The central cells of the papilla form the hair matrix, which lies deep within the subcutaneous fat. The cells of the matrix (which divide every 24 to 72 hours during anagen) form the hair shaft and surrounding structures. Melanocytes are found in the hair

---

HAIR GROWTH

Hair is in a constant state of growth, which follows a discernable pattern.

The growth process can be divided into three distinct phases: *anagen*, *catagen*, and *telogen*. Anagen (the growing phase) begins with mitotic activity in the hair bulb and dermal papilla. Catagen (regression of the hair follicle) lasts approximately 2 to 3 weeks. In this phase all mitotic activity stops. The outer root sheath degenerates, and the lower portion of the hair shaft retracts to form a club hair. Telogen (the resting phase) is characterized by cessation of all activity. The club hair formed in the catagen phase remains solidly in place during this time, until anagen begins again in the follicle, forcibly pushing the club hair out.

Hair growth is neither cyclic nor seasonal; rather, it has a mosaic pattern. At any given time, approximately 85% to 90% of the hairs on a person's body are in the anagen phase, and 10% to 15% are in the telogen phase. Normally, a person loses 50 to 100 head hairs a day.

matrix. The melanosomes are deposited in the cortical and medullary cells. Hair color is determined by the amount of melanin incorporated into the hair as it grows.

A mature hair follicle consists of a hair shaft, two surrounding sheaths, and a germinative bulb. The hair follicle is divided into three sections, the infundibulum, the isthmus, and the inferior segment. The infundibulum extends from the skin's surface to the sebaceous gland duct; the isthmus extends from the duct down to the insertion of the erector muscle; and the inferior segment extends from the muscle insertion to the base of the matrix.

Hair is dead protein and is formed by tightly packed cells covered by a cuticle of platelike scales. The hair shaft, which is formed in the hair bulb, has an outer cuticle, a cortex, and in some cases an inner medulla. The function of the cuticle is to protect the hair shaft. Cortex cells synthesize and accumulate proteins while in the lower regions of the hair follicle.

Three types of hair can be found on the body. Lanugo, the fine hair found on a fetus, is similar to the fine hairs (vellus hairs) found on adults. Terminal hairs are thick and pigmented and are found on top of the head and in the beard, axillae, and pubic area. Terminal hairs are influenced by androgens and become prominent during puberty.

The pilosebaceous unit, comprising the sebaceous gland and the arrector pili muscle, is found in conjunction with the hair follicle. As previously stated, the sebaceous gland empties sebum onto the skin via the hair follicle.

NAILS

Nails are found at the dorsal ends of the distal phalanges of each digit. The nails are formed of hard plates of tightly packed, specialized keratin. They protect the end of the digit and serve as a grasping tool. The components that make up the structure of the nail are the nail plate, cuticle (nail fold, or eponychium), paronychium, matrix, and lunula (Figure 1-6).

The nail plate is translucent and is surrounded on three sides by the cuticle (nail folds). The cuticle is made of the skin surrounding the lateral aspect (paronychium) and the proximal aspect (eponychium) of the nail plate. The nail matrix lies under the proximal nail fold; its keratin layer extends onto the proximal nail plate and forms the cuticle. The vasculature in the proximal nail fold includes capillary loops at the tip, which usually cannot be seen. The capillaries become apparent with such diseases as systemic lupus erythematosus (SLE) and scleroderma. The nail matrix epithelium synthesizes 90% of the nail plate. The lunula is the white, crescent-shaped area at the end of the proximal nail fold. It marks the end of the nail matrix and is the site of mitosis and nail growth.

FUNCTIONS OF THE SKIN

As mentioned previously, the skin has distinct and important functions: protection, maintaining homeostasis, thermoregulation, tissue repair, vitamin D synthesis, sensory perception, and psychosocial function. It protects the body against a hostile environment by creating a physical barrier against the invasion of bacteria, viral pathogens, foreign substances, and physical trauma. Invasion of microorganisms is retarded by the intact, dry stratum corneum and the skin's immune system, with the primary line of defense being an intact stratum corneum. Sebum, which is secreted onto the skin via the hair follicles and by the sebaceous glands, provides an acid coating with a pH between 4 and 6.8. This acidity, in conjunction with natural antibacterial substances in the sebum, retards the growth of microorganisms. The glandular secretions, which wash away microorganisms from the pores, and colo-

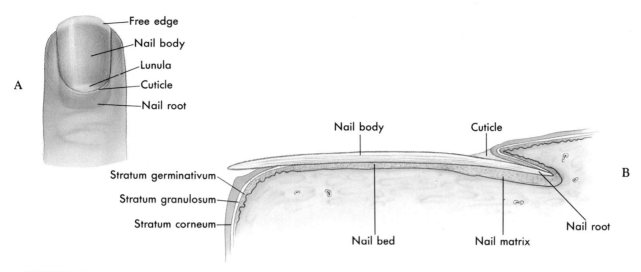

FIGURE 1-6
Structures of the nails. **A,** Fingernail viewed from above. **B,** Sagittal section of fingernail and associated structures. (From Thibodeau and Patton.[62])

nies of nonpathogenic bacteria (normal flora) on the skin help keep bacterial growth down through bacterial interference. The lymphatic and vascular tissues in the dermis respond to injury, inflammation, and infection. Langerhans' cells (antigen-presenting cells) of the epidermis are active in protection. Macrophages, which ingest and digest bacteria, and mast cells, which contain histamine, are found in the dermis and are also active in the protective function of the skin. Hairs in the nose, ears, anogenital area, eyebrows, and eyelids act as barriers against the entry of foreign materials. The keratin of the epidermis provides protection against corrosive materials, and strong intracellular bonds give skin mechanical strength. Thickening of the stratum corneum, dispersion of ultraviolet radiation, and increased melanin production protect deoxyribonucleic acid (DNA) from damage. Collagen, elastin, and ground substance in the dermis also function to protect. The subcutaneous tissue acts as a shock absorber.

As part of its barrier function, the skin impedes water loss and thus dehydration and maintains homeostasis. The epidermis, with its low permeability to water and electrolytes, provides a rate-limiting barrier to the diffusion of water, electrolytes, and nonpolar substances. The secretions from the sebaceous glands, in addition to preventing water loss, help waterproof the skin's surface, preventing absorption of water during immersion.

Thermoregulation is a function of both the epidermis and the dermis and is accomplished through circulation and sweating. Sweating activity is the function of both apocrine and eccrine sweat glands, although apocrine sweat glands do not play a significant role in thermoregulation (Figure 1-7). In the epidermis, the eccrine sweat glands allow dissipation of heat through evaporation of sweat secreted onto the skin's surface. The evaporation of sweat provides a cooling effect. This activity is controlled by the nervous system, which responds to both temperature and emotions. The cutaneous vasculature in the dermis aids thermoregulation through dilation or constriction. Dilation promotes heat conduction at the skin's surface through conduction, convection, radiation, and evaporation. Vasoconstriction inhibits heat conduction, thereby preserving body heat. The action of the arrector pili muscle, in conjunction with vasoconstriction, makes the hair stand vertically, causing shivering and "goose bumps."

Wound healing, or tissue repair, is an extremely important function of the skin. Wounds in the epidermis or dermis can heal by regeneration, because the epithelial, endothelial, and connective tissue can regenerate. Wounds through the dermis heal by scar formation, because deeper structures, hair follicles, glands, and subcutaneous tissue do not have the capacity to regenerate.

Key mediators in wound healing are found in the skin. These include epithelial cells (keratinocytes) in the epidermis and platelets, macrophages, and connective tissue in the dermis. A chemical substance found in the malpighian cells of the epidermis, 7-dehydrocholesterol, is synthesized into vitamin D (which is important in the mineralization of bone) through pho-

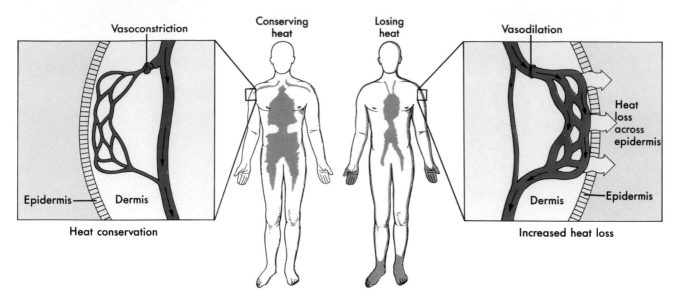

FIGURE 1-7
The skin as a thermoregulatory organ. When homeostasis requires that the body conserve heat, blood flow in the warm organs of the body's core increases *(left)*. When heat must be lost to maintain the stability of the internal environment, flow of warm blood to the skin increases *(right)*. Heat can be lost from the blood and skin by means of radiation, conduction, convection, and evaporation. (From Thibodeau and Patton.[62])

toconversion in the presence of sunlight.

All three layers of the skin are involved in sensory perception. A neuroreceptor system is present in the epidermis, a network of free and encapsulated nerve endings is found in the dermis, and large pressure receptors are present in the subcutaneous tissue. Sensations of pain, touch, temperature, and pressure are picked up by receptors in the skin and transmitted to the cerebral cortex of the brain. Burning, tickling, and itching are the results of a combination of these four basic sensations.

The psychosocial function of the skin is extremely important to a person's overall well-being. Changes in the skin, either acute or chronic, can be the source of considerable morbidity. Changes in body image associated with generalized skin diseases such as psoriasis can be extremely debilitating. Adolescents have a great deal of difficulty dealing with body image, and acne becomes most prevalent during puberty, leading to difficulty with socialization in some cases. Skin diseases and disorders are visible and therefore for the most part unacceptable in our skin- and beauty-conscious society.

EXERCISE AND THE SKIN

Excess heat produced by the skeletal muscles during exercise increases the core body temperature far beyond the normal range. Because blood in vessels near the skin's surface dissipates heat well, the body's control centers adjust blood flow so that more warm blood from the body's core is sent to the skin for cooling. During exercise, blood flow in the skin can be so high that the skin takes on a redder coloration.

To help dissipate even more heat, sweat production increases to as much as 3 L per hour during exercise. Although each sweat gland produces very little of this total, the skin has more than 3 million individual sweat glands. Sweat evaporation is essential to keeping the body temperature in balance, but excessive sweating can lead to a dangerous loss of fluid. Because normal drinking may not replace the water lost through sweating, it is important to drink more nonalcoholic fluids during and after any type of exercise to prevent dehydration.

From Thibodeau and Patton.[62]

ALTERATIONS IN SKIN AND ITS FUNCTIONING

Many factors can affect the skin and its functioning. Aging leads to decreased sensory perception, increased dryness, thinning, decreased vitamin D synthesis, and a decrease in the number of Langerhans' cells (altering immune response, increasing the risk of infection and skin cancer, and decreasing the ability to heal). The skin's thermoregulatory functioning is also decreased due to diminished vascularity, decreased subcutaneous tissue, and a decrease in the number of sweat glands.

Exposure to ultraviolet radiation can have many harmful effects on the skin. It promotes the formation of skin cancer, accelerates the aging process, and decreases the number of Langerhans' cells, which compromises the immune response in the skin. Hydration of the skin is extremely important for maintaining the barrier function, and sebum production is important in maintaining skin hydration. As sebum production decreases (as in aging and some diseases), maintaining adequate skin hydration becomes difficult. Relative humidity also affects the hydration of the skin. As skin hydration decreases, the barrier function of the skin becomes impaired.

Alkaline soaps can adversely affect the stratum corneum. The normal skin pH is 5.5, and alkaline soaps disturb this normal acid mantle, altering bacterial resistance. Excessive bathing or use of soaps and detergents interferes with the water-holding capacity of the skin, which also interferes with bacterial resistance.

Alcohol and acetone are also harmful to the barrier function of the skin.

A balanced diet is imperative to maintaining healthy skin. Protein, carbohydrates, fats, vitamins, and minerals are essential in a diet. With some diseases or skin disruptions, dietary intake of certain substances may be necessary. For example, with exfoliative erythroderma, increased amounts of protein and iron may be required to offset that being lost. For wound repair, dietary protein and carbohydrates may need to be increased.

Topical and systemic drugs also can directly affect the integrity of the skin. It is well known that corticosteroids interfere with epidermal regeneration and collagen synthesis. Antibacterial and antihypertensive drugs, analgesics, tricyclic antidepressants, antihistamines, antineoplastic agents, antipsychotic drugs, diuretics, hypoglycemic agents, sunscreens, and oral contraceptives all can affect the skin.

Alterations in the skin can be a considerable source of morbidity, and in some cases mortality. Normal changes that occur over the life span can increase a patient's susceptibility to certain problems. External and internal factors can elicit changes that will manifest in the skin. All of these factors must be taken into consideration when assessing a patient who presents with a skin disorder. Correlation of patient history and physical findings is essential in drawing correct conclusions regarding diagnosis and for planning the appropriate interventions for care.

CHAPTER 2

Assessment

Because the skin is the most visible organ of the body, it is accessible for careful examination without the use of sophisticated technologic devices or tests. As with any organ system, a careful history is taken, and a physical examination is done. The skin is assessed with an observant eye and critical thinking, to correlate the visible signs and the symptomatic history given by the patient. The skin is the mirror of the internal milieu and often the first indicator of diseases that involve more than the integument.

HISTORY

A clear, thorough history provides information that is vital to determining the cause of a cutaneous manifestation and to assessing the patient's general physical condition.

Important historical data for assessing the skin are outlined in the health history box. Careful inspection and palpation, in conjunction with accurate description of findings, constitute the physical component of skin assessment.

CURRENT PROBLEM

Often a patient will seek medical help for a skin problem that, although acute in onset, may be several days or weeks old. Therefore the current presentation may not readily lead the nurse to a conclusion as to the

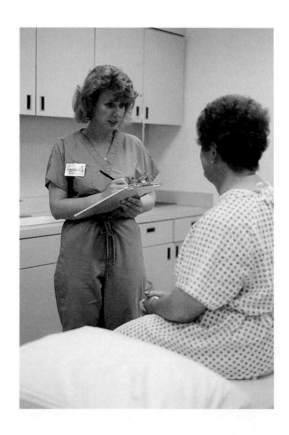

HEALTH HISTORY

Demographic data

   Name, address, phone number, birthdate, sex, race, marital status, occupation, education, religious preference

Chief complaint/reason for visit

What is the skin problem?
Define in patient's own words

Current problem/current health status

   What is the patient's perception of what the abnormality looks like? What are the symptoms (including pruritus, stinging, burning, tingling, numbness, pain, or tenderness to touch)? When did the problem begin? How have the lesions changed over time? Have the lesions spread? What was the pattern of spread? Is this a sudden onset or has the problem been chronic (present for an extended time or since birth)? Has the patient experienced this or a similar problem before? How often and how recently? Is there any definable relationship to an event or cause? Does anything make the condition worse or better?

Family background

   Is there a genetic disorder? Are there other skin disorders in the family? Is there a history of asthma or hay fever?

Medical history

Chronic illnesses
Recent infections (including sinuses and teeth), fever, malaise, upper respiratory or gastrointestinal problems
Previous skin problems
Allergies to medicine, food, or other substances (e.g., plants, cosmetics, chemicals)
Trauma to the skin

Medication history

Current prescription medications (systemic/topical)
Over-the-counter medications (particularly laxatives, cold remedies, and similar drugs)

Family health status

   Does anyone in the immediate family have a skin condition? Does anyone in the family have an allergy? If so, to what?

Development considerations

Pediatric patients:
   Feeding history—breast-fed or formula; types of foods currently eaten
   Diaper history—cleansing routine, type of diaper used
   Types of clothing and washing practices
   Bath practices—bathing routine, including frequency and soaps or oils used
   Dress habits—types and amounts of clothing used
   Temperature and humidity in the home
   Infant's habits—rubbing of head or extremities on mattress, rug, or some other object
   Child in day care; older school-aged children in the home
   Exposure to pets
School-aged children:
   Dietary habits
   Exposure to communicable diseases
   Known allergies
   Exposure to pets
   Outdoor exposures (e.g., plants, bugs)
   Trauma to the skin (cuts, abrasions)
   Nervous habits (biting/picking of nails, twisting/manipulation of hair/eyelashes, picking at skin lesions)
Adolescents:
   All of the above and:
   Use of cosmetics
   Cleansing agents
   Over-the-counter acne preparations

Continued.

HEALTH HISTORY—cont'd

Older adults:
  Increased/decreased sensation to touch
  Generalized pruritus
  Exposures (detergents, soaps, lotions, chemicals)
  Susceptibility to infection
  Condition of skin (friable, dry, thin)
  Healing response
  History of falls
  Underlying medical conditions (diabetes, hypertension, peripheral vascular disease, malignancy)
  Drug history (including over-the-counter medications)
  Hair loss (acute, pattern)

Social history

Type of employment
Nutritional status
Recreational activities
Exposure to chemicals/toxins (at work or through a hobby)
History of travel (especially outside the United States)
Basic hygiene (including oral hygiene)
Use of alcohol/recreational drugs

---

underlying problem. Well-directed questions help the patient relate the onset, progression, and symptoms of the problem. Probing questions, including onset and a description of the initial lesion, prodrome, or incident, give the nurse data that are useful in determining not only the possible cause but also the interventions needed. Review of related history should include the following as outlined.

GENERAL CONSIDERATIONS

Regardless of the presenting symptoms, several general considerations should be explored with every patient. Paramount to any history are the patient's skin care habits. The patient should be questioned about cleansing routines and the types of soaps, oils, lotions, or topical products used on a regular basis. Types of cosmetics and home remedies or preparations used, sun exposure patterns and history, use of sunscreens, or recent changes in the skin care routine should be explored. The nurse should also elicit information about hair and nail care habits. The patient should be asked about types of shampoos, rinses, or pomades used. The frequency of hair care and whether the hair has been subjected to permanent waves, dyes, peroxides, or other agents should be determined. The

patient's nail care routine should be ascertained (use of polish and artificial nails, frequency of trimming, and instruments used), as well as any habits such as chronic picking or biting of nails.

As important as ascertaining skin care habits is eliciting a medication history. This one aspect of the history may be the most informative. Questions about medication use may have to be asked several times before a complete and useful history is obtained. It is important to remember that many individuals do not consider over-the-counter drugs, topical agents, or home remedies to be medications; therefore the nurse may need to explain the questions. If appropriate, a history of recreational drugs should be obtained. Information about exposure to environmental or occupational hazards, such as chemicals, known toxins, or plants, or about frequent sun exposure is important in the history. More important in assessing the skin than for any other organ system is a history of any recent psychologic or physiologic stress. Many times cutaneous manifestations are the result of an emotional episode in the patient's life rather than a true physiologic state. It must be remembered that regardless of the underlying cause, the condition is still a concern for the patient.

THE SKIN

Before exploring the presenting symptoms, the nurse should ask the patient to describe the usual condition of her skin (e.g., oily, dry, thin). This will help in determining the actual or perceived change. Changes in the skin may be related as dryness, oiliness, pruritus, specific sores (lesions), rashes, lumps, a change in color or texture, increased or decreased hair, increased or decreased perspiration, a change in a mole or wart, or a lesion that does not heal or is chronically irritated.

It is crucial to the assessment to have the patient relate the sequence of the condition. This must include the initial onset, the evolution of the condition (how long between the onset and the presenting condition), if the onset was sudden or gradual, and if this is a recurrence of a previous or similar condition.

Prevailing symptoms should be assessed. The condition may have associated pain, pruritus, exudate, bleeding, or color change (without any other physical signs). The patient should be questioned about whether the condition is associated with climatic variations or seasonal patterns.

It is extremely important to determine the distribution of the lesion or lesions, because many conditions manifest in classic patterns. The patient should be asked where the first lesion appeared and, if it spread, to give a history of the pattern of spread. Lesions can be either localized or generalized, and skin folds and flexor or extensor surfaces may be involved. Whether the lesions are asymmetric or symmetric is also a clue to some disease processes.

Associated symptoms such as high fever or a systemic disease may give a clue as to what is presenting on the skin. The patient should be asked about stressful situations that may have occurred. Leisure activities, particularly hobbies that require the use of chemicals or toxins, should be explored. Occupational exposure should be determined, including whether the hands are frequently immersed in water. A travel history should be obtained, particularly if the patient has done recent international traveling. A sun exposure history should be obtained, particularly if skin cancer is suspected.

The patient should be questioned about what treatment, either prescribed or over the counter, has been used. Many times treatment modalities change the appearance of lesions and confuse the diagnosis. The patient should be asked about the response to any previous treatment. If the condition is a recurrence, the patient should be asked whether anything used in the past either improved or aggravated the condition. During the taking of a history, it is important to determine how the patient is adjusting to the skin problem, as well as how compliant she is likely to be with a treatment regimen.

THE HAIR

Problems with hair may be directly correlated with skin lesions or may develop without skin lesions. To determine whether the problem with the hair is associated with other skin problems, the patient should be asked about significant changes in the hair, such as an increase or decrease in the amount, a change in texture or color, or abnormal distribution (e.g., facial hair in women, which could be related to an endocrine disorder, or patchy baldness, which may be a symptom of syphilis). The onset of the problem, whether sudden or gradual, should be established. Whether the problem is symmetric or asymmetric is also important in establishing the cause.

Associated symptoms must be identified. These may include pruritus, pain, lesions, a history of high fever, pregnancy, psychologic or physiologic stress, or systemic disease. Current drug therapy for any conditions should be explored, as well as any exposure to environmental or occupational toxins or chemicals. Use or overuse of commercial hair care chemicals also may be the cause of (or may be contributing to) the presenting problem. Because conditions involving the hair may be directly related to dietary habits, the patient's nutritional status should be explored (e.g., fad dieting, vitamin deficiency). As with any other problem, the patient should be asked how the condition has been treated and what the response has been.

THE NAILS

Changes in the nails not only can cause disfigurement and pain, they may be a sign of systemic disease (e.g., cardiovascular disorders, lymphatic disease, endocrine disease, metabolic and congenital disorders, and infection). Changes may include splitting, discoloration, breaking, ridging, thinning, thickening, or actual separation from the nail bed. The patient may report pain, swelling, or exudate with the physical signs. The nurse should determine whether fever, underlying systemic disease, recent physiologic or psychologic stress, or physical trauma is a factor. The use of chemicals in the form of nail polish, other nail preparations, or artificial nails should be ascertained.

As with any cutaneous symptom the onset, acute or gradual, should be established, as well as the evolution of the problem. Any relationship to exposure to drugs, environmental hazards, chemicals, or toxins, or a history of prolonged immersion in water should be explored.

MEDICAL HISTORY

An assessment is not complete without obtaining a complete medical history from the patient (Figure 2-1). Information about past and present systemic illnesses, recent infections, fever or malaise, past skin

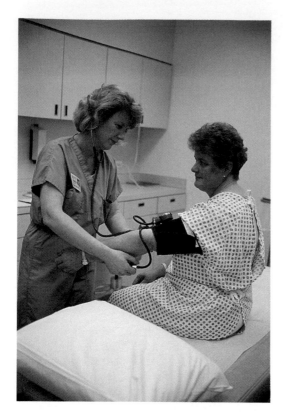

FIGURE 2-1
The patient's general health has a bearing on the condition of the skin. Taking the patient's blood pressure is an important step in the physical assessment.

problems, traumas affecting the skin, and current medications should be obtained. A complete allergy history should be taken, including not only drug allergies but also known or suspected allergies to foods, plants, or chemicals. It is always important to take the patient's age into consideration when obtaining a medical history.

FAMILY HISTORY

In exploring the family history, it is extremely important to focus on any history of skin disease, hay fever, or asthma (the last two have been shown to be directly related to atopic eczema). Unfortunately, because skin disease is not a socially acceptable problem, the patient may not be aware of a chronic skin disease in the family, particularly if it is not apparent in the immediate family. Careful documentation of any findings is paramount to assessing the patient's current problem.

PERSONAL AND SOCIAL HISTORY

Skin problems may be directly related to a person's life-style, making the personal and social history a crucial part of the assessment. The patient should be questioned about her occupation to ascertain whether she has a stressful working environment (stress can

manifest as a skin problem), whether she comes in contact with chemicals or toxins at work (industrial workers, roofers, hair stylists), or if she is required to have her hands in water frequently (nurses, dishwashers). Individuals who work with animals or plants may have skin problems directly related to this activity.

Along with the occupational history, the patient's recreational habits should be investigated. Recreational activities that place the patient in the sun for extended periods may lead to the development of skin cancer or may elicit a photo-induced reaction in conjunction with a systemic medication. Hobbies that require the use of chemicals may elicit skin rashes. Patients who work with ceramics or paints may experience skin problems.

Dietary habits should be explored with the patient. This is particularly important if a food allergy or nutritional deficit is suspected as the cause of the skin problem. A patient's travel history should be explored, particularly if it involves international travel. The patient should be questioned about where she traveled, how long she was there, what foods she ate, and any known exposure to endemic disease.

As part of the assessment, the patient should be questioned about hygiene habits. Patients who bathe frequently (more than once a day) may be causing problems by washing away the normal oils on the skin's surface, leading to pruritus and scratching. Continuous rubbing and scratching of the skin may cause rashes and open lesions. The use of alcohol and recreational drugs should be explored as indicated (e.g., lesions in the antecubital fossa that might be signs of drug use, unusual bruising caused by frequent falls).

PHYSICAL ASSESSMENT

ENVIRONMENT AND EQUIPMENT

The skin is examined after the history has been taken. Ideally the patient should be examined in a warm, private, well-lighted room. Generally only a sharp eye, a sensitive touch, a small flexible ruler, and a hand-held magnifying glass are needed for the examination. A flashlight may be used if closer inspection or better illumination of a lesion is needed. If a fungal infection is suspected, a Wood's lamp can be used to fluoresce lesions (Figure 2-2). Fungus displays a characteristic blue-green color under a Wood's lamp.

PHYSICAL EXAMINATION

Have the patient partly or completely disrobe so that the entire surface of the skin may be assessed. Trying to peek through scant openings in clothing is not an

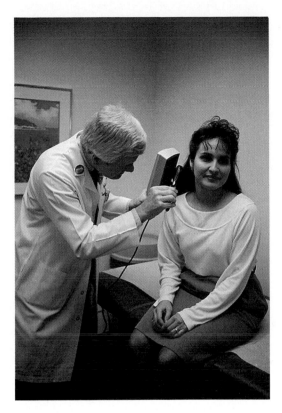

FIGURE 2-2
Using a Wood's lamp to determine if a fungal infection is
present.

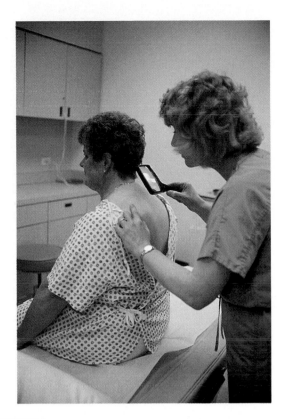

FIGURE 2-3
Inspecting the skin.

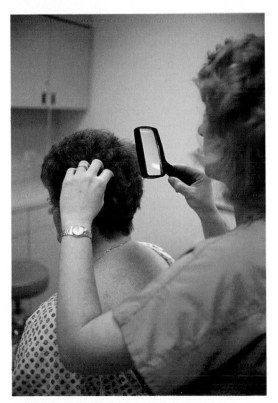

FIGURE 2-4
Inspecting the hair.

acceptable technique for skin examination. The examination should be thorough and systematic to encompass the skin's entire surface, including the hair, nails, and mucosal membranes (Figures 2-3 to 2-5).

Begin by making a brief but thorough overall visual sweep of the entire body. This gives a good idea of the distribution and extent of any lesions. It allows you to observe skin symmetry, to detect differences between body areas, and to compare areas of the body exposed to the sun to those that are not. Be alert for conditions that will require further attention as the examination progresses.

Because adequate exposure of the skin is necessary, it is essential to remove clothing and to fully remove drapes as each section of the body is examined. Look carefully at areas not usually exposed, such as the axillae, buttocks, perineum, backs of thighs, and inner upper thighs. Pay careful attention to intertriginous surfaces, especially in elderly and bedridden patients. As you complete the examination for each area, redrape the patient. Begin by inspecting the skin and mucous membranes (especially oral) for color and uniform appearance, thickness, symmetry, hygiene, and lesions.

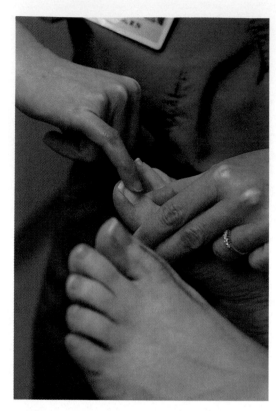

FIGURE 2-5
Inspecting the toenails.

The range of normal skin color varies from dark brown to light tan, with pink or yellow overtones. Color should be uniform overall, but some areas may be sun darkened, and the skin around the knees and elbows may be darker. Callused areas may appear yellow. Vascular flush areas (cheeks, neck, upper chest, and genital area) may appear pink or red, especially with anxiety or excitement. Keep in mind that skin color may be enhanced by cosmetics and tanning agents. Look for localized areas of discoloration. Several variations in skin color that occur in almost all healthy adults and children include nonpigmented striae (silver or pink "stretch marks"), freckles in sun-exposed areas, some birth marks, and some flat and raised nevi in various shades of brown, tan, or near-skin color. Adult women frequently have chloasma (also called melasma), areas of hyperpigmentation on the face and neck associated with pregnancy or the use of hormones. This condition is more noticeable in darker-skinned women.

Lesions

Inspection of the skin is directed at identifying abnormalities (lesions). Skin lesions are divided into two major categories, *primary lesions* and *secondary lesions*. Primary lesions are those present at the initial onset of the problem; secondary lesions are the results of change over time due to disease progression, manipulation (scratching, rubbing, picking), or treatment. The nurse must be able to distinguish between a primary lesion and a secondary lesion. These lesions are described, with clinical pictures, on pp. 22-26.

After the lesions have been categorized as primary or secondary, the next important step is to describe them (see the box above). Note the characteristics, pattern of arrangement, location and distribution, and whether exudates are present. The box on page 19 presents modifying terms that can be used in describing skin lesions.

Skin lesions may appear in a variety of colors, ranging from red/salmon pink, brown/black, blue/purple, to bone white/slate gray or yellow. The color of the lesion may be a clue to the underlying cause.

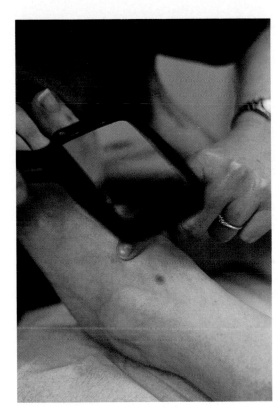

FIGURE 2-6
Palpating a lesion to determine its consistency.

KINDS OF SKIN LESIONS

Name	Description
Eczematous	Vesicles with oozing crust
Herpetiform	Closely grouped vesicles (herpeslike)
Reticulated	Netlike array
Round	Arcuate (arc shaped)
	Circinate (circular)
	Guttate (droplike)
	Iris (bull's eye)
	Nummular (coin shaped)
	Ovoid (oval)
Serpiginous	Snakelike
Telangiectatic	With dilated blood vessels
Verrucous	Rough, wartlike
Zosteriform	Similar to shingles, follows along a nerve root dermatome

After the initial visual inspection, palpate the lesions to determine their consistency and to test for tenderness (Figure 2-6). Lesions may vary from soft to rubbery to rock hard. Rock hard lesions are characteristic of metastatic tumors or cutaneous calcification. Tenderness on palpation may be a sign of infection (either bacterial or viral), tumors, or a vascular disorder. Most other skin lesions are not painful.

While inspecting the skin for lesions, note moisture (or lack thereof), temperature, texture, turgor, and mobility. Pay particular attention to intertriginous areas (fungal infections and maceration are most prominate here). Normal skin temperature may range from cool to warm. Using the dorsal surface of the fingers or hands is the best way to assess skin temperature. When assessing texture, note whether the skin has rough spots. Generally the skin should feel smooth, soft, and even. Turgor and mobility are assessed by gently pinching a small section of skin (generally on the forearm or in the sternal area) and releasing. If the skin does not return to its previous state, skin turgor is poor. Dehydration, edema, and connective tissue diseases (scleroderma) affect skin turgor and mobility.

Hair and Nails

Assessment of the hair and nails is essential to any skin examination. Hair should be checked for texture, color, quantity, and distribution. Dryness or brittleness of the hair could be a sign of a systemic problem such as thyroid disease. The quantity and distribution of hair are determined by heredity, but in some cases abnormal quantity or distribution can suggest systemic problems. Diffuse hair loss could be a side effect of some drugs. Excessive hair in women, with or without other signs of virilization, could be a sign of an endocrine disorder. Patchy hair loss could suggest syphilis, and hair loss with evidence of broken hair shafts could be due to manipulation, either chemical (dyes or peroxide) or mechanical (trichotillomania). Because male pattern baldness is symmetric, asymmetric hair loss in men may indicate an underlying systemic condition.

The nails should be inspected for length, color, configuration, symmetry, cleanliness, thickness, and any obvious malformations. Nails that have been bitten or picked down to the quick or are dirty or generally unkempt may be an indication of the patient's feelings of self-worth (patients with low self-esteem may not comply with the prescribed therapy). The color of the nail should be a variation of pink. In darker-skinned individuals hyperpigmented bands may be present; these are inconsequential unless they appeared suddenly. A hyperpigmented band that appears suddenly should be investigated to rule out malignant melanoma. Psoriasis and fungal infections give the nail a yellow appearance. Individuals with pulmonary disease and smokers (due to nicotine) may have yellow or

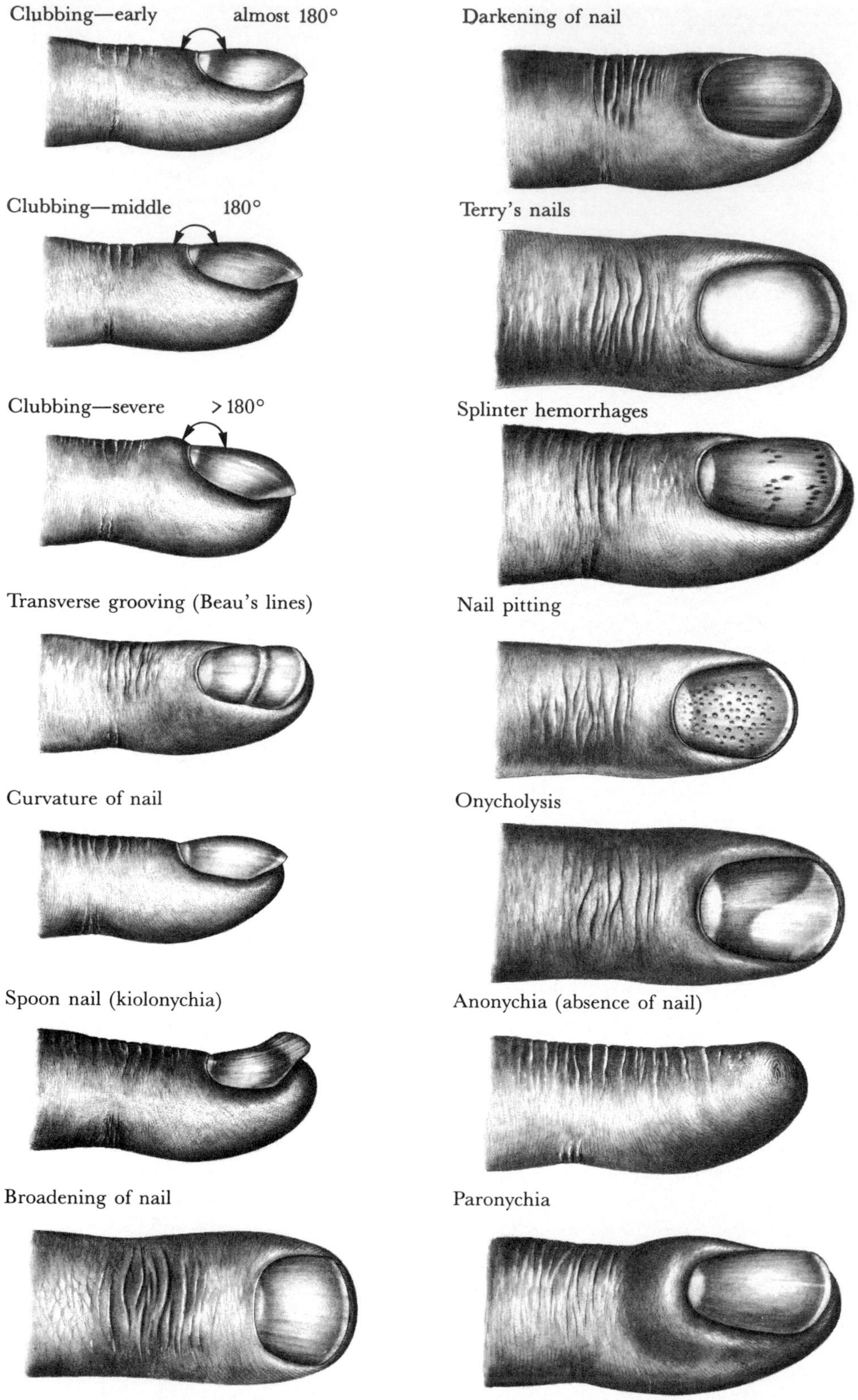

Clubbing—early   almost 180°

Darkening of nail

Clubbing—middle   180°

Terry's nails

Clubbing—severe   >180°

Splinter hemorrhages

Transverse grooving (Beau's lines)

Nail pitting

Curvature of nail

Onycholysis

Spoon nail (kiolonychia)

Anonychia (absence of nail)

Broadening of nail

Paronychia

FIGURE 2-7
Nails: unexpected findings and appearance. (From Seidel et al.[59])

brown nails. Many drugs can affect the color of the nail; antimalarial drugs may cause the nail to darken. Infection or trauma can produce a green-black color. Nail pitting is characteristic of psoriasis, as are splinter hemorrhages. Figure 2-7 shows some common disorders and findings for the nails.

An accurate, complete description of all findings should be documented. The description should include all parameters previously discussed (characteristics, exudates, pattern of arrangement, location, distribution) as well as color.

DIAGNOSTIC PROCEDURES

Even though assessment of the skin is based primarily on visual inspection and palpation, occasionally additional techniques are needed. These generally range from a simple potassium hydroxide (KOH) preparation (Figures 2-8 to 2-10) to a skin biopsy or possibly some type of laboratory workup. Discerning the evolution of existing skin lesions is essential to a good assessment; this is achieved through a thorough history and careful visual inspection.

Pages 22 through 26 provide a pictorial review of vascular, primary, and secondary skin lesions. Full-color drawings are accompanied by physical descriptions and possible causes of many different lesions.

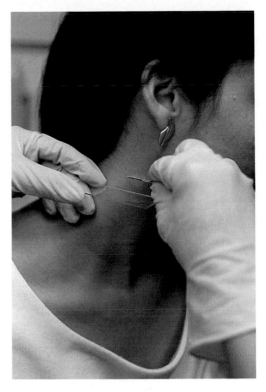

FIGURE 2-8
Scraping a suspected fungal lesion for preparation with KOH for microscopic examination.

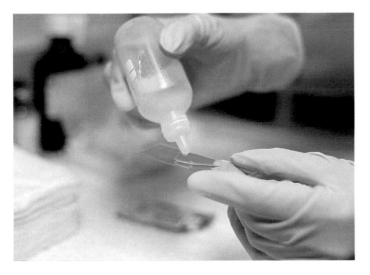

FIGURE 2-9
Preparation of slide with KOH for microscopic examination.

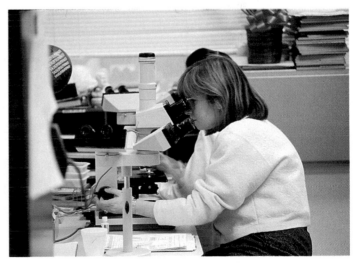

FIGURE 2-10
Microscopic examination of KOH-prepared scraping.

Pictorial Review of Skin Lesions

CHARACTERISTICS AND CAUSES OF VASCULAR SKIN LESIONS

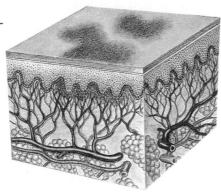

Spider angioma—red central body with radiating spiderlike legs that blanch with pressure to the central body
Cause: Liver disease, vitamin B deficiency, idiopathic

Purpura—red-purple nonblanchable discoloration greater than 0.5 cm diameter.
Cause: Intravascular defects, infection

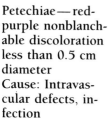
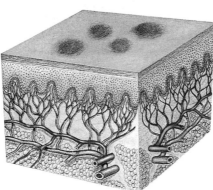

Venous star—bluish spider, linear or irregularly shaped; does not blanch with pressure
Cause: Increased pressure in superficial veins

Petechiae—red-purple nonblanchable discoloration less than 0.5 cm diameter
Cause: Intravascular defects, infection

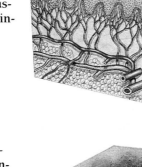
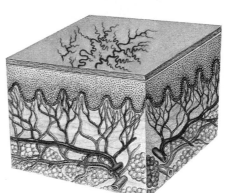

Telangiectasia—fine, irregular red line
Cause: Dilation of capillaries

Ecchymoses—red-purple nonblanchable discoloration of variable size
Cause: Vascular wall destruction, trauma, vasculitis

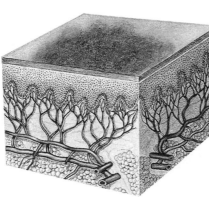

Capillary hemangioma (nevus flammeus)—red irregular macular patches
Cause: Dilation of dermal capillaries

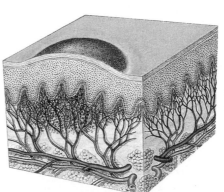

DESCRIPTIONS AND CHARACTERISTICS OF PRIMARY SKIN LESIONS

From Seidel et al.[59]

Plaque—elevated; flat topped; firm; rough; superficial papule greater than 1 cm in diameter; may be coalesced papules
Examples: Psoriasis; seborrheic and actinic keratoses

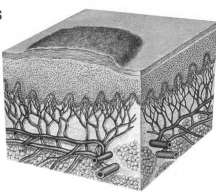

Macule—flat; nonpalpable; circumscribed; less than 1 cm in diameter; brown, red, purple, white, or tan in color
Examples: Freckles; flat moles; rubella; rubeola

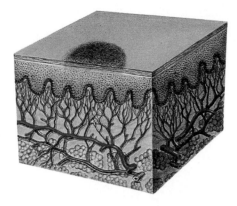

Wheal—elevated, irregular-shaped area of cutaneous edema; solid, transient, changing, variable diameter; pale pink with lighter center
Examples: Urticaria; insect bites

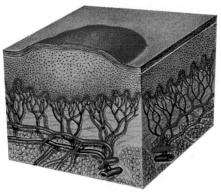

Patch—flat; nonpalpable; irregular in shape; macule that is greater than 1 cm in diameter
Examples: Vitiligo; port-wine marks

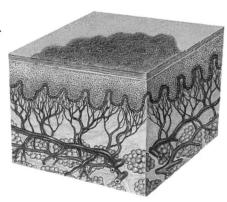

Nodule—elevated; firm; circumscribed; palpable; deeper in dermis than papule; 1 to 2 cm in diameter
Examples: Erythema nodosum; lipomas

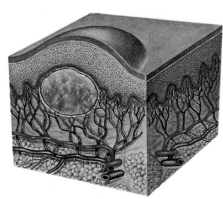

Papule—elevated; palpable; firm; circumscribed; less than 1 cm in diameter; brown, red, pink, tan, or bluish red in color
Examples: Warts; drug-related eruptions; pigmented nevi

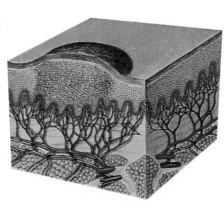

Tumor—elevated; solid; may or may not be clearly demarcated; greater than 2 cm in diameter; may or may not vary from skin color
Example: Neoplasms

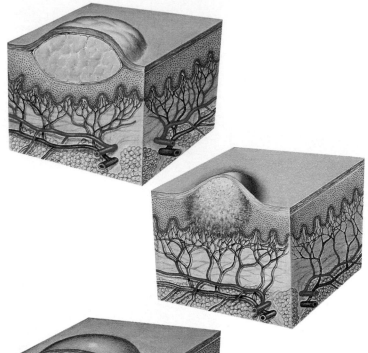

Pustule—elevated; superficial; similar to vesicle but filled with purulent fluid
Examples: Impetigo; acne; variola

Vesicle—elevated; circumscribed; superficial; filled with serous fluid; less than 1 cm in diameter
Examples: Blister; varicella

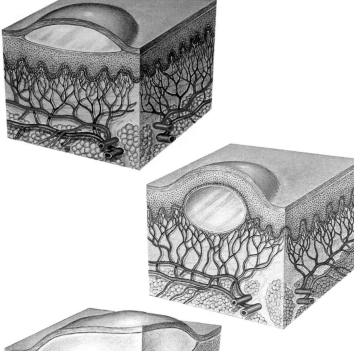

Cyst—elevated; circumscribed; palpable; encapsulated; filled with liquid or semi-solid material
Example: Sebaceous cyst

Bulla—vesicle greater than 1 cm in diameter
Examples: Blister; pemphigus vulgaris

DESCRIPTIONS AND CHARACTERISTICS OF SECONDARY SKIN LESIONS

From Seidel et al.[59]

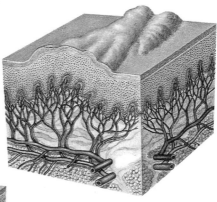

Scar—thin to thick fibrous tissue replacing injured dermis; irregular; pink, red, or white in color; may be atrophic or hypertrophic
Example: Healed wound or surgical incision

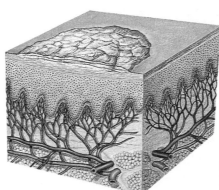

Scale—heaped-up keratinized cells; flaky exfoliation; irregular; thick or thin; dry or oily; varied size; silver, white, or tan in color
Examples: Psoriasis; exfoliative dermatitis

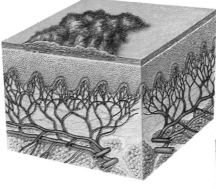

Crust—dried serum, blood, or purulent exudate; slightly elevated; size varies; brown, red, black, tan, or straw in color
Examples: Scab on abrasion; eczema

Keloid—irregularly shaped, elevated, progressively enlarging scar; grows beyond boundaries of wound; caused by excessive collagen formation during healing
Example: Keloid from ear piercing or burn scar

Excoriation—loss of epidermis; linear or hollowed-out crusted area; dermis exposed
Examples: Abrasion; scratch

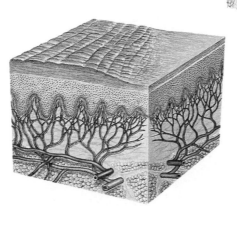

Lichenification—rough, thickened epidermis; accentuated skin markings caused by rubbing or irritation; often involves flexor aspect of extremity
Example: Chronic dermatitis

Fissure—linear crack or break from epidermis to dermis; small; deep; red
Examples: Athlete's foot; cheilois

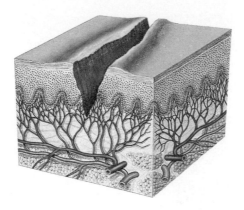

Erosion—loss of all or part of epidermis; depressed; moist; glistening; follows rupture of vesicle or bulla; larger than fissure
Examples: Varicella; variola following rupture

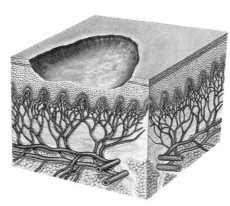

Ulcer—loss of epidermis and dermis; concave; varies in size; exudative; red or reddish blue
Examples: Decubiti; stasis ulcers

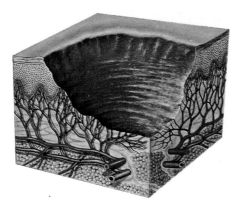

Atrophy—thinning of skin surface and loss of skin markings; skin translucent and paperlike
Examples: Striae; aged skin

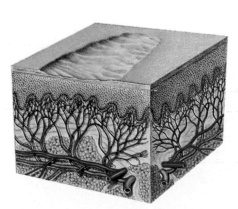

CHAPTER 3

Diseases of Epidermal Origin

Eczema

Eczema is not a specific disease. "Dermatitis" and "eczema" are terms that may be used interchangeably to describe a group of diseases with a characteristic appearance. A few examples of eczema are allergic contact dermatitis (eruptions caused by allergy to poison ivy, sumac, or oak, or a proven allergen, such as nickel); irritant dermatitis (eruption caused by direct contact with cosmetics, chemicals, dyes, or detergents); nummular eczema (coin-shaped, oozing, crusting patches); seborrheic dermatitis (yellowish-pink scaling of the scalp, face, and trunk); and atopic dermatitis (characteristic distribution of eczema in individuals with a family history of allergic disease).

Eczema/dermatitis has three primary stages: acute, subacute, and chronic; different types of eczema may manifest in any one of the three stages, or all three stages may manifest at one time.

Acute dermatitis is characterized by extensive erosions with serous exudate or by intensely pruritic, erythematous papules and vesicles on an erythematous base. Subacute dermatitis is characterized by erythematous, excoriated, scaling papules or plaques that are either grouped or scattered over erythematous skin. The scaling often is so fine and diffuse that the skin acquires a silvery sheen. Chronic dermatitis is characterized by thickened skin and increased skin marking secondary to rubbing and scratching (lichenification); excoriated papules, fibrotic papules, and nodules (prurigo nodularis); and postinflammatory hyperpigmentation and hypopigmentation.

Atopic Dermatitis

Atopic dermatitis is a chronic, relapsing, pruritic type of eczema that usually occurs in individuals with a personal or family history of allergic diseases. The word "atopic" refers to a group of three associated allergic diseases: asthma, allergic rhinitis (hay fever), and atopic dermatitis. There is no single distinguishing feature; the clinical diagnosis of atopic dermatitis is based on a combination of historical and morphologic findings. Atopic dermatitis is a common disease, affecting 0.5% to 1% of the people in all parts of the world, with a prevalence of 5% to 10% in children.

PATHOPHYSIOLOGY

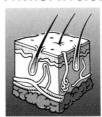

The exact cause of atopic dermatitis is unknown. Dry, lackluster skin is a hallmark of the disorder and is often, but not always, associated with ichthyosis vulgaris. Compared to normal skin, the dry skin of atopic dermatitis has a reduced water-binding capacity, a higher transepidermal water loss, and a decreased water content. Water loss leads to further drying and cracking of the skin, which leads to more itching. Rubbing and scratching of itchy skin cause many of the clinical changes seen in the skin.

CLINICAL MANIFESTATIONS

Atopic dermatitis can appear at any age but usually manifests between 2 and 6 months of age and may continue into young adulthood. The rash develops in a characteristic distribution on the body that varies according to the patient's age. When this disease occurs in infancy, it is called acute dermatitis. The red, oozing, crusting rash appears primarily on the face and scalp; however, it can develop in other areas, especially on the extensor surfaces of the extremities (see Color Plate 55 on page xxi). The rash is extremely itchy. In more than 50% of infants and toddlers with atopic dermatitis, the disease clears by 2 years of age and does not recur.

Almost 50% of infants still have the disease after 2 years of age. The skin tends to show the chronic form of dermatitis with a thickened, dry texture, brownish-gray color, and scale. The rash tends to localize to the large folds of the extremities as the patient becomes older. It is found mainly on elbow bends, backs of the knees, neck, sides of the face, eyelids, and backs of the hands and feet. In approximately half of these patients, the condition resolves almost completely by adolescence, but in the remaining group it is likely to persist through adulthood.

In adults the pattern remains the same as in adolescence. In general, the more severe and long-lasting the atopic dermatitis, the more likely it is that the disease will persist. Hand and foot dermatitis becomes a significant problem in some patients.

Pruritus is the major symptom of atopic dermatitis and causes the greatest morbidity. The urge to scratch may be mild and self-limiting, or it may be intense, leading to severely excoriated lesions, infection, and scarring.

NURSING CARE

See pages 33 to 38.

MEDICAL MANAGEMENT

The goal of therapy is to break the inflammatory cycles that cause excessive drying and cracking, as well as the itching and scratching. Primary prevention begins with good daily skin care that hydrates and lubricates the skin. The health care team's understanding of each patient's disease pattern, as well as discovering and reducing exacerbating factors, is crucial to effective management of this chronic disease. Other factors that must be considered are irritants, allergens, physical environment, and emotional stress.

DRUG THERAPY

Topical corticosteroids: Used to suppress inflammation and pruritus; best absorbed if applied immediately after the skin has been saturated with water.

Tar compounds: Useful as adjunctive therapy in patients with chronic dermatitis to achieve steroid-sparing effect.

Sedative antihistamines: Often used to suppress pruritus, allay anxiety, and allow sleep through sedating effects.

Oral antibiotics: Often required to treat clinical or subclinical secondary *Staphylococcus aureus* infections.

Systemic corticosteroids (PO or IM): Used only rarely.

Etretinate, thymopentin, and interferon-gamma: Immune-response modifiers that have shown promising results in research trials for patients with severe, recalcitrant disease.

GENERAL MANAGEMENT

Hydration is the key to management. The primary means to correct dryness is to add water to the skin and then immediately apply an occlusive substance.

Moisturizers or emollients relieve skin irritability and protect the skin. They should be applied frequently between applications of topical corticosteroids and to areas of resolving dermatitis (Figure 3-1).-

MEDICAL MANAGEMENT—cont'd

Wet wraps and occlusion, used immediately after soaking and application of topical drugs, can optimize hydration and topical therapy (Figure 3-2).

Ultraviolet light therapy (PUVA or UVB) can be helpful in some patients with recalcitrant, chronic, atopic dermatitis (Figure 3-3).

Allergen avoidance is helpful when specific triggers can be identified; however, blanket restrictions are unjustified.

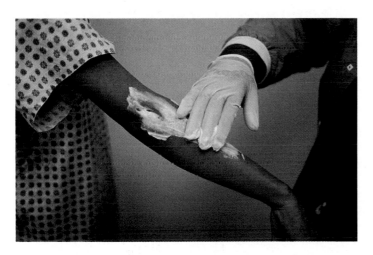

FIGURE 3-1
Clinician applying topical cream to patient's arm.

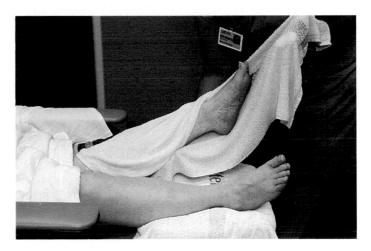

FIGURE 3-2
Clinician applying wet wrap to patient's leg.

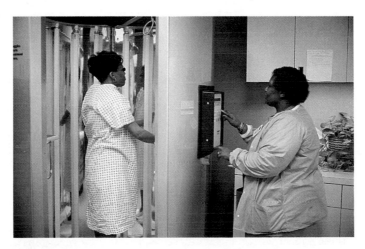

FIGURE 3-3
Patient receiving phototherapy.

Psoriasis Vulgaris

Psoriasis vulgaris is a chronic, recurrent, erythematous, inflammatory disorder involving keratin synthesis. Pruritus can be severe. Psoriasis occurs in both sexes, usually commencing in early adulthood. About 1% to 3% of the U.S. population has psoriasis.

The cause of psoriasis vulgaris is unknown. However, changes in cyclic nucleotides and prostaglandins and possible immunologic abnormalities have been noted. Genetic predisposition is also possible.

PATHOPHYSIOLOGY

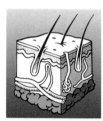 Rapidly proliferating epidermal cells form small, scaly patches of skin that develop into erythematous, dry, scaling patches of various size. Psoriasis vulgaris follows a prolonged and unpredictable course. Anxiety and stress often precede flare-ups, and exacerbations and remissions are common. The disease usually manifests at intervals, lasting for increasingly longer periods with each episode. Spontaneous clearing is uncommon. Patients with psoriasis have greater than normal colonization of *Staphylococcus* organisms on plaques. Patients who also are infected with the human immunodeficiency virus (HIV) are at high risk of infection from self-inoculation.

CLINICAL MANIFESTATIONS

Psoriatic patches are covered with silvery white scales. The eruptions, which usually are symmetric, commonly occur on the scalp, elbows, and knees and in sacral regions. The appearance of lesions at the site of a previous injury is known as Koebner's phenomenon. A generalized eruption may occur with severe psoriasis vulgaris. A rare form of psoriasis (pustular psoriasis) produces generalized, sterile cutaneous pustules. Severe systemic involvement can be fatal. Another form of pustular psoriasis, which is localized to the palms and soles, is not associated with systemic disease. About 15% to 20% of patients with psoriasis have psoriatic arthritis, which primarily affects the distal joints and may be deforming. Nail dystrophies and pitting occur in approximately 30% to 50% of clients.

NURSING CARE

See pages 33 to 38.

MEDICAL MANAGEMENT

Management of psoriasis depends on its type and severity. Mild involvement can be treated locally with natural sunlight or topical therapy, or both. Care consists of removing scales and treating inflammation. Tar preparations or keratolytic agents, or both, followed by topical corticosteroids are useful. Often steroids must be used under occlusive dressings to enhance percutaneous absorption. There is no consistently effective treatment of psoriatic involvement of the nails. The scalp and nails usually improve with remission of psoriasis on the body surface.

DRUG THERAPY

Topical corticosteroids: Used to suppress inflammation and pruritus; best absorbed if applied immediately after the skin has been saturated with water.

Injected corticosteroids: Used to suppress inflammation and stop pruritus. Injecting small, diluted amounts of corticosteroids (e.g., triamcinolone acetonide) into or just below a lesion gives a high drug concentration to a localized site. Possible localized side effects include atrophy, hypopigmentation, infection, and, in rare cases, ulceration.

Tar compounds: Used for antimitotic and antiinflammatory effect.

Keratolytic agents (e.g., salicylic acid): May remove scale and allow greater penetration of topical agents.

Anthralin: An effective topical therapy for psoriasis with widespread, discrete lesions consisting primarily of thick plaques.

MEDICAL MANAGEMENT—cont'd

Sedative antihistamines: Often used to suppress pruritus, allay anxiety, and allow sleep through sedating effects.

Oral antibiotics: Often required to treat clinical or subclinical secondary *Staphylococcus aureus* infections.

Etretinate: An immune-response modifier that has proved useful in pustular and erythrodermic psoriasis but is not as useful in chronic, plaque-type psoriasis; because of the drug's teratogenicity and extremely long half-life, it is used much less often in women of childbearing age and only with great caution.

Antimetabolites (e.g., methotrexate): Useful in small doses to inhibit DNA synthesis. Methotrexate is a folic acid antagonist used to treat psoriasis that does not respond to any topical therapies. Because the drug is potentially toxic to the renal, hepatic, and hematopoietic systems, it is reserved for the most severe cases.

GENERAL MANAGEMENT

Moisturizers or emollients: Used to soothe and relieve skin irritation and to protect the skin if applied frequently. They are used between applications of topical corticosteroids, or on areas of resolving psoriasis.

Ultraviolet light therapy (PUVA or UVB): Can be helpful in guttate psoriasis, psoriasis vulgaris, and fistular forms of psoriasis. Widespread involvement requires whole-body irradiation with ultraviolet light (UVL). Goeckerman regimen uses UVB irradiation with topical application of crude coal tar and emollients. Modified Goeckerman method uses topical steroids in conjunction with UVB irradiation, tar derivatives, and emollients. Photochemotherapy (PUVA) combines an oral photoactive drug with UVL; it is used for patients with extensive disease that does not respond to other treatment. Ingram's (methoxsalen) method (using anthralin paste with UVL) is limited to patients with large psoriatic plaques.

Wet wraps and occlusion: Used immediately after lubricating bath and application of topical drugs, they can optimize hydration and topical therapy.

Exfoliative Dermatitis (Erythroderma)

Exfoliative dermatitis is the term used to describe large skin surfaces that are covered with a scaly, erythematous dermatitis. Secondary effects on other organs can be debilitating.

PATHOPHYSIOLOGY

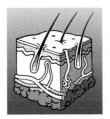

Exfoliative dermatitis always arises from another disorder, occurring secondary to underlying cutaneous or systemic disease. The release of chemicals that act as cutaneous toxins or suppress normal immunologic responses may cause this generalized, swollen, scarlet, desquamative condition. Desquamation can affect the conjunctivae and mucous membranes of the upper respiratory tract, and extensive hair loss may occur. Some diseases that may evolve into exfoliative dermatitis include severe psoriasis, atopic and seborrheic dermatitis, scabies, contact dermatitis, drug eruptions, and lymphoma. Exfoliative dermatitis in association with another cutaneous disorder increases the risks of secondary bacterial infection and metabolic effects.

CLINICAL MANIFESTATIONS

Exfoliative dermatitis may have an acute onset, but a gradual progression is more common. The disease is characterized by erythematous, scaling papules or plaques, often with generalized excoriations, over almost the entire body. Fever, chills, malaise, fatigue, skin tightness, and intolerable pruritus result from compromised skin integrity and blood flow changes through the skin. Because epidermal keratinization increases, water and protein losses cause dehydration and negative nitrogen balance. People with exfoliative dermatitis may have indications of cardiac failure, dyspnea, and edema stemming from the incease in cutaneous blood flow.

NURSING CARE

See pages 33 to 38.

COMPLICATIONS OF DISEASES OF EPIDERMAL ORIGIN

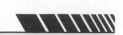

Cutaneous dryness (from skin's inability to hold moisture in stratum corneum)

Uncontrolled heat loss (from loss of barrier function)

Pruritus (from dry skin, external irritants, stress)

Infection (from excoriated skin and impaired resistance to cutaneous viral, fungal, and staphylococcal organisms)

Protein and iron loss (with exfoliation)

DIAGNOSTIC STUDIES AND FINDINGS IN DISEASES OF EPIDERMAL ORIGIN

Diagnostic Test	Findings
Serum IgE	Elevated in most patients with severe atopic dermatitis
Skin biopsy	*Atopic dermatitis:* Findings insufficient to differentiate disorder from other eczematous eruptions (e.g., contact dermatitis, nummular eczema, seborrheic dermatitis)
	Psoriasis: Psoriasiform epidermal thickening present, but histology often is not diagnostic
Skin prick tests	*Atopic dermatitis:* Immediate-wheal skin test responses to common protein allergens (e.g., foods or aeroallergens) in most patients
Patch tests	May be helpful to perform delayed hypersensitivity testing to evaluate for contact allergies

MEDICAL MANAGEMENT

Hospitalization for support and expert nursing care make up the best treatment. The goals of treatment are to reduce skin irritability, decrease inflammation, repair the skin barrier, and promote rest. Laboratory studies or history of cutaneous disease determines the underlying disorder. Close monitoring of the patient for systemic complications is important, especially with cardiac-compromised or elderly people.

DRUG THERAPY

Topical corticosteroids: Used to suppress inflammation and pruritus; best absorbed if applied immediately after the skin has been saturated with water. Topical corticosteroids are more effective if used under occlusion or wet wraps, but care must be taken to avoid excessive percutaneous absorption and secondary bacterial infection.

Sedative antihistamines: Often used to suppress pruritus, allay anxiety, and allow sleep through sedating effects.

Systemic antibiotics: Often required to treat clinical or subclinical secondary bacterial infection.

Systemic corticosteroids: May be needed, depending on the underlying cause of the erythroderma; dosing must be done with great care.

MEDICAL MANAGEMENT—cont'd

GENERAL MANAGEMENT

Emollients: Used to soothe and relieve skin irritability and to provide a temporary barrier. They are used between applications of topical corticosteroids, or on areas of resolving dermatitis.

Ultraviolet light therapy (PUVA or UVB): Can be helpful in some patients with recalcitrant, widespread disease.

Wet wraps and occlusion: Used immediately after lubricating bath and application of topical drugs, they can optimize hydration and topical therapy.

1 ASSESS

ASSESSMENT	OBSERVATIONS
History	*Atopic dermatitis:* Personal or family history of asthma, hay fever, or eczema *Psoriasis:* May have family history of psoriasis
Skin	May have xerotic, scaly skin with excoriations and lichenification: age-dependent distribution in atopic dermatitis; symmetric distribution of silvery, scaly patches in psoriasis; generalized distribution in exfoliative dermatitis
General complaints	Frequent complaints of pruritus; patient often can identify triggers of pruritus (e.g., sweating, rapid changes in temperature, contact with various irritants or allergens, stress)
Secondary infection	Purulent drainage; fever, tenderness; regional lymphadenopathy
Psychosocial	Difficulty coping with body image and self-esteem issues; inability to sleep because of pruritus

2 DIAGNOSE

NURSING DIAGNOSIS	SUBJECTIVE FINDINGS	OBJECTIVE FINDINGS
Impaired skin integrity related to pathologic process and mechanical factors	Reports skin discomfort and cutaneous dryness	Red, dry, flaky, scaly skin; excoriations from scratching
High risk for impaired skin integrity (pruritus) related to inflammatory process	Reports dry skin; reports feeling stressed; reports that skin is easily irritated to the point of itching	Scratches skin frequently; has excoriations from scratching; reports trouble sleeping because of itching

NURSING DIAGNOSIS	SUBJECTIVE FINDINGS	OBJECTIVE FINDINGS
Impaired skin integrity related to uncontrolled heat loss caused by loss of barrier function	Reports skin discomfort and constant shivering	Clothes appear warmer than temperature requires; visibly shivering; family reports patient sleeps in heavy pajamas, socks, and robe under several blankets
High risk for secondary infection related to skin excoriation	Reports skin discomfort and itching	Infectious lesions with pustules, exudate, and crusting
Body image disturbance related to skin lesions	Reports fear of rejection by significant others because of appearance and low self-esteem because of skin lesions	Clothes cover almost all skin; avoids eye contact; rarely socializes outside home
Psoriasis: **Social isolation** related to alterations in physical appearance	Reports fear that psoriasis is contagious and that others won't want to be around her	Family reports withdrawal from family members

3 PLAN

Patient goals

1. Patient will maintain well-hydrated skin, and inflammation will be reduced.
2. Pruritus will be alleviated.
3. Patient's skin will retain body heat.
4. Patient will be free of infectious lesions.
5. Patient will develop a positive self-concept.
6. Patient with psoriasis will be able to socialize.

4 IMPLEMENT

NURSING DIAGNOSIS	INTERVENTION	RATIONALE
Impaired skin integrity related to pathologic process and mechanical factors	Note lesions' characteristics, distribution, and severity.	To determine extent of disease.
	Stress the importance of adhering to therapeutic regimen; help patient set up overall schedule for managing regimen on daily basis.	To maximize therapeutic value and alleviate patient's frustration.
	Give written instructions for using topical preparations, tar baths, and shampoos.	To reinforce patient's understanding and increase adherence to therapeutic regimen.
	Teach patient how to apply occlusive dressings.	To increase patient's comfort and promote adherence to therapeutic regimen.

NURSING DIAGNOSIS	INTERVENTION	RATIONALE
	Instruct patient to scrub crusted lesions gently with antibacterial soap during daily bath.	To debride skin.
	Instruct patient in handwashing and good hygiene.	To prevent secondary infection.
	Instruct patient to cut fingernails short.	To reduce trauma and possibility of secondary infection.
	Explore stress factors affecting patient and alternatives for dealing with stress.	To help prevent exacerbations.
	Instruct patient not to apply keratolytics and tar to unaffected areas.	To avoid precipitating new lesions.
High risk for impaired skin integrity (pruritus) related to inflammatory process	Apply cool compresses for wet skin or oil compresses for dry skin.	To soothe itching and discomfort.
	Instruct patient in use of antipruritics.	To relieve itching.
Impaired skin integrity related to uncontrolled heat loss caused by loss of barrier function	Teach patient strategies to reduce heat loss: maintain room temperature at 21° C (70° F); prevent drafts by shielding patient's bed with curtain; provide warmth at night by layering bed linens and clothing patient in soft, warm pajamas, robe, and socks; keep extra blankets within reach.	To alleviate uncontrolled shivering, easy chilling, and poor tolerance to temperature changes.
	Closely monitor and document patient's oral temperature; notify physician if oral temperature is over 38.5° C (101.3° F).	Elevated temperature could be caused by thermal instability or infection.
High risk for secondary infection related to skin excoriation	Explain the signs of infection.	To ensure patient will know when to seek medical care.
	Make sure patient understands the importance of medical reevaluation with each recurrence of infection.	To ensure patient will not self-medicate with home medication remaining from the previous outbreak.
	Make sure patient knows that once an antibiotic is prescribed, it must be used on schedule and until the entire course of treatment is completed.	To maximize therapeutic value.
Body image disturbance related to skin lesions	Encourage patient to express feelings about body, appearance, or fear of rejection by others.	To begin process of realistic self-evaluation.

NURSING DIAGNOSIS	INTERVENTION	RATIONALE
	Encourage patient to develop other attributes and interests.	To support positive self-image, feelings of worth, and self-confidence, so that skin condition does not become focus of existence.
	Facilitate initiation of individual or group therapy.	If patient is unable to adjust to appearance.
Psoriasis: **Social isolation** related to alterations in physical appearance	Involve family members in treatment regimen, and encourage them to share feelings with each other about patient's appearance and chronic nature of the skin disease.	To provide patient support and prevent unidentified fears and concerns from hindering interpersonal relationships.
	Reinforce patient's sense of identity and personal competence by encouraging self-management of eczema.	Allowing patient to determine need for treatment modalities, such as when to initiate wet wraps, promotes positive self-concept.
	Refer patient for counseling.	If patient is socially disabled by disease.

5 EVALUATE

PATIENT OUTCOME	DATA INDICATING THAT OUTCOME IS REACHED
Skin is well hydrated, and inflammation has been reduced.	Patient reports greater skin comfort; flaking, scaling, and redness have decreased; there are fewer excoriations from scratching, and previous areas of breakdown have healed.
Pruritus has been alleviated.	There are fewer areas of excoriation; observed and reported scratching is reduced; patient reports increased skin comfort and fewer sleep interruptions.
Patient's skin retains body heat.	Patient reports greater skin comfort; shivering has decreased noticeably, and patient is more tolerant of change in temperature.
Patient is free of infectious lesions.	Patient's skin shows no sign of pustules, exudate, or crusting; body temperature is normal.
Patient exhibits a positive self-concept.	Patient expresses feelings of importance and self-worth.
Patient with psoriasis is able to socialize.	Patient resumes activities and enjoys social interactions.

PATIENT TEACHING

Teach strategies to promote skin hydration

1. Bathe at least once every day, soaking for 15 to 20 minutes. Immediately upon leaving the bath, apply an appropriate emollient or prescribed topical agent. Bathe more often when signs and symptoms increase. (Bathing has often been discouraged because of its alleged drying effect. Soaking for 15 to 20 minutes allows the stratum corneum to become saturated with water. Drying is the result of failure to *immediately* apply the appropriate occlusive moisturizer and allowing evaporation to occur. Applying an emollient or some occlusive agent within 2 to 4 minutes of leaving the bath is critical to prevent evaporation of water from the hydrated epidermis. Vigorously rubbing the skin dry removes more water from the skin and increases vasodilation.)
2. Use warm water—not hot. Hot water causes vasodilation, which increases pruritus.
3. Use superfatted soaps (e.g., Dove, Basis) or soaps for sensitive skin (e.g., Neutrogena, Aveeno, Oilatum, Purpose). Avoid bubble baths.
4. Apply occlusive topical agent (Vaseline, Aquaphor ointment, Eucerin cream, Vanicream, Moisturel cream), emollient (Moisturel lotion, Neutrogena emulsion), or prescribed topical preparation two or three times a day, particularly immediately after a bath or shower. (Ointments and creams seal in water and thereby hydrate the skin. The emollient selected depends on the degree of xerosis, the patient's preference, and whether the ingredients in the base, such as preservatives, stabilizers, and fragrances, are irritants or allergens to that patient).

Teach strategies to reduce inflammation

1. Apply topical steroids (available as lotion, solution, gel, cream, or ointment) to affected areas twice a day or as directed. (Topical corticosteroids reduce skin inflammation and relieve itching and are used to control flare-ups of dermatitis and psoriasis. The proper preparation depends on the location and severity of the lesions. The patient should be informed of the topical steroid's strength and possible side effects. Topical steroids should be applied only to active lesions and not to normal skin.)
2. Apply tar preparations (available as lotion, solution, gel, cream, ointment, or shampoo) to affected skin as directed. Tar preparations may also be added to the bathwater. (Before the advent of topical steroids, extracts of crude coal tar were used to reduce skin inflammation. The antiinflammatory properties of tars are not as quick acting as topical steroids, but the effect lasts longer, and fewer side effects arise.

Tars may be used alone or in conjunction with other topical agents. Using tar preparations on acutely inflamed skin may cause burning or irritation.)
3. Undergo ultraviolet light therapy for widespread involvement or recalcitrant disease. (UVB or PUVA therapy under professional supervision can be highly effective. The side effects include sunburn and possibly skin cancer; however, with severe disease, the potential benefits usually far outweigh the risks. Phototherapy is contraindicated in patients with photoexacerbated dermatoses.)
4. Use anthralin products as directed with widespread discrete lesions consisting primarily of thick, psoriatic plaques. (With all the various methods of applying anthralin, it is important to apply the medication only to the affected lesions for the prescribed period of time, avoiding contact with normal surrounding skin. Wash hands immediately after applying, and remove drug by showering or bathing.)

Teach signs and treatment of infection

1. Teach the patient the signs of infection—for example, erythema, warmth, and pain—and emphasize that development of these signs indicates a need for medical treatment.
2. Make sure the patient understands the importance of reevaluation with each outbreak, and that self-treatment with leftover medication at home should not be undertaken.
3. Emphasize that once an antibiotic has been prescribed, it is important to take it on schedule and until the entire course is completed.

Teach ways to reduce exposure to external irritants

1. Wash all new clothes before wearing to remove formaldehyde and other chemicals, and do not use fabric softeners. (Pruritus often is precipitated by an irritant or the allergic effects of certain chemicals or components of fabric softeners.)
2. Residual laundry detergent in clothing may be irritating. Changing to a milder detergent may help, but adding a second rinse cycle to ensure removal of soap is better. (The particular laundry soap used is not the key factor; rather, it is that all soap is rinsed out.)
3. Wear garments that allow air to pass freely to the skin. Open-weave, loose-fitting, cotton blend clothing may be most suitable. Avoid overdressing, rough or wool fabrics, and tightly woven fabrics. (Light, cotton blend clothing allows air to circulate and minimizes perspiration, reducing the risk of pruritus.)

4. Work and sleep in comfortable surroundings with a fairly constant temperature and humidity level. Air conditioning in the home, particularly the bedroom, may be beneficial. (Temperature extremes cause pruritus, frequently secondary to vasodilation and increased cutaneous blood flow. Besides providing a cooler environment, air conditioning decreases aeroallergen exposure, giving additional relief to patients with aeroallergen-induced symptoms.) Using a cool-mist humidifier at bedside will help increase humidity.

5. Keep fingernails very short, smooth, and clean to prevent damage and infection to the skin.

6. Take antihistamines to reduce itching.

7. Use sunscreen regularly. (Besides preventing flare-ups of disease caused by sunburn, sunscreen prevents photodamage and reduces the risk of skin cancer.)

8. Take a shower or bath immediately after swimming. Wash with a mild soap from head to toe to remove any residual chlorine or bromine from the skin. Apply an appropriate moisturizer.

CHAPTER 4

Bullous and Vesicular Diseases

Pemphigus

Pemphigus is an autoimmune process that involves the skin and mucous membranes. It may take either a superficial or a deep form and can be subclassified into two types, **pemphigus vulgaris** and **pemphigus foliaceus.**

PATHOPHYSIOLOGY

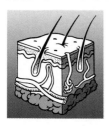

Pemphigus vulgaris is the more common form of the disease, and until the advent of corticosteroids, it was universally fatal. It is most commonly seen in the fourth, fifth, and sixth decades of life, although cases have been reported in children as young as 18 months of age and in individuals as old as 70. There is neither a predilection for sex nor a preponderant geographic region.

Clinically, pemphigus vulgaris manifests with flaccid, weeping, bullous lesions. The bullae may arise on skin that appears normal or on an erythematous base. The bullae rupture easily, leaving large denuded areas that develop crusts. Because the primary lesion, the bulla, is friable, crusting may be the only lesion present when the patient seeks diagnosis and treatment. Mucous membranes commonly are involved and may show the only apparent symptoms for weeks or months.

If pemphigus is suspected but no bullae are apparent, Nikolsky's sign (dislodging the epidermis by applying lateral finger pressure) will be positive.

Bullae may develop gradually and may be localized. If left untreated, the lesions generalize. Bullae vary in size, from 1 cm to several centimeters. The most commonly affected areas are the head, scalp, trunk (particularly intertriginous areas), and mucous membranes (including the conjunctiva). Photophobia, irritation, and pain are common with conjunctival involvement.

The patient may experience pruritus, burning, and local discomfort when the bullae first appear. As the lesions rupture, pain becomes the predominant symptom. Malodorous lesions are characteristic of untreated disease. Protein is lost through the fluid in the bullae, and with involvement of the oral mucosa, the patient is unable to maintain nutrition, compounding the protein depletion. Left untreated, the disease leads to malnutrition, excessive protein loss, and eventually death.

Pemphigus foliaceus, also known as *Cazenave's pemphigus* or *idiopathic pemphigus,* is a benign form of superficial pemphigus. The cause is unknown. The disease follows a variable course, which is punctuated by periodic flare-ups. It is diagnosed through observation and skin biopsy. Pemphigus foliaceus generally is seen after 70 years of age or during the preadolescent years. It is equally common in males and females. Pemphigus foliaceus has been reported in association with other autoimmune diseases such as rheumatoid arthritis, Sjögren's syndrome, and bullous pemphigoid.

Pemphigus foliaceus occurs in two forms, generalized and localized. The generalized form appears as a general exfoliative dermatitis. The localized form manifests as scattered lesions over the scalp, the butterfly area of the face, and the upper trunk. Either type may transform into the other. The initial lesion may be a scaling papule or plaque, or in some incidences a vesicle or bulla. The lesions generally first appear on the face, neck, or upper trunk and evolve slowly for 6 months. Generalization may occur within a few weeks, although this is unusual.

The primary lesion is a flaccid vesicle or bulla on normal-appearing skin or on an urticarial base. Bullae and vesicles rupture easily, releasing fluid and forming a crust from the roof of the vesicle or bulla. As the crust is forming centrally, the lesion may extend peripherally. These lesions may coalesce, extending to large areas. In contrast to pemphigus vulgaris, mucous membrane involvement in pemphigus foliaceus is transient. Pemphigus foliaceus may become chronic, manifesting as keratotic plaques, nodules, or hyperpigmentation.

Symptomatic complaints include pain, burning, and pruritus. With involvement of the intertriginous areas of the neck and axillae, symptoms increase. As in pemphigus vulgaris, the lesions have a characteristic odor. The lesions of pemphigus vulgaris are particularly malodorous, whereas those of pemphigus foliaceus have a musty smell.

COMPLICATIONS

Impaired skin integrity related to bullous lesions
Pain related to erosions of the skin's surface and oral lesions
Altered nutritional status related to oral lesions
High risk for infection related to compromised integument

The Tzanck test, conducted on the contents of the bulla, confirms the diagnosis of pemphigus. To obtain fluid for the test, the roof of the bulla is carefully removed, and the base is gently scraped with a curette or scalpel blade. The specimen is placed on a microscope slide, stained, and examined.

Immunofluorescent microscopic examination of tissue may be done to detect tissue-bound and/or circulating anti–intracellular substance antibodies. The tissue is obtained by skin biopsy. Skin biopsy also shows the level of blistering, which corroborates the diagnosis. The bullae form because cohesion of the epidermal cells below the basal cell layer is lost.

Increasingly severe anemia and increased leukocytosis are characteristic of advanced pemphigus; these laboratory values indicate a poor prognosis. Eosinophilia may be present, but it decreases as the disease progresses. Serum electrophoresis shows decreased albumin and increased alpha-1 and alpha-2 globulins. As the disease progresses, sodium, chloride, and calcium are depleted, with an associated rise in potassium. This electrolyte imbalance is very similar to that seen with severe burns.

Routine laboratory tests are of no particular benefit in the diagnosis of pemphigus foliaceus, because the patient's general health usually is not affected by the disease. Peripheral eosinophilia may be seen in patients with extensive, prolonged involvement. Both direct and indirect immunofluorescent techniques are used to detect anti–intercellular substance autoantibodies in skin biopsy specimens from individuals with pemphigus foliaceus.

Pemphigus foliaceous, generalized and of the mucous membrane, is illustrated in Color Plates 38 and 39 on pp. xviii and xix.

DIAGNOSTIC STUDIES AND FINDINGS

Diagnostic Test	Findings
Skin biopsy	Intraepidermal bulla, acantholysis (separation of epidermal cells near the blister following dissolution of the intercellular cement), mild to moderate eosinophilia; direct or indirect immunofluorescence demonstrates IgG antibodies
Tzanck test	Confirms acantholytic process
Complete blood count (CBC)	Severe anemia suggests the disease is progressive and indicates a poor prognosis; leukocytosis increases with severity; eosinophilia decreases with disease progression
Electrolytes	As disease progresses, sodium, chloride, and calcium decrease; potassium increases
Serum protein electrophoresis	Decreased albumin, increased alpha-1 and alpha-2 globulins

MEDICAL MANAGEMENT

GENERAL MANAGEMENT

Topical treatment: Sulfadiazine cream; topical antibiotic ointments for blisters or erosions. Mouthwashes: Cepacol, Benadryl Elixir, viscous Xylocaine. *It is important to maintain oral hygiene during outbreaks.* Supportive treatment: Patients with pemphigus foliaceus cannot tolerate topical ointments; creams, lotions, and dusting powders are more acceptable forms of delivering treatment.

Antimalarial drugs: Chloroquine, hydroxychloroquine, or a combination of these two has been used to treat pemphigus foliaceus; however, the risk-benefit trade-off for this therapy should be carefully considered.

DRUG THERAPY

Systemic corticosteroids: The mainstay of medical management; usually given orally but occasionally administered parenterally; used to suppress widespread involvement that includes mucous membranes

Immunosuppressants: Methotrexate, azathioprine (Imuran), or cyclophosphamide (Cytoxan) generally is used as an adjunct to steroid therapy.

Sulfone: Dapsone, alone or in combination with high-dose steroids.

OTHER MEDICAL MANAGEMENT

Plasmapheresis: May be used to eliminate circulating antibodies.

Extracorporeal photochemotherapy and oral cyclosporine: Currently under investigation as a therapeutic regimen.

---

1 ASSESS

ASSESSMENT	OBSERVATIONS
Current health status	May report presence of lesions in glabrous (hairless) skin or mucous membranes for weeks or months; may complain of inability to maintain adequate nutrition because of oral lesions; may report weight loss, decreased energy, and dry skin
Skin	**Early stage:** May have flaccid bullae ($\leq$1 cm in diameter), which may be generally distributed or may be confined to the head, trunk, and mucous membranes **Late stage:** Intact bullae or raw, denuded areas, or both scaling and crusting may be evident
Nikolsky's sign	Avulsion of outermost epidermal layers with application of lateral pressure is indicative of pemphigus
Odor	Offensive odor may be present
Oral mucosa	May have vesicular lesions on the gums; ragged ulcerative lesions may be present secondary to inadvertent biting of tissue

→ › ›

ASSESSMENT	OBSERVATIONS
Discomfort	May complain of pruritus, burning, and local discomfort, particularly with onset of new lesions
Pain	Usually a major symptom after bullae have ruptured; extensive involvement of tongue, cheeks, and oropharynx produces extreme pain

2 DIAGNOSE

NURSING DIAGNOSIS	SUBJECTIVE FINDINGS	OBJECTIVE FINDINGS
Impaired skin integrity related to skin lesions	Reports finding lesions	Localized or generalized flaccid bullae and/or erosions
Altered nutrition: less than body requirements related to oral lesions	Complains of inability to eat because of painful oral lesions	Lesions on oral mucosa; decreased food intake, decrease in total serum protein
Pain related to erosions on skin's surface and/or oral lesions	Complains of pain in involved area and of being unable to wear clothes comfortably	Facial expression indicates pain; reports pain during skin examination
High risk for infection related to compromised integument	Impairment of skin's barrier function increases potential for microbial invasion	Large denuded areas of skin

3 PLAN

Patient goals

1. The barrier function of the skin will be restored.
2. The patient will maintain adequate nutrition.
3. The patient will be free of pain.
4. The patient will be free of infection.

4 IMPLEMENT

NURSING DIAGNOSIS	NURSING INTERVENTIONS	RATIONALE
Impaired skin integrity related to skin lesions	Provide temporary barrier with topical medications or dressings.	Body must be protected from invasion by microorganisms while skin is healing.

NURSING DIAGNOSIS	NURSING INTERVENTIONS	RATIONALE
Altered nutrition: less than body requirements related to oral lesions	Offer mouthwash before eating; maintain good oral hygiene.	Mouthwashes containing topical anesthetics ease pain of lesions, allowing patient to eat.
	Offer high-protein milkshakes.	High-protein milkshakes are easily ingested and help replace protein lost through compromised skin.
Pain related to erosions on skin's surface and/or oral lesions	Assess pain, and administer pain relief medication as needed.	Degree of pain indicates disease progression.
High risk for infection related to compromised integument	Observe for clinical signs of infection.	To gauge extent of immunosuppression and loss of barrier function.

5 EVALUATE

PATIENT OUTCOME	DATA INDICATING THAT OUTCOME IS REACHED
Skin's barrier function has been restored.	Lesions have healed or are in an advanced stage of healing.
Patient's nutritional status has improved.	Patient's energy level has increased; skin's hydration has improved; laboratory values are normal.
Patient has no pain.	Patient reports increased level of comfort; need for pain medication has decreased.
Patient has no infection.	Patient shows no signs of local or systemic infection.

PATIENT TEACHING

1. Explain the need for a healthy, balanced diet to enhance healing.
2. Teach the patient about the disease and its course.
3. Teach the patient about the different types of treatment. *For patients taking systemic steroids:* Explain the need to have serum electrolytes monitored; explain that a latent infection may be reactivated, that a current one may be aggravated, or that gastrointestinal bleeding may develop; explain that steroid-induced diabetes is possible. *For patients receiving immunosuppressant therapy:* Give explicit instructions about the possible side effects of these drugs, including reversible neutropenia, alopecia, cystitis, and bleeding from an inflamed bladder.
4. Emphasize the need to comply with all provisions of the treatment regimen; advise the patient to be conscientious about follow-up visits to the physician.

Pemphigoid

Bullous pemphigoid, also known as **pemphigus vulgaris chronicus, pemphigus vulgaris benignus,** or **localized pemphigoid,** is a benign blistering disease of unknown cause. It is characterized histologically by subepidermal bullae and is seen primarily in adults past middle age.

PATHOPHYSIOLOGY

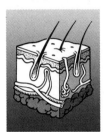 The underlying cause of pemphigoid is unknown, but some theorize that it may be associated with an underlying malignancy, even though the incidence of malignancy in affected individuals has not proved to be higher. Internal malignancy should always be considered in the workup of a patient with pemphigoid. Other researchers think the disease is somehow associated with ingestion of certain drugs, but this, too, is currently just a theory. Bullous pemphigoid has been reported in association with pemphigus vulgaris and pemphigus foliaceus. No immunologic significance has been shown with this association.

The disease is characterized by bullae that range in size from 5 to 10 cm. The bullae may arise from skin that appears normal or from erythematous or urticarial plaques. The bullae are recurrent and may remain localized to the trunk or extremities, showing a predilection for the intertriginous areas (in contrast to the bullae of pemphigus, which have a predilection for the scalp and chest). These recurrent lesions may last for weeks, or they may spread rapidly (within 1 or 2 weeks) to generalized distribution. Pemphigoid is generally self-limiting, remitting 2 to 6 years after onset. Pemphigus, in contrast, has a more protracted, lifelong course.

See Color Plates 8 and 9 on p. xiv for examples of bullous pemphigoid.

A pemphigoid bulla is filled with clear serum and is very tense (the bullae in pemphigus are flaccid). The contents may become purulent, and occasionally hemorrhagic, after 48 to 72 hours, and the bullae rupture easily. Severe pruritus and burning usually are the symptomatic complaints. Unlike in pemphigus, Nikolsky's sign (dislodging the epidermis with lateral finger pressure) is negative in pemphigoid. Oral lesions are less common and less severe than those seen with pemphigus.

Recognizing the clinical presentation of pemphigoid is paramount to diagnosis, because no laboratory findings other than skin biopsy lead to diagnosis. The occurrence of tense bullae on an erythematous or urticarial base, located on the trunk and proximal part of the lower extremities in a patient past middle age, should alert the clinician to rule out pemphigoid. The oral mucosa should always be examined for lesions, even though they are rarely present. In pemphigoid the patient's general health remains good, which is a good prognostic sign. Therefore, a thorough patient history, skin assessment, and skin biopsy generally make the diagnosis of pemphigoid.

COMPLICATIONS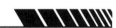

Impaired skin integrity
Severe pruritus
Infection
Debility, particularly in the elderly, secondary to generalized involvement

DIAGNOSTIC STUDIES AND FINDINGS

Diagnostic Test	Findings
Skin biopsy	Subepidermal blister, inflammation, edema of the papillary dermis; blister contains a mixture of eosinophils and polymorphonuclear leukocytes

MEDICAL MANAGEMENT

GENERAL MANAGEMENT

Topical treatment: Medicated tub baths using a 1:16,000 solution of potassium permanganate or Aveeno (oil-ated oatmeal) help relieve the pruritus and irritation. Local symptoms can be alleviated by applying wet dressings using 0.25% to 0.50% aluminum subacetate (Burow's solution) after the bath continuously for 24 hours, changing q 2-3 h to prevent drying, followed by application of a drying lotion (e.g., zinc oxide shake lotion). Tap water, wet dressings, and topical steroids are also useful when the disease flares.

DRUG THERAPY

Systemic corticosteroids: Usually given orally and generally at lower doses than those used in pemphigus. Maintenance therapy may be required for years, and exacerbations are treated by increasing the dosage.

Sulfa or sulfone: Sulfapyridine or dapsone sometimes is beneficial, but they should be given only after determining that kidney function is normal.

Immunosuppressive drugs: Azathioprine is used to help withdraw corticosteroid as maintenance therapy; in some instances pemphigoid may be managed by using azathioprine alone. Cyclophosphamide may be used in patients who develop complications from corticosteroids; it is given in combination to lower the dose of corticosteroid. Methotrexate may be used as an adjunct to corticosteroid therapy. Insulin-dependent diabetics tend to respond better to immunosuppressant therapy alone than to combination therapy with corticosteroids.

1 ASSESS

ASSESSMENT	OBSERVATIONS
Current health status	May report blisters on trunk and extremities and in intertriginous areas; may report severe pruritus or burning sensation
Skin	Tense bullae may be found on trunk and proximal extremities and in intertriginous areas; bullae may have erythematous or urticarial base ranging in size from 5 to 10 cm; bullae may be intact, or erosions secondary to rupture may be present
Nikolsky's sign	Negative
Oral mucosa	Lesions rarely present

2 DIAGNOSE

NURSING DIAGNOSIS	SUBJECTIVE FINDINGS	OBJECTIVE FINDINGS
Impaired skin integrity related to skin lesions	Reports finding lesions	Lesions on trunk, proximal extremities, and/or intertriginous areas

NURSING DIAGNOSIS	SUBJECTIVE FINDINGS	OBJECTIVE FINDINGS
Pain (pruritus) related to skin lesions	Complains of itching	Evidence of scratching; facial expression indicates discomfort
High risk for infection related to compromised integument	Complains of fever, pain, and presence of drainage	Erosions on skin secondary to rupture of bullae

3 PLAN

Patient goals

1. The barrier function of the skin will be restored.
2. The patient will be free of pruritus.
3. The patient will have no infection.

4 IMPLEMENT

NURSING DIAGNOSIS	NURSING INTERVENTIONS	RATIONALE
Impaired skin integrity related to skin lesions	Provide temporary barrier function with topical medications and dressings	Body must be protected from invasion by microorganisms while the skin is healing
Pain (pruritus) related to skin lesions	Assess pruritus and administer antipruritics as needed for comfort; use cool wet dressings and medicated baths for symptomatic relief	Assessment of pruritus will give an indication of disease progression
High risk for infection related to compromised integument	Observe for signs of clinical infection	Immunosuppression and loss of barrier function increase the potential for infection

5 EVALUATE

PATIENT OUTCOME	DATA INDICATING THAT OUTCOME IS REACHED
Skin's barrier function has been restored.	Lesions have healed or are in an advanced stage of healing.
Patient is free of pruritus.	Patient reports increased level of comfort; need for antipruritic drugs has decreased.

PATIENT OUTCOME	DATA INDICATING THAT OUTCOME IS REACHED
Patient has no infection.	Patient shows no clinical signs of infection.

PATIENT TEACHING

1. Teach the patient about the disease and its course.
2. Teach the patient about the types of treatment (see Patient Teaching for pemphigus).
3. Emphasize the need to comply with all provisions of the treatment regimen; advise the patient to be sure to keep follow-up visits with the physician.

CHAPTER 5

Cutaneous Manifestations of Systemic Disease

Many systemic diseases may produce cutaneous lesions, either as a primary sign or as secondary manifestations. Cutaneous manifestations can be divided into several categories: rheumatology, hematology/oncology, endocrinology/metabolic, infectious disease, and general reactions to cutaneous disease. The rheumatologic diseases that have distinct cutaneous manifestations are lupus erythematosus, dermatomyositis, and scleroderma.

Lupus Erythematosus

Lupus erythematosus (LE) is a chronic, multisystem, autoimmune, inflammatory disorder characterized chiefly by antibody formation directed against autologous tissues and serum factors.

LE can range from a benign, self-limited cutaneous presentation to a severe, often fatal systemic disease. Lupus is classified as discoid, subacute cutaneous, or systemic.

PATHOPHYSIOLOGY

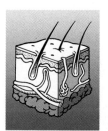

Discoid lupus erythematosus (DLE) is limited entirely to the skin and has a predilection for women, generally in the fourth decade of life. Lesions manifest as violet-red papules or plaques with thick adherent scale and hyperpigmented margins. The underside of the scale has a characteristic carpet tack appearance, seen when the scale is lifted off its erythematous base. This is caused by penetration of the scale into the orifices of hair follicles. Telangiectasia, hypopigmentation, and central atrophy are characteristic. Hypopigmented scars remain after the initial lesions resolve. The lesions characteristically are asymmetric and are most commonly found on the face, neck, scalp, and backs of the hands, although **Various manifestations of discoid lupus erythematosus are depicted in Color Plates 12 to 17 on pp. xiv to xv.** they may appear on any body surface. Scalp lesions may leave permanent alopecia (hair loss) when they resolve. The lesions may be initiated by trauma or exposure to ultraviolet light. Oral ulcers are a possible nonspecific manifestation. Evidence of systemic lupus erythematosus is seen in 5% to 10% of patients with DLE. Polymorphous light eruption and lichen planus should be ruled out during the workup for DLE.

Subacute cutaneous lupus erythematosus (SCLE) is seen in women between the ages of 35 and 45. The characteristic lesions are violet-red papules or plaques arranged in a polycyclic or annular distribution. Telangiectasia and scale are also present. The lesions are distributed in areas of the trunk, upper extremities, and shoulders that are exposed to the sun. Facial involvement is less than in DLE, and the lesions of SCLE are symmetric rather than asymmetric (in contrast to those of DLE). The lesions may resolve with hypopigmentation but without scarring. Nonspecific skin manifestations include periungual telangiectasia, photosensitivity, oral lesions, nonscarring alopecia, and livedo reticularis. In contrast to DLE, however, SCLE has systemic manifestations; fever, arthralgia, and malaise are seen in conjunction with the cutaneous lesions. In some cases renal involvement, serositis, and central nervous system (CNS) disease may be seen. These manifestations generally are less severe than with systemic lupus erythematosus. Differential diagnosis includes psoriasis, eczema, erythema multiforme, photodrug eruption, and dermatomyositis.

Systemic lupus erythematosus (SLE) is an autoimmune disorder of unknown origin characterized by the production of antibodies against host tissue. Antigen antibodies form against self-antigens. This leads to trapping of immune complexes in tissues, causing a generalized inflammatory response and widespread damage to organs. Besides autoimmunity, predisposition and drugs have been suggested as possible causes. SLE is known as the great imitator, because it can mimic many diseases. Because its symptoms may be transitory, joint and muscle pain, fatigue, chills, and occasional fever may be misdiagnosed as flu or rheumatoid arthritis, and respiratory infections may be attributed to pneumonia. The disease is more prevalent in women than men by a ratio of 8:1. The characteristic lesions are violet-red, indurated plaques that may have fine scale. The lesions seen in the sun-exposed areas of the face (malar area and nose) are known as the butterfly rash of lupus. Generalized erythema may be present in some cases. Oral ulcers, periungual telangiectasia, palpable purpura, livedo reticularis, urticaria, Raynaud's phenomenon, nonscarring alopecia, and panniculitis are nonspecific skin manifestations. Purpura, petechiae, leg ulcers, digital gangrene, urticarial lesions, and diffuse, transient rashes may also be cutaneous expressions of SLE. Systemic complaints include fever, arthralgia, and malaise. The differential diagnosis should include erysipelas, acne rosacea, and seborrheic dermatitis. The established criteria for diagnosing systemic lupus erythematosus are listed in the box on page 50. Four of the 11 criteria should be present before the diagnosis of SLE is made.

Symptoms and cutaneous presentations that mimic lupus may be seen in drug-induced lupus syndrome. This is most often the case with use of penicillamine, hydralazine, and procainamide. **Color Plates 29 to 32 on p. xvii illustrate a variety of systemic lupus erythematosus manifestations.** The lesions are distributed in a sun-exposed pattern, and patients may complain of fever, myalgia, arthralgia, serositis, rash, and CNS disturbances. Renal manifestations are rare. The cutaneous and systemic manifestations are related to liver metabolism of the drug. Up to 10% of patients will have chronic cutaneous lesions. The symptoms improve when the drug is withdrawn.

COMPLICATIONS

Photosensitivity
Atrophic scarring (DLE)
Painless oral or nasopharyngeal ulceration
Arthritis involving two or more peripheral joints
Serositis
Persistent proteinuria
Seizures
Hemolytic anemia, leukopenia, lymphopenia, thrombocytopenia
Fatigue

CRITERIA FOR CLASSIFICATION OF SYSTEMIC LUPUS ERYTHEMATOSUS

The 1982 revised classification of SLE is based on the 11 criteria defined below. For the purpose of identifying patients in clinical studies, a person should be said to have SLE if any four or more of the 11 criteria are present, serially or simultaneously, during any interval of observation.

Malar rash: fixed erythema, flat or raised, over malar eminences, tending to spare nasolabial folds

Discoid rash: erythematous raised patches with adherent keratotic scaling and follicular plugging; atrophic scarring may occur in older lesions

Photosensitivity: skin rash as a result of unusual reaction to sunlight, based on patient's history or physician's observation

Oral ulcers: oral or nasopharyngeal ulceration, usually painless, observed by physician

Arthritis: nonerosive arthritis involving two or more peripheral joints, characterized by tenderness, swelling, or effusion

Serositis: pleuritis—convincing history of pleuritic pain or rub heard by a physician or evidence of pleural effusion—or pericarditis—documented by electrocardiogram, rub, or evidence of pericardial effusion

Renal disorder: persistent proteinuria greater than 0.5 g/day or greater than 3+ if quantitation is not performed or cellular casts—may be red cell, hemoglobin, granular, tubular, or mixed

Neurologic disorder: seizures in the absence of offending drugs or known metabolic derangements (such as uremia, ketoacidosis, or electrolyte imbalance) or psychosis in the absence of offending drugs or known metabolic derangements

Hematologic disorder: hemolytic anemia with reticulocytosis or leukopenia—less than 4,000/mm^3 total on two or more occasions or lymphopenia—less than 1,500/mm^3 on two or more occasions or thrombocytopenia—less 100,000/mm^3 in the absence of offending drugs

Immunologic disorder: positive LE cell preparation or anti-DNA—antibody to native DNA in abnormal titer or anti-Sm—presence of antibody to Sm nuclear antigen or false-positive serologic test for syphilis known to be positive for at least 6 months and confirmed by *Treponema pallidum* immobilization or fluorescent treponemal antibody absorption test

Antinuclear antibody: abnormal titer of antinuclear antibody by immunofluorescence or equivalent assay at any point in time and in the absence of drugs known to be associated with drug-induced lupus syndrome

From Thompson et al.[61]

DIAGNOSTIC STUDIES AND FINDINGS

Diagnostic Test	Findings
Antinuclear antibody (ANA)	Positive in titers 1:80
Anti-double-stranded DNA antibody (ds-DNA)	Positive in titers >1:80
Rapid plasma reagin (RPR)	False positive
Antibody absorption (FTA-ABS)	Negative
Complement (C3 and C4)	Decreased during flare-ups, indicative of inflammation; otherwise within normal limits
Skin or muscle biopsy	Evidence of inflammation with or without tissue necrosis; deposits of immunoglobulin and complement at dermal-epidermal junctions
Kidney biopsy	Focal or diffuse proliferative nephritis; also membranous or interstitial disease
Complete blood count	Pancytopenia or selective deficits; lymphopenia during flare-ups
C-reactive protein	Elevated during flare-ups, indicative of inflammatory state
Erythrocyte sedimentation rate	Elevated during flare-ups, indicative of acute inflammatory state

Diagnostic Test	Findings
Coombs' test	Positive with hemolytic anemia because of autoantibody production against erythrocytes
Coagulation profile	Prolonged prothrombin time and partial thromboplastin time if circulating anticoagulant antibodies are present
Rheumatoid factor (RF) (anti-IgG antibody)	Usually positive in titer >1:40
Circulating immune complexes	Present during flare-ups
Urinalysis	Abnormal casts and sediment associated with renal damage

MEDICAL MANAGEMENT

The goal of treatment is to reduce inflammation.

GENERAL MANAGEMENT

Nutrition: A balanced diet is indicated for all patients, regardless of type or stage of LE; salt-restricted diet is indicated for patients receiving systemic corticosteroids.

Activity: Exercise should be balanced with adequate rest and should be avoided during flare-ups.

Sun exposure: Photosensitivity is a complication of LE in all stages; sunscreens, appropriate clothing, and staying out of the sun should be encouraged.

Miscellaneous: Patients diagnosed with LE should not use birth control pills.

DRUG THERAPY

Nonsteroidal antiinflammatory agents: Acetylsalicylic acid, given daily; indomethacin (Indocin), given daily in divided doses for symptomatic relief of joint pain.

Antimalarial drugs: Hydroxychloroquine (Plaquenil) or chloroquine, used after failure to respond to topical steroids; effective in the treatment of all forms of cutaneous LE; dosage is kept at daily recommended dosage until resolution of lesions, then reduced to lowest possible dosage.

Systemic corticosteroids: Prednisone, given in low to high doses depending on stage of disease; used for antiinflammatory effect.

Topical steroids: Generally used first in the treatment of all forms of cutaneous LE; grade I to grade V steroid (see topical steroid potency chart) is applied directly to lesions three times a day to control cutaneous lesions.

Intralesional corticosteroids: Triamcinolone (Kenalog) mixed with equal parts lidocaine or saline may be injected directly into the lesions of DLE; usually used after failure to respond to topical steroid application.

Antineoplastic agents: Azathioprine (Imuran), cyclophosphamide (Cytoxan, Neosar), chlorambucil (Leukeran) are drugs of choice.

Sulfones: Effective alternative to antimalarial drugs; Dapsone is the drug of choice.

Systemic corticosteroids: Used in patients who have failed trials of antimalarial drugs, topical steroids, and Dapsone; other drugs are discontinued before therapy is begun.

OTHER MEDICAL MANAGEMENT

Plasmapheresis: Used to decrease circulating immune complexes and autoantibodies.

Peritoneal dialysis or hemodialysis: Indicated for patients with renal insufficiency or failure.

POTENCY RANKING OF COMMON TOPICAL STEROIDS*

Group	Brand name	Generic name
1	Diprolene Creme	Betamethasone dipropionate
	Diprolene Ointment	Betamethasone dipropionate in optimized vehicle
	Psorcon Ointment	Diflorasone diacetate
	Temovate Cream/Ointment	Clobetasol propionate
	Ultravate Cream/Ointment	Halobetasol propionate
2	Cyclocort Ointment	Amcinonide
	Diprolene AF Cream	Betamethasone dipropionate
	Diprolene Ointment	Betamethasone dipropionate
	Elocon Ointment	Mometasone furoate
	Florone Ointment	Diflorasone diacetate
	Halog Cream	Halcinonide
	Lidex Cream/Gel/Ointment	Fluocinonide
	Maxiflor Ointment	Diflorasone diacetate
	Maxivate Ointment	Betamethasone dipropionate
	Topicort Cream/Ointment	Desoximethasone
3	Aristocort Cream	Triamcinolone acetonide
	Diprosone Cream	Betamethasone dipropionate
	Florone Cream	Diflorasone diacetate
	Halog Ointment/Solution	Halcinonide
	Lidex-E Cream	Fluocinonide
	Maxiflor Cream	Diflorasone diacetate
	Maxivate Cream	Betamethasone dipropionate
4	Aristocort Ointment	Triamcinolone acetonide
	Cordran Ointment	Flurandrenolide
	Elocon Cream	Mometasone furoate
	Kenalog Ointment	Triamcinolone acetonide
	Synalar Cream (HP)/Ointment	Fluocinolone acetonide
	Topicort LP Cream	Desoximethasone
5	Cordran Cream	Flurandrenolide
	Diprosone Lotion	Betamethasone dipropionate
	Elocon Lotion	Mometasone furoate
	Kenalog Cream/Lotion	Triamcinolone acetonide
	Locoid Cream/Ointment	Hydrocortisone butyrate
	Maxivate Lotion	Betamethasone dipropionate
	Synalar Cream	Fluocinolone acetonide
	Westcort Cream	Hydrocortisone valerate
6	DesOwen Cream/Lotion/Ointment	Desonide
	Aclovate Cream/Ointment	Aclometasone dipropionate
	Synalar Solution	Fluocinolone acetonide
	Tridesilon Cream	Desonide
7	Nutracort Cream/Lotion	Hydrocortisone

Other topicals with hydrocortisone, dexamethasone, flumethalone, prednisolone, and methylprednisolone

*Group 1 is most potent, with Group 7 being the least potent.

1 ASSESS

ASSESSMENT	OBSERVATIONS
Skin and mucous membranes	Facial erythema; butterfly rash; diffuse, transient rash; urticarial lesions; discoid lesions; classic sun-exposed distribution of lesions; photosensitivity; oral and nasal ulcerations; purpura; petechiae; demarcated, annular, erythematous plaques with atrophy, scaling, and telangiectasia; periungual erythema; digital gangrene; leg ulcers; edema; periorbital edema; alopecia; Raynaud's phenomenon; livedo reticularis; adherent scale that "plugs" dilated hair follicles (carpet tack appearance)
Neuropsychiatric	Visual disturbances; facial weakness; vertigo; nystagmus; trigeminal neuralgia; aphasia; hemiparesis; headache; peripheral neuropathies; anxiety; depression; mania; insomnia; confusion; hallucinations; disorientation; emotional lability; psychosis
Musculoskeletal	Arthralgia; arthritis; Baker's cysts; diffuse myalgia; aseptic bone necrosis or myopathy; pseudothrombophlebitis
Gastrointestinal	Acute abdomen; dysphagia; gastric and duodenal ulcerations
Hematologic	Anemia: autoimmune hemolytic anemia, iron-deficiency anemia, chronic anemia; granulocytopenia; leukocytosis; lymphocytopenia; thrombocytopenia; lymphadenopathy; splenomegaly; hepatomegaly; coagulopathies
Cardiovascular	Diffuse vasculitis; dysrhythmias; thrombophlebitis; endocarditis; pericarditis; myocarditis
Pulmonary	Pleurisy; pleural effusion; pneumonitis; decreased pulmonary function; pulmonary hypertension; pulmonary emboli
Renal	"Lupus nephritis"; hypertension; electrolyte imbalances

2 DIAGNOSE

NURSING DIAGNOSIS	SUBJECTIVE FINDINGS	OBJECTIVE FINDINGS
Impaired skin integrity related to cutaneous manifestations	Reports presence of lesions and rash	Facial erythema; butterfly rash; diffuse, transient rash; urticarial lesions; discoid lesions; involvement of sun-exposed areas; photosensitivity; oral and nasal ulcerations; purpura; petechiae; demarcated, annular, erythematous plaques with atrophy, scaling, and telangiectasia; periungual erythema; digital gangrene; leg ulcers; edema; periorbital edema; alopecia; Raynaud's phenomenon
Ineffective individual coping related to organic brain syndrome associated with SLE or difficulty dealing with diagnosis and its implications	Exhibits signs of poor coping, disorientation; family or significant other reports decrease in mentation	Disoriented to person, place, time; poor attention span; exhibits poor coping mechanisms; emotionally labile

→ > >

NURSING DIAGNOSIS	SUBJECTIVE FINDINGS	OBJECTIVE FINDINGS
Impaired physical mobility related to arthritis and general weakness	Reports decreased mobility, increased pain and weakness	Decreased range of motion, increased swelling over joints; unable to complete routine daily activities
Decreased cardiac output related to reduced ventricular filling (most commonly due to pericarditis)	Reports dizziness; palpitations; shortness of breath; chest pain	Irregular apical pulse; pericardial friction rub on auscultation; peripheral edema
Ineffective breathing pattern related to pulmonary complications	Reports difficulty breathing; chest pain	Abnormal respiratory rate and rhythm; abnormal breath sounds
Altered renal tissue perfusion related to renal complications	Reports ankle swelling, weight gain, or anorexia and nausea	Hypertension; abnormal urinalysis; peripheral edema; increased fluid weight gain (>2 g/48 h)
Altered nutrition: less than body requirements related to anorexia, electrolyte imbalance, or chemotherapy side effects	Reports decrease in appetite; fatigue	Low serum albumin and protein; delayed wound healing; decreased body weight
Body image disturbance related to multisystem involvement of SLE, including skin changes	Family or significant other reports decreased socialization; patient reports fear of rejection by others because of appearance	Does not make eye contact; poor hygiene is evident; most skin is hidden under clothes
High risk for infection related to disease process and/or treatment	Complains of skin rash and difficulty breathing	Skin lesions; patient is taking systemic corticosteroids

3 PLAN

Patient goals

1. Skin's barrier function will be maintained.
2. Patient will develop appropriate coping mechanisms and be able to identify resources for support.
3. Patient will attain optimum mobility.
4. Cardiac status will be maximized.
5. Respiratory status will be maximized.
6. Renal status will be maximized.
7. Patient will maintain adequate nutrition.
8. Patient will have a positive and realistic body image.
9. Patient will be free of infection.
10. Patient will achieve an adequate level of comfort.

4 IMPLEMENT

NURSING DIAGNOSIS	NURSING INTERVENTIONS	RATIONALE
Impaired skin integrity related to cutaneous manifestations	Assess skin and mucous membranes; palpate while noting color, vascularity, size, configuration, and distribution of lesions.	To establish a baseline for further assessment and to monitor for extension of disease or infection.
Ineffective individual coping related to organic brain syndrome associated with SLE or difficulty dealing with diagnosis and its implications	Assess changes in neurologic status; assess patient's ability to cope; provide emotional support; encourage verbalization; include family or significant other in care planning.	To identify source of ineffective coping (organic or psychologic) and to identify support mechanisms available; verbalization allows patient to vent feelings.
Impaired physical mobility related to arthritis and general weakness	Assess degree of movement; assess for swelling, atrophy, or deformity.	To establish baseline for assessment of progress.
	Encourage range of motion (ROM) as tolerated.	To maintain joint integrity.
	Consult with physical therapist.	To plan for beneficial interventions.
	Provide rest and support to affected joints.	To stabilize and reduce stress and discomfort.
	Help patient analyze daily tasks and effect of decreased mobility.	To help patient maintain normal routines.
Decreased cardiac output related to reduced ventricular filling (most commonly due to pericarditis)	Assess cardiac status (subjective and objective data); institute prescribed medical regimen.	To initiate appropriate interventions in a timely manner and prevent cardiac complications.
Ineffective breathing pattern related to pulmonary complications	Assess pulmonary status; auscultate lungs for decreased breath sounds, rhonchi, or crackles.	To detect or prevent respiratory compromise and to determine adequacy of gas exchange, effectiveness of breathing, and areas of congestion and atelectasis.
	Monitor respiratory rate and rhythm.	To determine the work of breathing.
	Monitor changes in activity tolerance.	Activity may induce dyspnea.
	Teach patient deep-breathing exercises, and encourage her to perform them as often as needed.	To facilitate deep breathing and to help manage or prevent pulmonary complications.
Altered renal tissue perfusion related to renal complications	Monitor fluid status, intake and output, daily weight, and blood pressure; check for edema and shortness of breath.	Increased fluid volume may indicate that kidneys are unable to handle excess fluid as a result of decreased renal function.

→ > >

NURSING DIAGNOSIS	NURSING INTERVENTIONS	RATIONALE
	Monitor urinalysis and 24-hour creatinine clearance (Crcl); normal Crcl is 80-120 ml/min.	Proteinuria of 500 mg/day and Crcl of 50 ml/min indicate decreasing renal function and require further evaluation.
	Monitor serum laboratory values, specifically elevations in blood urea nitrogen (BUN), creatinine (Scr), potassium, and phosphorus (alterations in calcium-phosphorus balance) and decreased hematocrit (Hct), hemoglobin (Hgb), and carbon dioxide.	To detect early signs of renal insufficiency.
Altered nutrition: less than body requirements related to anorexia, electrolyte imbalance, or chemotherapy side effects	Weigh patient daily.	To obtain baseline and ongoing data on adequacy of nutritional intake.
	Measure fluid intake and output.	To determine fluid balance and whether weight gain is true weight gain or fluid.
	Monitor albumin, transferrin, and serum protein.	These indicate whether protein intake is adequate.
	Measure midarm circumference and triceps skinfold.	These indicate protein and fat stores, respectively.
	Encourage patient to eat small, frequent meals and to take vitamin supplements.	To promote adequate nutritional intake.
Body image disturbance related to multisystem involvement of SLE, including skin changes	Assess patient's perception of body image; investigate what aspects are not pleasing and how changes are perceived as deviating from social norms; determine what personal, social, or community resources are available.	To adequately assess the disturbance to body image and the specific threat, and to guide therapeutic interventions.
	Help patient explore and express feelings about changes in body image.	To help patient realize what changes in body image imply for her.
	Teach patient ways to improve body image (e.g., improved personal hygiene, wearing makeup, change in clothes, protecting skin from sun).	To help patient create a better feeling about her appearance by trying new looks.
	Offer opportunities for social contact, and encourage participation in self-help groups.	Introducing different contacts and services can help patient gain new skills and confidence.
	Acknowledge and give positive reinforcement whenever patient attempts to improve body image.	To demonstrate support and acceptance and to assist in developing patient's self-confidence and a positive body image.
	Encourage patient to participate actively in usual roles and responsibilities.	To maintain independence, a positive outlook, and an active role within the family.

NURSING DIAGNOSIS	NURSING INTERVENTIONS	RATIONALE
	Encourage family members to maintain open communication with patient.	Open communication may minimize stress of role performance, assist family in modifying roles, and Identify and support strengths related to adequate role performance.
High risk for infection related to disease process and/or treatment	Assess and monitor temperature, vital signs, and WBC.	Fever, tachycardia, tachypnea, and an elevated WBC are indicators of infection.
	Assess breakdown in integument, including mucosa.	Infection is resisted through the body's defense mechanisms, the skin being the prime mechanical barrier; disruption in wound healing and oral candidal infections are common with high-dose steroids.
	Encourage sanitation and hygiene practices (e.g., routine mouth care, daily bath, good handwashing).	To help keep skin and mucous membranes intact and to decrease risk of proliferation and transmission of infectious organisms.
	Use aseptic technique when providing care; wash hands thoroughly before and after contact with patient.	To prevent introduction of microorganisms.

5 EVALUATE

PATIENT OUTCOME	DATA INDICATING THAT OUTCOME IS REACHED
Skin's barrier function is maintained.	Skin integrity has been restored; lesions do not progress.
Patient has developed appropriate coping mechanisms and has identified sources of support.	Patient verbalizes feelings about disease and altered body image related to skin lesions; patient has sought outside support.
Patient has attained optimum mobility.	Patient can perform activities of daily living and enjoys an acceptable level of independence.
Cardiac status has been maximized.	Patient is free of cardiac symptoms.
Respiratory status has been maximized.	Patient is breathing without difficulty; arterial blood gases (ABGs) are normal; vital capacity measurements are optimum for patient.
Renal status has been maximized.	Patient is normotensive; appetite is adequate; weight is stable; urine/plasma ratio is normal; BUN, creatinine, Hct, and electrolytes are normal.

→ > >

PATIENT OUTCOME	DATA INDICATING THAT OUTCOME IS REACHED
Patient maintains adequate nutrition.	Patient's diet will be assessed to make sure dietary needs are being met.
Patient has a positive and realistic body image.	Patient will verbalize feelings about body image and ability to cope with changes.
Patient is free of infection.	There are no signs or symptoms of infection.
Patient has achieved adequate level of comfort.	Patient reports increased level of comfort; need for pain medication has decreased.

PATIENT TEACHING

1. Teach the patient about the disease and its course.
2. Teach the patient about the treatment regimen and the importance of compliance.
3. Emphasize the need for frequent assessment of health status and early intervention when problems are identified.
4. Emphasize the need to maintain a good level of mo-

bility by using medications to decrease pain from arthritis and arthralgia; by using range-of-motion exercises; and by alternating exercise with rest.
5. Emphasize the need for adequate rest to prevent symptoms from flaring up.
6. Teach the patient the warning signs of infection.
7. Discuss the need for adequate nutrition.

Dermatomyositis

Dermatomyositis is a rare necrotizing disease of striated muscle with associated inflammatory cutaneous lesions. Skin lesions may be the first sign of the disease or may develop after other symptoms have appeared.

Myositis can be detected by testing the strength of the proximal muscle groups (hip, thigh, arm, and shoulder). Muscle biopsy, an abnormal electromyogram, and elevated serum enzymes (SGOT, aldolase, and creatine phosphokinase) confirm the diagnosis (see the box on p. 59).

PATHOPHYSIOLOGY

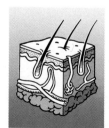

The cause of dermatomyositis is not fully known, but the disease is thought to be the result of immune-mediated vessel injury in which complement is bound and activated to completion in the intramuscular arterioles and capillaries. Dermatomyositis may be grouped with either connective tissue or autoimmune diseases, because many of the presenting characteristics are similar to those noted in the two categories (rheumatic symptoms, cutaneous manifestations, abnormal blood val-

---

DIAGNOSTIC CRITERIA FOR DERMATOMYOSITIS

Symmetric proximal weakness
Compatible muscle biopsy
Myopathy or inflammatory myositis
Compatible electromyogram
Elevated skeletal muscle enzymes (e.g., creatine phosphokinase, aldolase, SGOT)
Compatible dermatologic features
    Heliotrope erythema of eyelids
    Gottron's papules
    Violet, scaling patches
    Periungual erythema and telangiectasia
    Poikiloderma

Adapted from Habif.[25]

---

ues). Dermatomyositis may affect either children or adults over 40 years of age. In adults, the disease can be associated with malignancy and collagen-vascular diseases. It may be acute, chronic, recurrent, or cyclic.

Patients who have proximal muscle weakness but **See Color Plate 4 on p. xiii for an example of dermatomyositis.** show no evidence of other symptoms may be diagnosed with polymyositis, but they are indistinguishable from patients with dermatomyositis. Weakness most often is prominent in the shoulder and girdle muscles (hips and thighs), making rising from a sitting position, walking, and lifting difficult. The onset is insidious. If the neck muscles become involved, the patient has difficulty raising the head. Progression of weakness to other muscle groups can lead to dysphagia (involvement of pharyngeal muscles), an increased risk of aspiration pneumonia, and respiratory difficulty.

Cutaneous signs of dermatomyositis, which are seen in only about 40% of patients, may precede or accompany the muscle weakness. Cutaneous signs include heliotrope erythema of the eyelids; Gottron's papules; violet, scaling patches; periungual erythema and telangiectasia; and poikiloderma.

Red-to-violet (heliotrope) edema of the eye area is a hallmark cutaneous manifestation of dermatomyositis. This discoloration may be the first cutaneous sign of dermatomyositis or a residual finding when diffuse erythema has faded. Gottron's papules are inflammatory papules found over the knuckles. They are 0.2 to 1 cm in diameter, smooth, violet to red, and flat topped. They can also be seen on the sides of the fingers and occasionally on the knees and elbows.

Localized or diffuse erythema, with or without scaling, is a characteristic cutaneous finding in dermatomyositis. In the localized form, the erythema is found symmetrically over bony prominences. Dermatomyositis typically involves the skin over knuckles and spares the skin over the phalanges (this presentation is reversed in lupus). The diffuse form of erythema appears dusky red or violet, and generally emerges in sun-exposed areas of the body initially. As the disease progresses, the erythema may be seen over the buttocks and legs, and it becomes confluent. Minimal scaling may develop. In patients with internal malignancy, the erythema takes on a deeper redness. Patients are photosensitive and should be cautioned about sun exposure. As the disease progresses and the erythema fades, the skin in the sun-exposed areas of the body takes on a characteristic look of hypopigmentation, hyperpigmentation, telangiectasia, and atrophy.

Prominent periungual telangiectasia and erythema are also a classic cutaneous manifestation of dermatomyositis. This phenomenon may be seen in other collagen-vascular diseases as well, but in dermatomyositis, unlike in other diseases, the cuticles have a moth-eaten appearance (thick, rough, hyperkeratotic, and irregular).

Dermatomyositis can be associated with malignancy in some cases (adults show a higher incidence of this combination.) When an associated malignancy is present, the patient has a myasthenia gravis–like syndrome, painless muscle weakness exacerbated by activity. The most common tumor sites are the breast and the lung. Dermatomyositis manifestations in children are similar to those in adults, but the course is more chronic. This leads to calcinosis of subcutaneous tissue, muscle atrophy, and contractures. Because an associated gastrointestinal vasculitis may be seen in children, they should be followed closely.

Dermatomyositis has four distinct patterns: acute, chronic, recurrent, and fluctuating. The acute pattern has a rapid onset, and severe weakness is characteristic. With an acute presentation, the patient may die within 2 years of onset, but some patients do well. Spontaneous remission, although rare, is possible. The chronic pattern is characterized by a slow onset and progression. Patients either improve gradually or die within 2 years of diagnosis. As with the acute form, spontaneous remission is possible. Recurrent dermatomyositis is marked by complete remission between exacerbations of myositis. Fluctuating dermatomyositis is characterized by exacerbations that occur when the dosage of systemic corticosteroids used for treatment is reduced. No preventive measures are known for this disease, but mortality has decreased as a result of corticosteroid therapy.

COMPLICATIONS

Muscle weakness	Arthralgia
Dysphagia	Muscle atrophy
Respiratory difficulty	Increased risk of malignancy
Aspiration pneumonia	Photosensitivity

DIAGNOSTIC STUDIES AND FINDINGS

Diagnostic Test	Findings
Muscle biopsy from proximal muscle groups	Widespread destruction of muscle fibers; cellular infiltrate of lymphocytes, plasma cells, and histiocytes
Electromyogram	Abnormal
Laboratory values: serum muscle enzymes (creatine phosphokinase, aldolase, transaminases, and SGOT)	Elevated
Antinuclear antibody (ANA)	May be positive
24-Hour urine collection for creatine	Elevated levels

MEDICAL MANAGEMENT

GENERAL MANAGEMENT

Activity: Bed rest is essential for strengthening when muscle involvement is active; an aggressive program of passive physical therapy should be initiated to keep muscle strength up, but it can be initiated only when muscle pain decreases.

Sun exposure: Photosensitivity is a complication of dermatomyositis; sunscreens, appropriate clothing, and staying out of the sun should be encouraged.

Nutrition: A balanced diet is indicated for all patients with dermatomyositis; a soft diet should be started if the patient has dysphagia.

DRUG THERAPY

Systemic corticosteroids: Treatment of choice, particularly in adults who show skin and muscle symptoms; initial dosage of 60 mg/day in divided doses with tapering, slowing to alternate day therapy; dosage is determined by clinical signs and muscle enzymes; used to treat inflammation.

Immunosuppressant agents: Methotrexate, 25-50 mg PO or IV; azathioprine, 2 mg/kg/day PO, may be used in patients unresponsive to systemic corticosteroid therapy; used to treat inflammation.

Topical corticosteroids: Group IV and group V topical steroids are used to reduce erythema of skin lesions.

Sunscreen: A sunscreen with a sun protection factor (SPF) of at least 15 should be used.

Antimalarial drugs: Hydroxychloroquine sulfate (Plaquenil), 200-400 mg/day, and chloroquine phosphate, 250-500 mg/day (if hydroxychloroquine sulfate fails), are helpful in the treatment of cutaneous lesions; these drugs have no effect on muscle disease.

Cyclosporine: Used to treat chronic active disease (present for an average of 3 years).

1 ASSESS

ASSESSMENT	OBSERVATIONS
Current health status	May have no somatic complaints and manifest only skin lesions; may complain of general muscle weakness, dysphagia, or difficulty breathing
Skin and mucous membranes	Heliotrope erythema of eyelids; Gottron's papules; localized or diffuse erythema, with or without scaling; periungual erythema and telangiectasia or poikiloderma; may complain of photosensitivity
Neuropsychiatric	Body image disturbance; depression
Musculoskeletal	Proximal muscle weakness; arthralgia; possible involvement of pharyngeal muscles, leading to dysphagia; contractures
Gastrointestinal	Guaiac-positive stools related to vasculitis, particularly in children
Pulmonary	Respiratory infections with involvement of respiratory and pharyngeal muscles
Renal	No involvement associated

2 DIAGNOSE

NURSING DIAGNOSIS	SUBJECTIVE FINDINGS	OBJECTIVE FINDINGS
Impaired mobility related to involvement of proximal muscles	Reports difficulty rising from sitting position, lifting, or walking	Unable to rise from a chair or walk without assistance
Impaired swallowing related to involvement of pharyngeal muscles	Reports increasing difficulty in swallowing	Abnormal swallowing on diagnostic testing
Increased risk of respiratory infection related to involvement of respiratory muscles	Complains of respiratory infections	Respiratory infection; aspiration pneumonia; poor quality of respiration
Increased risk of high cardiac output failure related to diffuse erythema	Complains of generalized redness, chills, increased heart rate	Generalized erythroderma; elevated heart rate due to general vasodilation and shunting of blood
Body image disturbance related to changes in appearance and decreased mobility	Expresses feelings about changes in appearance and decrease in activity	Social interaction is inappropriate

→ ❯ ❯

NURSING DIAGNOSIS	SUBJECTIVE FINDINGS	OBJECTIVE FINDINGS
Impaired skin integrity related to disease process	Reports rash; erythema; heliotrope; and smooth, violet-to-red papules over knuckles and on sides of fingers	May have localized or diffuse erythema; purple discoloration around eyes; Gottron's papules present

3 PLAN

Patient goals

1. Patient will reach maximum mobility.
2. Patient will maintain adequate nutritional status and have fewer episodes of aspiration pneumonia.
3. Pulmonary function will be maximized.
4. Cardiac function will be maximized.
5. Patient will develop appropriate coping mechanisms and be able to identify sources of support.
6. Skin integrity will be maintained.

4 IMPLEMENT

NURSING DIAGNOSIS	NURSING INTERVENTIONS	RATIONALES
Impaired mobility related to involvement of proximal muscles	Assess joint function and mobility; perform ROM exercises; ambulate regularly; plan rest periods; urge bed rest during exacerbation.	To assess degree of limitation; to maintain highest level of functioning.
Impaired swallowing related to involvement of pharyngeal muscles	Assess swallowing.	To note dysphagia and degree of involvement.
Increased risk of respiratory infection related to involvement of respiratory muscles	Monitor respiratory rate and depth; assess patient for dyspnea and shortness of breath; assess breath sounds.	To determine pulmonary involvement; to note condition of lungs and possible respiratory complications.
Increased risk of high cardiac output failure related to diffuse erythema	Continuously monitor patient's cardiac status during erythrodermic states.	To determine compromise of cardiac system related to vasodilation and shunting of blood.
Body image disturbance related to changes in appearance and decreased mobility	Assess patient's concerns about the effects of disease on body image and self-esteem.	To determine patient's ability to cope with disease.
Impaired skin integrity related to disease process	Assess skin for erythema or open lesions.	To determine whether barrier function is impaired.

5 EVALUATE

PATIENT OUTCOME	DATA INDICATING THAT OUTCOME IS REACHED
Patient maintains maximum mobility.	Patient can achieve maximum mobility within limitations of the disease.
Patient maintains adequate nutritional status and has fewer episodes of aspiration pneumonia.	Patient has adequate diet based on stage of disease and ability to swallow.
Patient is free of respiratory infection.	Patient shows no signs of respiratory infection.
Cardiac status is maintained.	Patient's erythroderma is aggressively treated to prevent cardiac difficulties.
Patient exhibits adequate coping mechanisms.	Patient can verbalize her feelings about disease and its course.
Skin's barrier function is protected during episodes of skin breakdown.	Open skin lesions are treated appropriately to provide temporary barrier function and decrease risk of infection.

PATIENT TEACHING

1. Explain the disease and its course.
2. Encourage the patient to participate in physical therapy and to adhere to a regimen of exercise and rest.
3. Explain the signs and symptoms of respiratory infection, exacerbation, and cardiac problems.
4. Explain the treatment regimen and possible side effects when appropriate.
5. Emphasize the importance of quickly seeking medical help at the first sign of respiratory or cardiac problems or exacerbation of the disease.

Scleroderma

Scleroderma is a chronic disease that manifests in two forms: localized (morphea) and systemic sclerosis (commonly referred to as systemic scleroderma).

Scleroderma is characterized by symmetric cutaneous lesions that show three phases of involvement: edematous, sclerotic, and atrophic. Systemic scleroderma is a progressive, fatal condition characterized by diffuse involvement of the connective tissue of the dermis, leading to induration and thickening of skin and fibrous deposition in certain organs. Skin changes generally precede visceral involvement, but there is no evidence that morphea (localized scleroderma) naturally evolves into systemic scleroderma.

PATHOPHYSIOLOGY

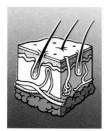

The cause of scleroderma has not been clearly established, but it is thought to be of autoimmune origin. Alteration and fibrosis of connective tissue in the skin and internal organs constitute the basic physiologic change seen. The disease predominantly appears in women of childbearing age and early menopause. A strong autoimmune cause is suspected, because the disease occasionally coexists with lupus erythematosus or dermatomyositis.

Localized scleroderma (morphea) manifests with one or more circumscribed areas of abnormal skin occurring in a variety of shapes, sizes, and distributions. At least three patterns of tissue injury may be seen: inflammation/edema, sclerosis (induration), or atrophy. The skin becomes thickened and swollen and has a tense, shiny appearance in the edematous phase. In the sclerotic stage the lesion becomes shiny and bound down, followed by atrophy. Lesions evolve from erythematous/edematous, to sclerotic, to hyperpigmentation or depigmentation and atrophy. Morphea manifests clinically as a white or yellow-ivory lesion with a violet border. It may be linear, plaquelike, guttate, or generalized. An atrophic epidermis is evident with fine wrinkling and shininess. Induration is felt in the dermis, and the skin lacks appendages in the area of involvement. Some patients report pruritus with the cutaneous lesions. Coinciding with or preceding the lesions, the patient may experience joint signs and symptoms such as arthralgia or acute synovitis.

Scleroderma and the CREST syndrome are depicted in Color Plates 42 to 44 on p. xix.

Systemic scleroderma has two subsets, diffuse scleroderma and CREST syndrome. Diffuse scleroderma may be rapidly progressive and fatal. Symmetric fibrous thickening and hardening of the skin, as well as fibrous and degenerative changes in the synovium, digital arteries, and certain internal organs, are seen in diffuse scleroderma. The organs most often affected other than the skin are the esophagus, intestinal tract, heart, lungs, and kidneys. Clinical symptoms of diffuse scleroderma include thickening of the skin of the hands or Raynaud's phenomenon, or both; rheumatic complaints; possible complaints of weakness; weight loss; easy fatigability; stiffness; edema; and diffuse musculoskeletal aching. In advanced stages of systemic scleroderma, these cutaneous changes give the face a masklike appearance and the fingers a sausagelike appearance. Movement of the hands is restricted. In the indurative phase, the skin becomes hard and "bound down," further restricting movement. With induration comes the loss of appendages, resulting in hair loss and anhidrosis. As the cutaneous lesions progress, telangiectasia and hypopigmentation or hyperpigmentation develop. With progressive involvement of the skin and fibrosis of connective tissue, the fingers develop a clawlike appearance (sclerodactyly). Distal bone is resorbed, leading to narrowing and tapering of the terminal phalanges. Raynaud's phenomenon, a vasospastic disorder precipitated by temperature change, is another sign of systemic scleroderma and may be the presenting symptom.

CREST syndrome, another subset of systemic scleroderma, is a more benign, chronic, and localized variant. The acronym CREST stands for the five manifestations of this form of systemic scleroderma: calcinosis, Raynaud's phenomenon, esophageal dysfunction, sclerodactyly, and telangiectasia. The syndrome manifests with the exact same three phases of skin involvement as morphea or diffuse scleroderma (edematous, indurative [sclerotic], and atrophic).

CREST SYNDROME	
C =	Calcinosis
R =	Raynaud's phenomenon
E =	Esophageal dysfunction
S =	Sclerodactyly
T =	Telangiectasia

Calcinosis is seen most often on the palmar aspects of the tips of the fingers. It may be present over bony prominences (knees, elbows, iliac crest, spine) as well. Clinically it manifests as firm subcutaneous nodules. These nodules may rupture, expelling calcium into the tissue and causing a foreign body reaction (redness and pain). Infection may result in conjunction with calcinosis.

Raynaud's phenomenon in CREST manifests exactly as it does in diffuse scleroderma. Esophageal dysfunction is characterized by hypomobility, dysphagia, reflux esophagitis, and fibrotic strictures. Gastroesophageal reflux is the major complaint from patients.

As the disease progresses, the skin of the fingers and hands becomes thin, shiny, smooth, and bound down, resulting in contracture of the fingers. With this contracture and resorption of distal bone, the fingers take on a sausagelike or clawlike appearance, referred to as sclerodactyly. The presence of telangiectasia completes the clinical manifestations of CREST. In scleroderma, telangiectasia manifests as flat collections of tiny vessels found mainly on the face, lips, palms, and backs of the hands.

COMPLICATIONS

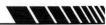

Systemic disease
Intolerance to cold
Gastrointestinal bleeding
Dysphagia
Dyspnea
Impaired mobility
Pain
Increased risk of infection
Renal involvement

DIAGNOSTIC STUDIES AND FINDINGS

Diagnostic Test	Findings
Antinuclear antibody (ANA)	Positive in >95% of patients
Erythrocyte sedimentation rate	Elevated in 60% of patients
Skin biopsy	Collagen bundle pattern of reticular dermis is obliterated; distinguishing between papillary and reticular dermis is difficult

MEDICAL MANAGEMENT

Treatment is palliative; physical therapy is the most important management therapy to be instituted.

GENERAL MANAGEMENT

Nutrition: Supplements are given to maintain adequate intake; soft diet is used when swallowing becomes difficult; fiber in diet is increased to aid elimination.

Physical therapy: A well-planned physical therapy regimen should be instituted, to help reduce peripheral edema and to increase overall strength. ROM exercises are needed to aid in activities of daily living (ADLs); adequate rest periods must be emphasized in the regimen.

DRUG THERAPY

Systemic corticosteroids: Given for the antiinflammatory effect; dosages are given as 40 to 60 mg in divided doses for an 8- to 12-week course.

Penicillamine: Blocks cross-linkages during collagen synthesis; decreases skin thickness and slows progression of visceral disease in some cases.

Cholinergic agents: Used before meals in patients with dysphagia.

Analgesic-antipyretic agents: Used to help alleviate joint symptoms.

Topical corticosteroids: Used for the treatment of morphea, even though results are not always rewarding.

OTHER MEDICAL MANAGEMENT

Complications and symptoms that develop secondary to the involvement of internal organs must be treated as they arise.

1 ASSESS

ASSESSMENT	OBSERVATIONS
Skin and mucous membranes	Swollen, tight, thickened skin on hands and face; sausage appearance of fingers; telangiectatic mats on face, palms, lips, and backs of hands; signs of Raynaud's phenomenon; In later stages, calcinosis, digital ulceration
Musculoskeletal	Arthralgia; limited mobility; weakness; diffuse muscle aches; stiffness; joint pain; easy fatigability; resorption of bone in the distal phalanges
Gastrointestinal	Dysphagia; problems with elimination; weight loss
Pulmonary	Impaired gas exchange; dyspnea, cough, shortness of breath; decreased breath sounds
Renal	Urinary output decreased due to renal involvement; renal hypertension
Neuropsychiatric	Body image disturbance; depression

2 DIAGNOSE

NURSING DIAGNOSIS	SUBJECTIVE FINDINGS	OBJECTIVE FINDINGS
Impaired skin integrity related to altered peripheral perfusion, changes in skin turgor, and Raynaud's phenomenon	Reports pain, numbness, and tingling in hands and fingers; complains that skin feels tight and leathery over entire body; reports intolerance to cold; pain, blanching of digits	Widespread telangiectasia; follicular hyperpigmentation or hypopigmentation; fingers cool to touch and have several small ulcerations; skin generally has hidebound appearance (tight and shiny) with loss of normal wrinkles and folds; blanching, cyanosis, and redness are initiated with exposure to cold
Impaired physical mobility related to muscle and joint involvement	Reports restriction in movement caused by joint pain or progression in loss of skin elasticity; reports stiffness, swelling, and weakness	Limited range of motion, particularly in hands, wrists, elbows, feet, knees, and hips; flexion contractions; muscle weakness and atrophy
High risk for aspiration related to difficulty swallowing and esophageal disease	Reports difficulty swallowing and heartburn	Coughing follows swallowing; barium studies show peristalsis of distal portion of esophagus and gastroesophageal reflux; delayed gastric emptying
Altered nutrition: less than body requirements related to esophageal reflux, difficulty swallowing, reduced mouth opening, and malabsorption	Complains of difficulty swallowing, midsternal discomfort when eating, loss of appetite, and intermittent diarrhea and constipation	Weight loss, inadequate intake of food and fluids, dysphagia, muscle atrophy, and wasting; steatorrhea, with bacterial overgrowth in the stool; x-rays show dilation of duodenum and possibly jejunum

NURSING DIAGNOSIS	SUBJECTIVE FINDINGS	OBJECTIVE FINDINGS
Impaired gas exchange related to pulmonary involvement (pulmonary fibrosis)	Reports shortness of breath, dyspnea, cough	Dyspnea and fatigue with minimal exertion; tachypnea; nonproductive cough; crackles in lower lung fields
Altered patterns of urinary elimination related to renal failure	Reports infrequent urination and small volume	Decreased urinary output with progressive disease, rising BUN and creatinine, proteinuria <1 g/day; elevated BP
Body image disturbance related to changes in appearance	Complains of feeling ugly and not looking the same	Masklike face; tight, hard skin; thin lips; drawn, wrinkled mouth; smooth, immobile forehead; wasted musculature; hands contracted; social interaction is inappropriate

3 PLAN

Patient goals

1. Skin's barrier function will be protected during episodes of skin breakdown.
2. Patient will maintain maximum mobility and be free of pain.
3. Patient will not aspirate.
4. Patient will maintain adequate nutritional status and elimination.
5. Pulmonary function will be maximized.
6. Patient will have adequate renal perfusion.
7. Patient will develop appropriate coping mechanisms to deal with change in appearance and will identify sources of support.

4 IMPLEMENT

NURSING DIAGNOSIS	NURSING INTERVENTIONS	RATIONALE
Impaired skin integrity related to altered peripheral perfusion, changes in skin turgor, and Raynaud's phenomenon	Assess and monitor extremities, particularly hands and fingers, for adequacy of peripheral arterial blood flow (e.g., skin color, pulses, capillary refill, sensation, temperature).	Severity of symptoms reflects degree of decreased arterial blood flow and guides therapy.
	Instruct patient to avoid exposure to cold (e.g., outdoors, frozen food section of grocery store, refrigerator).	To prevent vasoconstriction and decreased tissue perfusion.
	Monitor for complaints of tingling, numbness, or burning.	These indicate lack of oxygenation, leading to ischemia.

NURSING DIAGNOSIS	NURSING INTERVENTIONS	RATIONALE
	Instruct patient in importance of routine skin care (i.e., using tepid water, mild soap, and patting completely dry).	To promote healing and maintain skin integrity.
	Protect affected areas (fingers and hands) from trauma; keep fingernails short to prevent scratching.	To promote healing; trauma may cause vasoconstriction and eventual ulceration.
Impaired physical mobility related to muscle and joint involvement	Assess joint function and mobility.	To assess degree of limitation and to guide therapeutic interventions.
	Perform ROM and strengthening exercises.	Routine exercise may minimize further contractures, increase strength, and improve circulation.
	Provide rest periods between activities.	To minimize weakness.
	Provide progressive increase in activity as tolerated.	As endurance improves, independence is facilitated.
High risk for aspiration related to difficulty swallowing and esophageal disease	Provide small, frequent meals.	To help manage esophageal hypomotility and reflux.
	Cut food into small pieces, and remind patient to take small bites and to chew food well before swallowing.	Lack of adequate chewing may cause aspiration of large pieces of food.
	Monitor for signs of coughing, gagging, nasal regurgitation, holding food in mouth, decreased breath sounds, or signs of air hunger.	These are signs of possible aspiration.
	Teach family members the Heimlich maneuver.	To use in emergencies if patient chokes.
Altered nutrition: less than body requirements related to esophageal reflux, difficulty swallowing, reduced mouth opening, and malabsorption	Assess dietary habits and needs; calculate for additional calories and nutrients if infection is present.	To guide therapeutic interventions and individualize diet.
	Document weight, and monitor daily.	To establish baseline and to monitor changes in weight.
	Help provide routine oral hygiene, particularly before meals.	To improve appetite and moisten skin that is tightly contracted around mouth.
	Provide small, frequent meals.	Esophageal hypomotility prevents intake of large amounts of food at one time; offering small, frequent meals promotes intake and absorption of nutrients.

NURSING DIAGNOSIS	NURSING INTERVENTIONS	RATIONALE
	Encourage fluids and foods high in fiber (e.g., fruits, cereals, grains).	To minimize constipation.
Impaired gas exchange related to pulmonary involvement (pulmonary fibrosis)	Observe breathing pattern for shortness of breath, nasal flaring, pursed-lip breathing, use of accessory muscles, and intercostal retraction.	To identify increased work of breathing.
	Inspect thorax for symmetry of respiratory movement.	To determine adequacy of breathing.
	Auscultate breath sounds.	To determine adequacy of air exchange.
	Encourage patient to use adaptive breathing techniques.	To decrease work of breathing.
Altered patterns of urinary elimination related to renal failure	Monitor BP q 2-4 h.	Hypertension may develop secondary to decrease in renal perfusion and activation of renin-angiotensin system.
	Monitor serum potassium, BUN, creatinine, and creatinine clearance.	These are indicators of renal function; an elevation in potassium, creatinine, and BUN and a decrease in creatinine clearance may suggest impaired renal perfusion and function.
	Monitor urinary protein.	Increases in urinary protein ($>$500 mg/24 h) indicate renal impairment, suggesting alteration in the glomerular basement membrane.
	Monitor intake and output, daily weight, central venous pressure (CVP), breath sounds, and degree of peripheral edema.	As indicators of fluid status; increase in daily weight, CVP, intake over output, and rales, or diminished or absent breath sounds suggest increasing fluid volume; peripheral edema may increase secondary to low albumin.
	Assess and monitor mental status.	Changes in mental status may indicate increasing azotemia or severe hypertension.
	If renal insufficiency requires dialysis or hemofiltration, work with nephrology nurse to provide patient and family with information about resources for these treatment modalities.	To increase patient's and family's knowledge about treatments for acute renal failure and to minimize fear and provide support.
Body image disturbance related to changes in appearance	Assess patient's concerns about body image.	To obtain an understanding of patient's specific concerns and to guide therapeutic intervention.

NURSING DIAGNOSIS	NURSING INTERVENTIONS	RATIONALE
	Encourage patient to express feelings about joint deformities, skin abnormalities, and facial changes; offer support and understanding of patient's feelings and concerns.	Ventilation helps patient resolve grief over physical changes and clarify feelings and concerns; support and understanding may help with process of regaining a positive body image.
	Consult medical cosmetologist, and teach patient strategies for improving body image (e.g., how to dress, apply makeup or wigs, improve hygiene).	Expert team members can help provide individualized care and promote a positive body image.
	Help significant others understand impact of disease limitation on patient, and elicit their help in identifying methods to promote patient's efforts toward a positive body image.	Significant others can play a pivotal role in helping patient regain a positive body image.
	Refer patient to community resources and self-help groups.	To provide access to individuals who may have effective alternative strategies and to provide ongoing support.

5   EVALUATE

PATIENT OUTCOME	DATA INDICATING THAT OUTCOME IS REACHED
Skin's barrier function is protected during episodes of skin breakdown.	Open skin lesions are treated appropriately to provide temporary barrier function and decrease risk of secondary infection.
Patient maintains maximum mobility and is free of pain.	Patient can perform self-care and ADLs within limitations of the disease; patient is free of pain.
Patient does not aspirate.	There is no evidence of aspiration; breath sounds are clear in all lobes; patient has no air hunger and appears well oxygenated.
Patient maintains adequate nutritional status and elimination.	Patient has appropriate diet based on stage of disease; bowel and bladder elimination is maximized.
Pulmonary function has been maximized.	Patient has no dyspnea with activity; respiratory rate is normal; breath sounds are clear on auscultation. Patient takes planned rest periods to help control periods of increased shortness of breath.
Patient's renal perfusion is adequate.	Patient is normotensive; BUN, creatinine, potassium, and creatinine clearance are normal or optimum for patient; urinary protein is <500 mg/24 h.

PATIENT OUTCOME	DATA INDICATING THAT OUTCOME IS REACHED
Patient has developed appropriate coping mechanisms to deal with change in appearance and has identified sources of support.	Patient verbalizes acceptance of limitations. She shows an effort to improve her appearance and participates in a self-help support group.

PATIENT TEACHING

1. Explain the disease and its course.
2. Encourage the patient to participate in physical therapy and to adhere to a regimen of exercise and rest.
3. Explain the signs of involvement of other organ systems (i.e., congestive heart failure, renal failure, pulmonary fibrosis).
4. Explain the treatment regimen and possible side effects where appropriate.
5. Emphasize the importance of obtaining medical help quickly when new symptoms arise or flare-ups occur.

CHAPTER 6

Infections

As the body's barrier against the environment, the skin is continuously exposed to many insults. As such, the most important function of the skin is to serve as a barrier against the invasion of microorganisms. Intact skin and mucous membranes, in conjunction with both resident and transient flora, provide that barrier. It is important to distinguish between resident and transient flora of the skin.

A resident organism is defined as one that can establish itself and multiply on the skin. Resident flora include coryneform bacteria (diphtheroids), staphylococci, micrococci B, *Propionibacterium* spp., and a few fungi. These organisms are not easily dislodged. Most resident flora are found in the superficial epidermis and the upper portion of the hair follicles. The ability of transient microorganisms to colonize on the skin's surface depends on many ecologic factors. Resident flora function as a defense against bacterial infection.

Colonization occurs when microorganisms contaminating the skin's surface multiply. Resident and transient bacteria can resist colonization by producing antibacterial substances or by competing for available nutrients. The infections commonly seen in the skin are bacterial, viral, or fungal types. Common bacterial infections of the skin are impetigo, cellulitis, furuncles, and toxic shock syndrome.

Bacterial Infections

PATHOPHYSIOLOGY

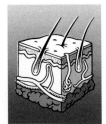

Impetigo, a common bacterial skin infection, is caused by beta-hemolytic streptococci or *Staphylococcus aureus,* or both. Impetigo is subclassified into two categories: impetigo contagiosa, caused primarily by group A beta-hemolytic streptococci, and bullous impetigo, caused primarily by group II *S. aureus. Impetigo contagiosa* is most often seen in children and is often endemic. Cases of impetigo are more prevalent in temperate climates. Clinically it manifests with early vesicular or pustular lesions. These lesions eventually evolve to the classic lesion with a honey-colored crust. The lesions most commonly develop on the legs; they are seen less frequently on the arms, face, and trunk. Systemic symptoms are uncommon. The infection is thought to originate from insect bites, infestation with scabies, or poor hygiene. Scratching or abrading the skin damages its integrity, allowing bacteria to enter. *Ecthyma* is an ulcerative form of impetigo.

Bullous impetigo is caused by group II *S. aureus.* The lesions begin as small vesicles; these rapidly develop into bullae that eventually rupture, leaving a shallow erosion. The lesions occur most often on the face but may be seen on the trunk and extremities.

Cellulitis is a diffuse, acute streptococcal or staphylococcal infection of the skin and subcutaneous tissue. It occurs most commonly in the lower extremities. The infection spreads locally as a result of the release of enzymes produced by the bacteria. These enzymes prevent the normal body responses that would reduce local spread of infection by walling off the site. Clinically the skin becomes erythematous, edematous (pitting edema, peau d'orange), hot, and tender to the touch. Lymphangitic streaks may develop proximal to the infection. **Erysipelas** is a distinctive type of acute cellulitis caused by group A beta-hemolytic streptococci.

Furuncles, commonly known as boils, are caused by an acute, localized, perifollicular, staphylococcal infection, which produces an abscess of the skin and subcutaneous tissue. Central necrosis and suppuration occur. Furuncles most often are caused by coagulase-positive *S. aureus.* Clinically the lesions begin in the area of a hair follicle or sebaceous gland. Obstruction of the sebaceous gland or ingrowth of hair may induce the condition. Secondary factors include scratching, friction, scabies, pressure from belts and clothing, chemical irritants, and hyperhidrosis. Lesions are seen most commonly on the back of the neck, face, buttocks, thighs, perineum, and breasts or in the axillae. Single or multiple lesions (furunculosis) may appear. Primary lesions are minute, painful, and indurated. As the lesions evolve, they become elevated, indurated, tender, shiny, and bright red. Intense, throbbing pain commonly marks these lesions. As the furuncle matures, it becomes boggy and fluctuant, developing a yellow or creamy white discharge as suppuration and central necrosis occur. The lesions may rupture spontaneously, but incision and drainage instantly relieve pain and speed healing. Systemic symptoms (e.g., fever, malaise, regional adenopathy) may accompany the cutaneous symptoms. A **carbuncle** is an aggregation of interconnected furuncles that drain through several openings in the skin.

Toxic shock syndrome (**TSS**) originally was seen principally in menstruating girls or women, but it now has been documented to be associated with a variety of surgical situations. These situations, which are unrelated to menses, include surgical wounds, tubal ligation, hysterectomy, laparotomy, mastectomy, bladder suspension, orchidectomy, uterolithotomy, hip osteoplasty, and knee surgery. The infection is thought to occur secondary to an exotoxin produced by *S. aureus.* The following box lists the case definition for toxic shock syndrome proposed by the Centers for Disease Control (CDC).

CASE DEFINITION FOR TOXIC SHOCK SYNDROME: CENTERS FOR DISEASE CONTROL GUIDELINES

1. Fever (>38.9° C [102° F])
2. Rash (diffuse macular erythroderma)
3. Desquamation, 1 to 2 weeks after onset of illness, particularly of palms and soles
4. Hypotension (systolic blood pressure <90 mm Hg for adults)
5. Involvement of three or more of the following organ systems:
   a. Gastrointestinal (vomiting or diarrhea at onset of illness)
   b. Muscular (severe myalgia or creatine phosphokinase twice the normal level)
   c. Mucous membranes (vaginal, oropharyngeal, or conjunctival hyperemia)
   d. Renal (blood urea nitrogen [BUN] or creatinine twice normal levels or more than five white blood cells per high-power field in the absence of urinary tract infection)
   e. Hepatic (total bilirubin, serum glutamic-oxaloacetic transaminase, or serum glutamic-pyruvic transaminase twice the normal level)
   f. Central nervous system (disorientation or changes in consciousness without focal neurologic signs)
6. Negative results if the following tests are performed:
   a. Blood, throat, or cerebrospinal fluid cultures
   b. Serologic tests for Rocky Mountain spotted fever, leptospirosis, or measles

TSS is a multisystem disease that may progress to profound shock and disseminated intravascular coagulation, renal failure, adult respiratory distress syndrome, or cardiac involvement. The cutaneous sign of TSS is a macular erythema that begins in the groin area. Superficial desquamation begins as the erythema fades. A prodrome develops (myalgia, headache, vomiting, diarrhea, pharyngitis, and hyperemic conjunctivae), which may progress rapidly to hypotension and multiorgan system dysfunction. In less severe cases prodromal features may not manifest and progression may not occur. Edema and erythema of the palms and soles with desquamation, hyperemia of oral and vaginal mucous membranes, and "strawberry tongue" are also seen in TSS. Beau's lines may develop in the nails as a secondary manifestation. Focal cutaneous pyodermas, surgical wound infections, postpartum infections, adenitis, bursitis, deep abscesses, primary bacteremia, and nasal packings may be associated with TSS. Early recognition and institution of appropriate therapy improve the prognosis.

COMPLICATIONS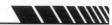

Acute glomerulonephritis (2% to 5% of patients with impetigo)
Scarring (ecthyma)
Local abscesses (cellulitis)
Systemic symptoms (fever, malaise, hypotension)
Bacteremia (carbuncles)
Thrombophlebitis with septic emboli or metastatic abscesses (carbuncles)
Central nervous system (CNS) infections (carbuncles on the head and neck)
Acute renal failure (TSS)
Adult respiratory distress syndrome (TSS)
Cardiac irritability (TSS)
Disseminated intravascular coagulation (TSS)
Long-term sequelae of TSS:
- Decreased renal function
- Prolonged weakness and fatigue
- Protracted myalgia
- Vocal cord paralysis
- Upper extremity paresthesia
- Carpal tunnel syndrome
- Arthralgia
- Amenorrhea
- Gangrene

DIAGNOSTIC STUDIES AND FINDINGS

Diagnostic Test	Findings
Bacterial culture	Positive for causative organisms
Gram's stain	Gram positive or negative
Blood culture	Only occasionally positive for causative organism
TSS	
White blood cell count	Increased
Blood urea nitrogen	Increased
Creatinine	Increased
Bilirubin	Increased
Serum glutamic-oxaloacetic transaminase (SGOT) and serum glutamic-pyruvic transaminase (SGPT)	Increased
Creatinine phosphokinase	Increased
Platelets	Decreased

MEDICAL MANAGEMENT

DRUG THERAPY

Impetigo contagiosa

Systemic antibiotics: oral phenoxymethyl penicillin, oral erythromycin, intramuscular benzathine penicillin G, or a mixture of intramuscular benzathine penicillin G and procaine G; cephalosporins are effective but expensive.

Cellulitis

Systemic antibiotics: penicillin V, penicillin G or benzathine penicillin, erythromycin, or penicillin G aqueous IV in severe cases; aspirin or acetaminophen alone or in combination with codeine for pain.

TSS

Systemic antibiotics: cefoxitin sodium (Mefoxin) IV, cefazolin sodium (Ancef) IV, cephalothin sodium IV, methicillin sodium (Staphcillin) IM, oxacillin sodium (Bactocill), cloxacillin sodium (Cloxapen), penicillin G (Bicillin) IM, dicloxacillin sodium (Dycill) PO, or methicillin sodium (Staphcillin) IM.

Corticosteroids: Hydrocortisone sodium succinate (Solu-Cortef) IV or IM.

OTHER MEDICAL MANAGEMENT

Furuncles

Surgery: Incision and drainage.

GENERAL MANAGEMENT

Impetigo

Remove crusts with soap and water and cool, moist compresses.

Nutritional therapy when indicated.

Appropriate therapy for underlying disease.

Cellulitis

Immobilization and elevation of affected limb.

Hospitalization as indicated.

Cool compresses for discomfort.

Warm compresses or soaks to increase circulation.

Appropriate therapy for underlying disease.

Toxic shock syndrome

Septic shock treatment as indicated.

Increased fluid intake unless contraindicated.

Treatment for fluid and electrolyte imbalance as indicated.

1 ASSESS

ASSESSMENT	OBSERVATIONS
Current health	
Impetigo/ecthyma	Appears healthy
Cellulitis/ erysipelas	Fever, chills, regional lymphadenopathy, headache, malaise
Furuncles/ carbuncles	Malaise, fever, regional lymphadenopathy
TSS	High fever, sore throat, headache, exhaustion
Skin and mucous membranes	
Impetigo/ecthyma	Vesicles, bullae, exudate present; honey-colored crust, possible ulceration, satellite lesions
Cellulitis	Local tenderness and pain, erythema, heat, lymphangitic streaking, edema (peau d'orange skin), purulence, abscess
Erysipelas	Tenderness and pain, erythema, heat, edema, raised plaque, vesicles, bullae, purulence
Furuncles/ carbuncles	Tenderness and pain, edema, erythema around infected follicle
TSS	Edema and impaired profusion in extremities; erythematous rash on palms and soles; non-purulent inflammation of conjunctivae; hyperemia and edema of oropharynx; vaginal hyperemia
Neuropsychiatric	
Impetigo/ecthyma	Body image disturbance; concern with possible spread of infection
Furuncles/ carbuncles	Body image disturbance; CNS infections with lesions on head and neck
TSS	Disorientation, intermittent confusion
Gastrointestinal	
TSS	Profuse, watery diarrhea
Hematologic	
Cellulitis/ erysipelas	Elevated WBC, decreased neutrophils, elevated eosinophils, elevated lymphocytes, elevated sedimentation rate
TSS	Elevated WBC, BUN, creatinine, bilirubin, SGOT/SGPT, creatinine phosphokinase; decreased platelets
Cardiovascular	
Cellulitis/ erysipelas	Tachycardia, hypotension
TSS	Rapid hypotension, orthostatic syncope, cardiac irritability, disseminated intravascular coagulation
Pulmonary	
TSS	Adult respiratory distress syndrome in severe cases
Renal	
TSS	Diminished urine output, acute renal failure, decreased renal function as a long-term sequela

2 DIAGNOSE

NURSING DIAGNOSIS	SUBJECTIVE FINDINGS	OBJECTIVE FINDINGS
Impaired skin integrity (impetigo/ ecthyma, cellulitis/ erysipelas, furuncles/ carbuncles, TSS) related to inflammatory process	Reports finding lesions	Involvement of skin and mucous membranes, with erosions, vesicles, or bullae; cutaneous signs of inflammation
High risk for impaired skin integrity (impetigo/ ecthyma, cellulitis/ erysipelas, furuncles/ carbuncles) related to exudates	Reports manipulation of lesions or poor hygiene	Macerated or abraded skin (from scratching); long fingernails; evidence lesions have been picked or squeezed
High risk for infection (impetigo/ ecthyma, cellulitis/ erysipelas, furuncles/ carbuncles, TSS) related to inadequate primary or secondary defenses	Reports practices that may increase risk of spreading infection or of secondary infection	Lacks knowledge of contagious aspect of disease; poor nutritional status; obese patient
Body image disturbance (impetigo/ ecthyma, cellulitis/ erysipelas, furuncles/ carbuncles) related to reaction of others to lesions	Reports lack of social activity; attempts to hide lesions	Unable to maintain eye contact; has difficulty discussing disease and talking about feelings
Pain related to infection (cellulitis/ erysipelas, furuncles/ carbuncles, TSS)	Reports discomfort	Guarding behavior, distraction behavior, facial expressions of discomfort
Impaired physical mobility (cellulitis/ erysipelas, TSS) related to pain and discomfort	Reports decreased mobility due to edema, pain, and myalgia	Limited range of motion (ROM); reluctance to move affected limb

NURSING DIAGNOSIS	SUBJECTIVE FINDINGS	OBJECTIVE FINDINGS
Altered renal, cerebral, cardiopulmonary, GI, and peripheral tissue perfusion (TSS) related to exchange problems associated with shock	Reports decrease in urinary output, periods of lightheadedness, rapid heartbeat, difficulty breathing, fever	Decreased output; abnormal results on renal function studies; altered level of consciousness; increased heart rate and respiratory rate; respiratory alkalosis in early stage with metabolic acidosis in later stage; elevated temperature

3   PLAN

Patient goals
1. Patient's skin integrity will be restored or maintained.
2. Patient will be free of infection.
3. Patient will regain and maintain a positive body image.
4. Patient will be free of pain.
5. Patient will achieve maximum physical mobility.
6. Patient's altered systems will be stabilized.

4   IMPLEMENT

NURSING DIAGNOSIS	NURSING INTERVENTIONS	RATIONALE
Impaired skin integrity (impetigo/ecthyma, cellulitis/erysipelas, furuncles/carbuncles, TSS) related to inflammatory process	Assess lesions for characteristics, inflammation; use good handwashing; remove crusts (impetigo/ecthyma) before applying prescribed topical medications; trim patient's nails as indicated; provide treatment as ordered; elevate and immobilize affected extremity (cellulitis/erysipelas).	To assess progression or resolution of infection; to prevent spread of infection; removal of crusts enhances delivery of topical medication; trimming nails decreases risk of damage to skin from scratching; elevation and immobilization help decrease edema and increase circulation.
High risk for impaired skin integrity (impetigo/ecthyma, cellulitis/erysipelas, furuncles/carbuncles) related to exudates	Trim patient's nails; use and instruct patient in good handwashing; use antibacterial soap.	To prevent autoinoculation and spread.
High risk for infection (impetigo/ecthyma, cellulitis/erysipelas, furuncles/carbuncles, TSS) related to inadequate primary or secondary defenses	Instruct patient to use antibacterial soap, to avoid predisposing factors such as oils (furuncles), and to observe insect control (impetigo) and judicious use of tampons; closely monitor patients with packing in a body cavity for signs of infection; maintain good nutritional status.	To reduce risk of recurrence; to eliminate source of infection; to reduce risk of exotoxin release with tampon use and packing materials; to maintain healthy status.

NURSING DIAGNOSIS	NURSING INTERVENTIONS	RATIONALE
Body image distur-bance (impetigo/ ecthyma, cellulitis/ erysipelas, furuncles/ carbuncles) related to reaction of others to lesions	Assess patient's perception of body image; give positive reinforcement; allow verbal-ization of feelings.	To effectively assist patient during treat-ment and recovery.
Pain related to infec-tion (cellulitis/ erysipelas, furuncles/ carbuncles, TSS)	Assess level of discomfort; administer ap-propriate medication and assess effect; elevate and immobilize affected limb as indicated; apply cool compresses to re-lieve pain, warm moist compresses to in-crease circulation.	To allow for appropriate medication to be given and to assess effect of current pain medication regimen; elevation and immo-bilization promote lymphatic drainage and decrease edema; cool compresses help with pain control; warm compresses in-crease circulation and aid suppuration.
Impaired physical mobility (cellulitis/ erysipelas, TSS) related to pain and discomfort	Assess restriction of movement; elevate and immobilize extremity.	To better evaluate effectiveness of inter-ventions; elevation promotes drainage and helps decrease edema.
Altered renal, cere-bral, cardiopulmo-nary, GI, and peripheral tissue perfusion (TSS) re-lated to exchange problems associated with shock	Assess for signs and symptoms of septic shock; impose complete bed rest; main-tain body temperature with warming blan-kets; keep accurate intake and output (I & O); administer parenteral therapies as or-dered; check vital signs, including periph-eral pulses, frequently; monitor blood gas levels frequently; maintain patent airway.	To be able to institute lifesaving measures immediately.

5 EVALUATE

PATIENT OUTCOME	DATA INDICATING THAT OUTCOME IS REACHED
Skin integrity has been improved or maintained.	Lesions have healed, and no new lesions or erythema is evident; patient understands prin-ciples of hygiene and infection.
No infection is evi-dent.	Skin and mucous membranes are free of any signs of infection; systemic infection is not evident through appropriate assessment.
Positive body image is evident.	Patient verbalizes feelings; defining characteristics are no longer evident.
Pain has been re-lieved.	Need for analgesics has decreased or is nonexistent.
Mobility has in-creased.	ROM has increased; patient can move without pain.

→ > >

PATIENT OUTCOME	DATA INDICATING THAT OUTCOME IS REACHED
Renal, cerebral, cardiopulmonary, GI, and peripheral tissue perfusion is normal.	All abnormalities have been corrected; vital signs and laboratory values are normal.

PATIENT TEACHING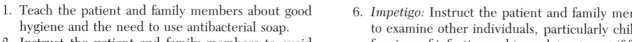

1. Teach the patient and family members about good hygiene and the need to use antibacterial soap.
2. Instruct the patient and family members to avoid sharing towels and washcloths when infection is present.
3. Instruct the patient and family members in the use of moist compresses.
4. Emphasize the importance of adhering to the prescribed medical regimen and the need to take all medications as instructed.
5. Explain to the patient and family members the negative aspects of picking or squeezing lesions.
6. *Impetigo:* Instruct the patient and family members to examine other individuals, particularly children, for signs of infection and to seek treatment if found.
7. Instruct the patient and family members in wound care as indicated.
8. Explain the need for immobilization and elevation of the affected limb as indicated.
9. Instruct a girl or woman with TSS to avoid using tampons until vaginal cultures are negative and the physician has approved use of tampons.
10. Inform girls and women about the need to change tampons regularly and frequently and to avoid wearing them overnight.

Viral Infections

Viruses are small particles that are not classified as living cells. They have six distinguishing characteristics: (1) they are unable to produce energy; (2) they depend on the ribosomes of infected cells to produce energy; (3) they do not contain enzymes needed to transform nutrients into energy; (4) they have either deoxyribonucleic acid (DNA) or ribonucleic acid (RNA), but not both; (5) their replication is directed by nucleic acid (DNA or RNA); and (6) replication involves an eclipse cycle.

Viruses may enter the body by many portals: the oral and respiratory tract (inhalation), the intestinal tract (ingestion) or urinary tract (or both), the genital tract (venereal contact), the skin or mucous membranes (percutaneous injection or direct inoculation), or the blood (inadvertent infusion). Intact skin and mucous membranes generally constitute a competent barrier against invasion by viruses. The cells of the stratum corneum may lack receptors for certain viruses, and mucus, sweat, and tears contain nonspecific virus inhibitors. Infection of the skin with certain viruses produces characteristic lesions, and based on the presentation, many viruses can be diagnosed without further testing needed (see the following box). Rubella, rubeola, the human papillomavirus, herpesviruses, and the human immunodeficiency virus (HIV) are all commonly seen in the skin.

PATHOPHYSIOLOGY

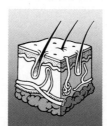

Rubella (German measles) is a mild, erythematous, infectious illness characterized by a few prodromal symptoms, including low-grade fever, coryza, malaise, headache, and conjunctivitis. Prodromal symptoms may precede the appearance of cutaneous signs by 1 to 5 days. The prodrome may not manifest at all in some cases, particularly in young children. The incubation period generally is 14 to 21 days from infection to onset of

CUTANEOUS PRESENTATIONS IN VIRAL INFECTIONS

Clinical manifestation	Virus
Macular/maculopapular lesions	Rubella, rubeola, roseola
Papular lesions	Molluscum contagiosum
Vesicular/vesiculopustular lesions	Varicella-zoster, herpes simplex

Adapted from Tyring.[63]

rash. Clinical cutaneous manifestations include a discrete, pink, maculopapular eruption that lasts up to 3 days, with associated lymphadenopathy in the suboccipital, posterior cervical, and posterior auricular lymph nodes. The exanthem begins on the face, then spreads centrifugally from the head toward the hands and feet. A low-grade fever may be associated with the exanthem, as may a mild pharyngitis and petechial lesions on the soft palate and uvula.

Viral invasion proceeds primarily through nasopharyngeal secretions but may also occur via blood, urine, and feces. Transplacental transmission of the virus may cause fetal death or congenital damage. The virus may be cultured from the throat 5 to 7 days before and up to 2 weeks after the onset of the disease. Rubella is seen more often in the winter and spring.

Rubeola (red measles) is an acute, highly communicable viral disease that results from respiratory (droplet) spread of paramyxovirus. The prodrome consists of fever, conjunctivitis, coryza, bronchitis, and Koplik's spots on the buccal mucosa. Three to 7 days after infection, a characteristic red, blotchy rash appears on the face. The rash becomes generalized and lasts from 4 to 7 days. A brawny desquamation may result as the rash clears.

Warts are benign epidermal growths caused by viruses. The *human papillomavirus (HPV)* is the most common cause of warts. Warts occur in both children and young adults but can occur at any age. Most resolve spontaneously after a variable course. Sites of trauma, hands, periungual regions (secondary to nail biting), and plantar surfaces are areas in which warts commonly develop. Warts can be transmitted simply by touch. It is not uncommon to see lesions on adjacent toes ("kissing lesions"). Cell-mediated immunity determines the severity and duration of warts. Individuals with acquired immune deficiency syndrome (AIDS), atopic dermatitis, and lymphomas and those taking immunosuppressive drugs have more severe warts when infected.

Common warts (verruca vulgaris) manifest as elevated, circumscribed lesions with irregular, hyperkeratotic, rough surfaces with minute papillary projections. They vary from pinhead size to more than 10 mm in diameter. Warts may proliferate and become confluent, and they range in color from brownish to grayish or may be flesh colored. Warts characteristically are found on the dorsa of the hands and on the fingers, but they can be found on the palms and soles. They generally manifest as multiple rather than single lesions.

Plane warts (verruca plana, flat warts, juvenile warts) are no larger than a pea. They are slightly raised with an irregular, smooth, or slightly hyperkeratotic surface. Multiple lesions with irregular distribution are the characteristic presentation. These warts show a preference for the dorsa of the hands and the face. Plane warts on the face are flat and generally flesh colored. On the dorsa of the hands, they are more hyperkeratotic and may be confluent. Plane warts are prevalent in immunocompromised patients.

Anogenital warts (condylomata acuminata) appear in cauliflower-like clusters and may involve large areas of the genitalia. In men they frequently are seen on the inner aspect of the prepuce, at the frenulum and coronal sulcus. They are seen less commonly on the shaft and the glans and within the urinary meatus. Perianal presentation is similar to the genital presentation in that large areas are involved. Condylomata acuminata in children may occur secondary to exposure to the virus while passing through the birth canal or secondary to sexual abuse.

Molluscum contagiosum is a benign tumor of the skin and mucous membranes caused by an unassigned poxvirus. In young adults it is spread most commonly through sexual contact. Autoinoculation in otherwise healthy individuals is common. If the lesions are widespread, an impaired immune system should be suspected. Clinically, the lesions of molluscum contagiosum appear as smooth, firm, spherical lesions with central umbilication. When manipulated, a cheesy white material can be expressed; this material contains the virus and should be handled carefully. Lesions may be seen on the face, especially around the eyes and mouth in children, and on the trunk and extremities. A linear configuration of lesions indicates autoinoculation. Lesions in the pubic region or on the genitalia, inner thighs, or lower abdomen indicate sexual transmission. Individuals with atopic dermatitis are at risk for widespread infection. The lesions resolve spontaneously over time.

Cold sores, fever blisters, genital herpes, and herpetic whitlow all are caused by *Herpesvirus hominis*. This category is subdivided into two closely related viruses, *herpes simplex virus type 1 (HSV-1)* and *herpes simplex virus type 2 (HSV-2)*. These viruses have both a

DIFFERENTIAL DIAGNOSIS IN GINGIVOSTOMATITIS

Aphthous ulcers
Streptococcal pharyngitis
Diphtheria
Infectious mononucleosis
Coxsackievirus infection
Severe candidiasis
Pemphigus vulgaris
Behçet's syndrome
Vincent's infection
Erythema multiforme (Stevens-Johnson syndrome)

primary and a secondary presentation. Primary infections generally are subclinical, but if they are clinically manifest, they are severe and can be life threatening. Secondary presentations (recurrences) generally are milder and of shorter duration.

Subclinical primary infections may manifest only small vesicles, which evolve into ulcerations, form crusts, and eventually heal within a few days or up to 3 weeks. Local pain and lymphadenopathy may be associated with the lesions of the primary presentation. Recurrences may have a prodrome of tenderness or tingling (or both) in the involved area.

The most common form of herpetic infection induced by HSV-1 is *gingivostomatitis*. It is characterized by painful vesicles and erosions of the tongue, palate, gingivae, buccal mucosa, and lips. Regional lymphadenopathy, fever, and general malaise are also associated with primary gingivostomatitis. Nutritional intake may become difficult as the lesions coalesce and become more painful. The infection is limited and usually resolves within 2 to 3 weeks. Primary herpes infection of the oral cavity and mucous membranes must be differentiated from other diseases of the oral cavity, as shown in the box below.

HSV-2 is the infective factor in genital herpes. Primary infection generally is seen 3 days to 2 weeks after exposure. It manifests as painful grouped vesicles on an erythematous base. Progression to ulceration usually occurs within 3 to 4 days. In men, lesions are most commonly seen on the glans, prepuce, and shaft of the penis. Perianal lesions are seen in homosexual men. Lesions in women are seen on the external genitalia, mucosa of the vulva, vagina, and cervix. Pregnant women with a history of genital herpes should be monitored carefully for signs of infection before delivery.

Headache, dysuria, vaginal and uretheral discharge, fever, malaise, and inguinal lymphadenopathy have been associated with infection. It takes up to 3 weeks for the lesions to heal completely. Recurrences can be induced by trauma, menses, sexual intercourse, and emotional stress; the recurrences generally are less severe and of shorter duration.

Herpetic infection of the hands is called *herpetic whitlow*. This type of infection, which is common in health care providers, generally is caused by HSV-1. The lesions are painful and manifest with erythema, vesicles, and swelling. An associated regional lymphadenopathy may be present. Primary infection lasts 2 to 6 weeks, whereas recurrences last 7 to 10 days. Differential diagnosis includes bacterial infections and dyshidrosis. Infection with the herpes simplex virus is always more severe in immunocompromised patients.

Other herpesvirus infections include *varicella (chickenpox)* and *herpes zoster*. Both infections are caused by *Herpesvirus varicellae*. Varicella is an acute, highly contagious infection that manifests a maculopapulovesicular exanthem that has centripetal distribution. The characteristic lesion, a singular vesicle on an erythematous base, is described as "a dewdrop on a rose petal." Because the lesions continue to develop in crops, the presentation shows some lesions resolving while new lesions are developing. Complete healing occurs in 2 weeks. Pruritus is the most troubling symptom. Varicella generally is self-limiting, but it is a life-threatening disease in immunocompromised patients.

Herpes zoster (shingles) is an acute vesicobullous eruption. Clinically it shows a dermatomal distribution (most commonly in thoracic dermatomes), with sharp demarcation at the midline. Zoster that crosses the midline, or disseminates, is a sign that the patient may be immunocompromised or may have an internal malignancy. Herpes zoster can be precipitated by trauma, x-rays, or ultraviolet light, or it may be associated with a malignancy. Pain or burning may develop 1 to 10 days before clinical lesions appear. Hyperesthesia is common in the involved dermatome. Headache and malaise may be associated with the infection, although they are unusual.

An increased susceptibility to both superficial and disseminated infections is a common complication in patients with *acquired immune deficiency syndrome (AIDS)*. Superficial infections that may be seen include scabies, molluscum contagiosum, a variety of papillomavirus infections, herpes simplex, herpes zoster, and cytomegalovirus. Other cutaneous manifestations seen in AIDS are Kaposi's sarcoma, psoriasis, and seborrheic dermatitis.

Nonspecific cutaneous problems also occur in AIDS patients, the most troublesome being chronic pruritic eruptions. This pruritic condition has been referred to as eosinophilic folliculitis of AIDS, papular eruption of AIDS, and pruritic eruption of AIDS. The cause is unknown, and treatment is only minimally effective. The infections are indolent, and other common skin diseases generally are chronic and manifest in atypical patterns. Bacterial and fungal infections are common, and malignant lesions develop at a much higher rate than in the general population.

COMPLICATIONS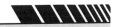

Rubella
  Arthritis/arthralgia
  Thrombocytopenic purpura
  Myocarditis/pericarditis (rare)
  Congenital rubella syndrome (CRS) (frequent)
    Deafness
    Growth retardation
    Cataracts
    Retinitis
    Meningoencephalitis
    Microcephaly
    Mental retardation
    Myocarditis
    Structural defects of the heart
    Death
Rubeola
  Photophobia
  Clear rhinorrhea
  Pharyngitis
  Gastrointestinal symptoms (diarrhea)
Warts
  Contagious
Herpes simplex
  Nutritional problems (gingivostomatitis)
  Contagious
  Recurrent

  Aseptic meningitis (seen in some primary infections of genital herpes)
  Possibly fatal in immunocompromised patients
Varicella
  Primary varicella pneumonia
  Superimposed bacterial infection
  Bacterial sepsis/focal abscesses (rare)
  Reye's syndrome
Herpes zoster
  Scarring
  Varicella pneumonitis
  Postherpetic neuralgia
  Motor weakness (with involvement of cranial nerves)
  Bell's palsy
  Conjunctivitis
  Iritis
  Corneal ulcers
  Blindness
AIDS
  Opportunistic infections
  Neoplasia
  CNS disease

DIAGNOSTIC STUDIES AND FINDINGS

Diagnostic Test	Findings
Rubella/rubeola	
Culture of pharyngeal secretions, blood, urine, stool (unstable and time consuming)	Positive for rubella virus 1 week before rash to 2 weeks after onset of rash
Complete blood count	Leukopenia
Hemagglutination inhibition	To detect long-lasting antibodies (used to determine immune status)
Complement fixation	To detect short-term antibodies during and shortly after rash
Herpes simplex	
Tzanck smear	Multinucleated giant cells
Viral culture	Isolation of virus
Enzyme-linked immunosorbent assay (ELISA), Western blot test, glycoprotein G−specific immunodot enzyme assay, solid-phase radioimmunoassay, indirect hemagglutination or indirect immunofluorescence	Used to quantitate type-specific antibodies to HSV-1 and HSV-2

Continued.

DIAGNOSTIC STUDIES AND FINDINGS—cont'd

Diagnostic Test	Findings
Varicella/varicella zoster	
Tzanck smear	Multinucleated giant cells
AIDS	
Complete blood count	
White blood cells	Depressed
Lymphocytes	Depressed
T cells	Number and function depressed
B cells	Number and function depressed
Cultures	Positive for microbial infections (fungal, viral, protozoal, bacterial)
Viral titers	To document exposure to HSV, hepatitis, Epstein-Barr virus, cytomegalovirus
Skin biopsy	Kaposi's sarcoma

MEDICAL MANAGEMENT

DRUG THERAPY

Rubella

Antipyretics: To control temperature.

Antibiotics: To treat otitis media.

Rubeola

Antiinfective drugs: To treat secondary infections.

Antipyretics: To control temperature.

Warts (human papillomaviruses)

Cryotherapy: Application of liquid nitrogen directly to the surface of the wart.

Surgical excision: Indicated for filiform and digitate cutaneous warts.

Electrocautery/electrodesiccation: Used for single lesions.

Topical medications: Equal parts of salicylic and lactic acid in flexible collodion; cantharidin; salicylic acid plasters; topical 5-fluorouracil; 20% trichloroacetic acid (for plantar warts); bleomycin for large, hyperproliferative, recrudescent hand warts; retinoic acid; resorcin solution; podophyllin.

Herpes simplex

Acyclovir: Oral, intravenous, topical; used to treat mucocutaneous HSV in immunocompromised adults and children and herpes genitalis in immunocompetent patients.

Vidarabine: Topical: To treat herpes keratoconjunctivitis/keratitis; may be given intravenously in severe cases.

Idoxuridine: Topical: To treat herpes keratoconjunctivitis/keratitis.

MEDICAL MANAGEMENT—cont'd

Varicella/varicella zoster

Idoxuridine: (Varicella) systemic administration with severe infections, particularly in immunocompromised patients.

Systemic corticosteroids: (Varicella zoster) may reduce postherpetic neuralgia.

Analgesics: To control pain.

AIDS

Cutaneous disease is treated aggressively according to the cause; use of antiviral medications to treat HIV has been disappointing.

OTHER MEDICAL MANAGEMENT

Rubeola/rubella

Management is supportive; tepid baths with cornstarch, Aveeno, or baking soda to help relieve pruritus; bed rest during febrile period.

Warts (human papillomavirus)

Laser treatment is used for anogenital lesions resistant to other forms of therapy (health care workers should take strict precautions to avoid inhaling vapor from laser, because papillomavirus could be inhaled).

Herpes simplex

Lesions must be kept clean and dry.

Varicella

Careful attention to cleanliness; tepid baths with cornstarch, Aveeno, or baking soda to help relieve pruritus.

AIDS

Supportive therapy.

1 ASSESS

ASSESSMENT	OBSERVATION
Current health	
Rubeola	Fever; cough, coryza, and conjunctivitis; lymphadenopathy
Rubella	Eye pain, sore throat, headache, fever, aches, cough, chills, anorexia, nausea; postauricular, postcervical, and occipital lymphadenopathy
Herpes simplex	Otherwise healthy
Varicella	Sudden onset of fever, mild malaise; pruritus with onset of rash; anorexia
Varicella zoster	Constitutional symptoms unusual but may include headache and malaise
AIDS	Malaise, fatigue, anorexia, weight loss, lymphadenopathy, diarrhea

ASSESSMENT	OBSERVATION
Skin and mucous membranes	
Rubella	Light pink to red, discrete macular rash evolving into papules; appears on face and trunk initially, moving to upper and lower extremities; fades in approximately 3 days; reddish spots on soft palate
Rubeola	Irregular macules on face and neck, appearing in postauricular areas initially; evolves into maculopapular rash and extends to trunk and extremities; rash becomes brownish as it fades; desquamation occurs; Koplik's spots present on oral mucosa; periorbital edema, conjunctivitis, photophobia
Warts	
Common warts	Elevated, circumscribed lesions with hyperkeratotic rough surface with papillary projections; found mainly on dorsa of hands and on fingers; palmar and plantar presentations seen
Plane warts	Slightly raised, irregular or slightly hyperkeratotic surface; irregularly distributed; usually localized on dorsa of hands and on face (especially chin, cheeks, and forehead)
Condylomata acuminata	Pink-red or white-gray raised lesions with lobulated surface; cauliflower-like clusters; involves large areas of genitalia; in men lesions found on prepuce, frenulum, and coronal sulcus; seen less frequently on shaft and glans and within urinary meatus; in women seen on labia majora, labia minora, and clitoris; extension to surrounding skin is common
Molluscum contagiosum	Smooth, firm papule with central umbilication; cheesy white material can be expressed; found on face, trunk, and extremities; sexually transmitted molluscum found in pubic region, on genitalia, inner thighs, and lower abdomen
Herpes simplex	Primary infection: small vesicles that ulcerate and form crusts; regional lymphadenopathy; keratitis; conjunctivitis
	Recurrent infection: grouped vesicles on an erythematous base that ulcerate and crust; may be hemorrhagic
Varicella	Macular eruption, usually on trunk, that becomes papular, then vesicular (characteristic "dewdrop on a rose petal"), then forms a crust; new crops of lesions continue to develop while others resolve
Varicella zoster	Hyperesthesia of involved dermatomes; grouped, edematous, erythematous papules in a dermatomal distribution; regional adenopathy; lesions rupture, then form crusts; scarring is common
AIDS	Superficial infections, Kaposi's sarcoma, psoriasis, seborrheic dermatitis; scabies, molluscum contagiosum, herpes simplex, varicella zoster, cytomegalovirus; stomatitis
Neuropsychiatric	
Rubella	Symptoms of encephalitis (rare)
Rubeola	Symptoms of encephalitis (rare); headaches, seizures, altered state of consciousness
Warts	Body image disturbance
Herpes simplex	Body image disturbance
Varicella	Headache, body image disturbance
Varicella zoster	Motor weakness with involvement of cranial nerves; body image disturbance
AIDS	Body image disturbance
Hematologic	
Rubella/rubeola	Leukopenia
AIDS	Decreased white cells, lymphocytes, T cells, and B cells
Pulmonary	
Rubella	Coryza, cough during prodrome
Rubeola	Dyspnea with secondary bacterial infection
Varicella	Lowered oxygen saturation secondary to primary varicella pneumonia
Varicella zoster	Pneumonitis (varicella pneumonitis) may occur
AIDS	Pulmonary infection, with resultant impaired gas exchange

ASSESSMENT	OBSERVATION
Musculoskeletal Rubella	Self-limiting polyarthritis (possible); pain in proximal interphalangeal and metacarpophalangeal joints of hands and knees and in ankle joints

2 DIAGNOSE

NURSING DIAGNOSIS	SUBJECTIVE FINDINGS	OBJECTIVE FINDINGS
Impaired skin integrity related to presence of lesions (herpes simplex, varicella, varicella zoster, AIDS)	Reports finding lesions	Characteristic lesions present
High risk for infection related to impaired skin integrity (herpes simplex, varicella, varicella zoster, AIDS)	Reports symptoms indicative of infectious process	Lesions showing signs of secondary infection; cultures positive for bacterial infection
Pain related to skin lesions (rubella, herpes simplex, varicella, varicella zoster)	Reports discomfort from cutaneous involvement	Guarding behavior, facial expressions indicating discomfort
Hyperthermia related to disease process (rubella, rubeola, herpes simplex, varicella, varicella zoster)	Reports feeling warm	Elevated body temperature; flushed skin that is warm to touch
Altered nutritional status related to presence of oral lesions (rubeola, herpes simplex, varicella, varicella zoster, AIDS)	Reports inability to take in adequate diet	Lesions on oral mucosa
Body image alteration related to presence of cutaneous lesions	Expresses concern about appearance; exhibits defining characteristics	Avoids eye contact; appears embarrassed

3 PLAN

Patient goals

1. Integrity of patient's skin will be restored or maintained.
2. Patient will be free of infection.
3. Patient will regain and maintain a positive body image.
4. Patient will be free of pain.
5. Patient will have adequate nutrition.
6. Patient will have a normal body temperature.

4 IMPLEMENT

NURSING DIAGNOSIS	NURSING INTERVENTIONS	RATIONALE
Impaired skin integrity related to presence of lesions (herpes simplex, varicella, varicella zoster, AIDS)	Assess extent of lesions; cleanse lesions as indicated; discourage scratching; maintain cool room temperature.	To allow early recognition of extension of lesions; to remove exudate as necessary; to prevent secondary infection; to prevent scarring; to increase comfort level.
High risk for infection related to impaired skin integrity (herpes simplex, varicella, varicella zoster, AIDS)	Assess for signs of secondary infection.	To allow early intervention.
Pain related to skin lesions (rubella, herpes simplex, varicella, varicella zoster)	Administer analgesics as needed; apply topical medications as ordered; apply compresses as indicated; maintain cool room temperature.	To relieve pain and increase comfort.
Hyperthermia related to disease process (rubella, rubeola, herpes simplex, varicella, varicella zoster)	Assess for fever; administer antipyretics; use sponge bath as necessary.	To assess severity of fever; to lower fever.
Altered nutritional status related to presence of oral lesions (rubeola, herpes simplex, varicella, varicella zoster, AIDS)	Assess nutritional needs; assess extent of oral lesions.	To establish appropriate diet; to establish need for mouthwashes to relieve pain and increase oral intake.
Body image alteration related to presence of cutaneous lesions	Assess patient's current perceptions and feelings.	To allow patient to express feelings and to assist patient during course of disease.

5 EVALUATE

PATIENT OUTCOME	DATA INDICATING THAT OUTCOME IS REACHED
Skin integrity is improved or has been maintained.	Lesions have healed, and no new lesions or erythema are evident; patient understands principles of hygiene and infection.
No infection is evident.	Skin and mucous membranes are free of any signs of infection; systemic infection is not evident through appropriate assessment.
Positive body image is evident.	Patient verbalizes feelings; defining characteristics are no longer evident.
Pain has been relieved.	Need for analgesics has decreased or is nonexistent.
Nutritional status has improved.	Oral lesions are healed; patient can resume normal diet.
Patient is afebrile.	Temperature is normal.

PATIENT TEACHING

1. Instruct the patient and family members in good hygiene.
2. Instruct the patient and family members in the use of moist compresses as a comfort measure.
3. Teach the patient and family members the signs of infection, and instruct them to seek treatment if infection develops.
4. Instruct the patient and family members in wound care as indicated.
5. Teach the patient and family members about the contagious aspect of the disease.

Fungal Infections

Fungal, or **dermatophyte,** infections (also known as tineas) are superficial infections of the skin. They account for the vast majority of skin, nail, and hair infections. Fungi infect and survive in the dead keratin of the stratum corneum, hair, and nails, causing a condition commonly called ringworm. Because a keratin layer does not form on mucosal surfaces, dermatophytes cannot survive in these areas. These infections rarely produce deep local invasion or multivisceral involvement except in immunocompromised patients. Laboratory confirmation of a fungal infection is necessary, because the lesions closely resemble other skin diseases.

Microsporum, Trichophyton, and *Epidermophyton* are the genera to which the ringworm fungi belong. Dermatophytes are further classified as anthropophilic, geophilic, or zoophilic, depending on their place of origin and the type of inflammation that results (Table 6-1).

Table 6-1

DERMATOPHYTE FUNGAL INFECTIONS

Classification	Origin	Inflammatory response
Anthropophilic	Human skin, hair, or nails	Mild
Geophilic	Soil	Brisk
Zoophilic	Animals	Brisk

PATHOPHYSIOLOGY

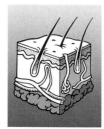 Dermatophyte (tinea) infections are classified by body region. The clinical presentation varies, depending on body location and species. However, even though species and presentation vary, all dermatophytes respond to the same topical and oral antifungal agents. All dermatophyte infections are characterized by an active border of infection. The lesions have an active border marked by scale with central clearing. Hyphae are most concentrated in the scale of the active, or advancing, border, making this the best area to obtain a culture specimen. If inflammation is severe, vesicles may be evident at the advancing border. Dermatophyte infections with inflammation on the palms and soles do not vesiculate. Table 6-2 lists the common tinea infections, their distribution, occurrence, and clinical features.

Refer to color plates 20 to 24 on p. xvi for examples of various tinea manifestations. **Pityriasis versicolor (tinea versicolor, tinea flava)** is a superficial, chronic fungal infection seen on the upper trunk or arms or on the neck. The infection is caused by a yeast, *Pityrosporum orbiculare.* The lesions appear as slightly scaling, papular, nummular, or confluent, and color varies from red to brown to white. Postpubertal and mature individuals are more susceptible to tinea versicolor. Lesions are found in the seborrheic, occluded areas of the body. Pruritus may be present, but the most common complaint is the cosmetic effect. The lesions become more prominent during the summer months because of sweating and tanning of surrounding skin. The lesions of tinea versicolor do not tan.

Candida albicans is the most common cause of candidiasis (moniliasis, thrush), an infection of the skin, mucous membranes, and, in rare cases, internal organs. Infection with *C. albicans* can result in *oral candidiasis, glossitis, paronychia, vaginitis/vulvovaginitis,* and candidal granuloma. Oral candidiasis manifests as white, cheesy patches or gray pseudomembranes on the oral mucosa. Glossitis is marked by intense erythema and

---

HOST SUSCEPTIBILITY IN CANDIDIASIS

Physiologic factors

Susceptibility increases during perinatal period, premenstrual period, and pregnancy

Genetic factors

Down syndrome
Acrodermatitis enteropathica
Candidal granuloma

Acquired factors

Chronic granulomatosis
Autoimmune endocrine disease

Other congenital or acquired endocrine imbalances

Diabetes mellitus
Hypoparathyroidism
Addison's disease
Malignancy (leukemia, lymphoma, Hodgkin's disease)
Anemia
Other debilitating diseases

---

denudation. Red, shiny, swollen nail beds are indicative of paronychia; proximal and lateral nail destruction and discoloration are also characteristic. Vaginitis is characterized by intense pruritus, white discharge, and white, patchy lesions on the vaginal wall. Cutaneous manifestations of vulvovaginitis include edema and erythema. Clinical manifestations of candidal granuloma include crusts and horns on the face and scalp. Chronic oral and paronychial candidiasis, as well as blepharitis, are also seen with candidal granuloma.

Candidiasis may develop at any age, in any susceptible host. Physiologic, genetic, or acquired factors can increase susceptibility (see the following box for a list of factors). Certain treatments also increase susceptibility (e.g., immunosuppressive drugs, protracted administra-

Table 6-2

SUMMARY OF TINEA

Type	Distribution	Occurrence	Clinical features
Tinea corporis	Nonhairy parts of body; face; neck; extremities	More common in hot and humid climates; more common in rural than in urban settings; occurs in both adults and children	Pruritus; papulosquamous annular lesions with raised borders; lesions expand peripherally with central clearing
Tinea cruris	Groin; inner thigh; scrotum or labia not involved	More common in adult men; tends to recur; flare-ups common in summer; aggravated by tight clothes, perspiration, and physical activity	Pruritus; hypopigmented, well-demarcated lesions; dryness and scaling; pustules present at margins; central clearing sometimes present; secondary bacterial or candidal infection and maceration common
Tinea capitis	Scalp	More common in children; contagious	Lesions vary; small, gray scaly patches with short broken hairs; mild, erythematous papules; raised, boggy, inflamed nodules dotted with perifollicular abscesses; thick, yellow, suppurative lesions; lesions may be small and coalesced or may cover entire scalp; hairless patches
Tinea pedis	Feet; begins in third and fourth interdigital spaces and spreads to involve plantar surface; may involve nails	Rare in children; not transmitted by simple exposure	Lesions vary; maceration, scaling, fissuring of interdigital space; vesicular scaling, erythema of plantar surface; chronic, noninflamed, diffuse scaling; nails brittle, discolored; pruritus
Tinea unguium	Toenails and (less commonly) fingernails	—	Nails thickened, lusterless, and discolored; subungual debris; nail plate crumbling or absent

tion of antibiotics or corticosteroids). In addition to the physiologic, genetic, or acquired factors, environment plays a role in susceptibility. Heat, humidity, and friction of skin surfaces increase the risk of developing candidal infections. Overweight individuals also are at higher risk of infection, particularly in intertriginous areas. Maceration of the skin from frequent handwashing, contact with urine or feces for prolonged periods (seen in infants and debilitated individuals), and other situations that moisten and macerate the skin increase the risk of infection.

COMPLICATIONS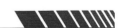

Secondary infection
Id reaction (cutaneous response elicited in other areas of the body distant from the primary infection)
Pruritus
Atypical, generalized, or invasive dermatophyte infection

DIAGNOSTIC STUDIES AND FINDINGS

Diagnostic Test	Findings
Potassium hydroxide wet mount (**KOH**)	Hyphae seen under magnification
Wood's lamp examination	Blue-green fluorescence of hair indicates infection with *Microsporum canis or Microsporum audouinii;* scale and skin do not fluoresce
Fungal culture	Positive

MEDICAL MANAGEMENT

DRUG THERAPY

Antiinfective agents: Griseofulvin (Fulvicin, Grisfulvin, Grisactin, Gris-Peg): Used in tinea capitis and in severe cases of other tineas.

Topical antifungal agents: Tolnaftate, miconazole, clotrimazole, econazole, or Ciclopirox olamine: Applied bid to tid for up to 3 weeks.

1   ASSESS

ASSESSMENT	OBSERVATION
Current health	Otherwise healthy; may be immunocompromised or have an underlying chronic disease
Skin and mucous membranes	See Table 6-2

2   DIAGNOSE

NURSING DIAGNOSIS	SUBJECTIVE FINDINGS	OBJECTIVE FINDINGS
Impaired skin integrity related to presence of lesions	Reports finding lesions	Characteristic lesions present
High risk for infection related to loss of skin protective barrier	Reports symptoms indicative of infectious process	Lesions show signs of secondary infection; cultures positive for bacterial infection
Pain related to skin lesions	Reports discomfort from cutaneous involvement	Guarding behavior, facial expressions indicating discomfort

3 PLAN

Patient goals

1. Integrity of patient's skin will be restored or maintained.
2. Patient will be free of infection.
3. Patient will be free of pain.

4 IMPLEMENT

NURSING DIAGNOSIS	NURSING INTERVENTIONS	RATIONALE
Impaired skin integrity related to presence of lesions	Assess extent of lesions; cleanse lesions as indicated; discourage scratching.	To allow early recognition of extension of lesions; to prevent secondary infection and increase comfort.
High risk for infection related to loss of skin protective barrier	Assess for signs of secondary infection.	To allow early intervention.
Pain related to skin lesions	Administer analgesics as needed; apply topical medications as ordered.	To relieve pain and improve comfort.

5 EVALUATE

PATIENT OUTCOME	DATA INDICATING THAT OUTCOME IS REACHED
Skin integrity has improved or has been maintained.	Lesions have healed, and no new lesions or erythema is evident.
No infection is evident.	Skin and mucous membranes are free of any signs of infection.
Pain has been relieved.	Need for analgesics has decreased or is nonexistent.

PATIENT TEACHING

1. Teach the patient and family members the signs of infection, and instruct them to seek treatment if such signs are found.
2. Instruct the patient and family members in the proper application of topical medications or appropriate dosing for oral medications; explain the possible side effects.
3. Teach the patient and family about transmission of the infection, recurrence, and reinfection.
4. Teach the patient how to avoid aggravating factors (e.g., tight clothing, excess moisture).

CHAPTER 7

Bites, Stings, and Infestations

Although more than 1 million species of insects have been identified, relatively few of them cause humans anything more than annoyance or irritation. People encounter insects in a wide variety of ways, resulting in an equally wide variety of consequences—and an array of treatments.

Because of the diversity of effects and treatments, this chapter is divided into two main sections. The first section discusses insects that bite or sting to protect themselves or their habitat. This group includes scorpions and spiders (which are "insects" only in the popular sense—they are actually arachnids); members of the order Hymenoptera (bees, wasps, hornets, and ants); and blood-sucking insects that feed on humans (ticks, fleas, mosquitos, chiggers, and bedbugs).

The second section of the chapter covers the ectoparasites (mites and lice).

Bites and Stings

Health care professionals are likely to see patients who have been stung or bitten by a venomous insect (e.g., bees, wasps, spiders). Table 7-1 gives the common skin manifestations of insect bites and stings. Nursing care includes teaching these patients how to avoid future painful encounters.

Stings or bites cause greater concern if the victim is atopic or has been stung or bitten before and is sensitized to the allergen. In the United States, allergic reactions to stings occur in about 1 million people, or 0.4% of the population. Most severe reactions are caused by hymenopteran venom. The venoms of bees, wasps, and hornets are closely related and therefore cause cross-sensitization.

Reactions generally are divided into three types: large local reactions (type I), systemic reactions (type II), and delayed, or serum sickness, reactions (type III).

A local reaction (type I) may involve immediate, sharp pain; edema; and pruritus that resolves in a few hours. A sting on the head or in the mouth may produce marked edema. More extensive local reactions that involve an entire extremity indicate a

Table 7-1

COMMON SKIN MANIFESTATIONS OF INSECT BITES AND STINGS

Insect	Characteristic lesion
Scorpion	Small puncture wound with local edema, discoloration, and sharp, burning sensation; area of paresthesia may develop at the site
Black widow spider	Small puncture wound centered in a 3 to 4 mm reddish papule, which may develop a small ulceration
Brown recluse spider	Tiny puncture site that develops a gray-blue surrounding halo with central ischemic necrosis
Hornet, paper wasp, honeybee	Red papule that becomes urticarial and edematous
Imported fire ant	Red papule that quickly becomes a vesicopustule with a reddish halo
Flea	Small red papule or wheal that may become petechial or bullous
Mosquito	Small, red, pruritic papule that may progress to wheals, bullae, and hemorrhagic areas
Tick	Small papule that may progress to painful ulcer; with Lyme disease, the papule enlarges in an annular fashion to as large as 50 cm in diameter, with central clearing and a firm, bluish-red border (erythema chronicum migrans); with Rocky Mountain spotted fever, the macular rash begins on the wrists and ankles and progresses toward the trunk with facial sparing; the rash becomes more petechial as it progresses and often involves the palms and soles
Chigger	Small, erythematous macule that progresses to 3 to 5 mm in diameter; an intensely pruritic lesion develops within 6 to 8 hours
Bedbug	Small red mark, often in pairs, that may progress to hemorrhagic bullae

greater risk of systemic reaction with future exposure to the antigen.

Systemic allergic reactions (type II) vary in severity. The symptoms of a mild reaction are caused by release of histamine, which causes diffuse pruritus, urticaria, distant edema, and flushing. More severe reactions involve laryngeal edema or bronchospasm, resulting in respiratory compromise. Profound hypotension may follow, resulting in myocardial infarction, brain damage, or renal failure. These systemic reactions are immediate hypersensitivity reactions mediated by immunoglobulin E (IgE) antibodies.

A delayed or serum sickness reaction (type III) may occur hours or weeks after envenomation. An influenza-like syndrome involving fever, myalgia, and chills may occur. Guillain-Barré syndrome, glomerulonephritis, and myocarditis have also been noted. Immune complexes between allergens and specific IgG- antibodies are thought to be responsible.

SCORPIONS

The scorpion helps to control insect populations. It has a forebody with six projecting legs and a hindbody. The *Centruroides* scorpion is common in Arizona and surrounding states and in northern Mexico. Scorpions use a hooked, caudal stinger, which projects from the hindbody, to inject venom.

In people, stings frequently occur on the legs, thighs, and buttocks, often because the unwary visitor was walking or sitting in the scorpion's territory. The sting is immediately painful, and the resulting symptoms may range in severity from pain at the site with local swelling, tenderness, and paresthesia, to life-threatening dysfunction of cranial nerves and somatic skeletal neuromuscular structures. Severe agitation, peripheral motor jerking, and hypersalivation are not uncommon in more severe reactions. An anaphylactic reaction may occur, with itching and swelling of the upper airway, convulsions, and collapse. Supporting the airway and breathing takes precedence over the actual skin wound, which often is no more than a puncture site that may ulcerate later.

Although it is not commercially available, a goat serum antivenin developed by Arizona State University has been shown to relieve symptoms in 1 to 3 hours; without the antivenin, symptoms last 9 to 30 hours. As with any serum, support must be available in case of an anaphylactic reaction.

SPIDERS

Scientists have identified about 30,000 species of spiders. In the United States, about 54 or 55 species bite people. With the vast majority of these species, a bite produces little more than a local skin reaction. However, four or five species have a bite that causes a more serious tissue response or necrosis, particularly if a secondary infection is present.

Black Widow Spiders

The black widow spider *(Latrodectus mactans)*, which is found in every U.S. state except Alaska, is one of two species of spiders whose bite has significant consequences, even in the absence of secondary infection.

Most people can describe the female black widow, with her coal-black body and characteristic red hourglass marking on the ventral surface of the abdomen. Like the scorpion, the black widow has a firm exoskeleton.

Although few people die from the bite of a black widow, small children and debilitated individuals should get immediate medical attention. With a significant bite, a potent neurotoxin is injected, and its effects are out of proportion to the relatively small volume of venom. The results are severe skeletal muscle pain and cramping, and an autonomic response that manifests as diaphoresis and hypertension. The typical skin lesion is a small puncture wound centered in a 3 to 4 mm reddish papule.

For neurologic symptoms, parenteral opioids are administered to control muscle, back, and abdominal pain. Benzodiazepines may also be needed. Nearly half of all victims are bitten on the leg or foot, which causes abdominal or back pain. A bite on the trunk, arm, or hand may produce chest cramping or pain.

A horse serum antivenin is available, but care must be taken to ensure that the patient is not sensitive to serums. Infusion of the serum relieves the pain, either immediately or within 2 hours. When the antivenin is not used, the symptoms persist for 24 to 48 hours.

All patients who are given the antivenin must be in-

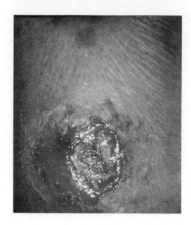

FIGURE 7-1
Brown recluse spider bite after 48 hours of treatment. (Courtesy Dr. William N. New, Dallas, Texas.)

structed in the signs and symptoms of delayed serum hypersensitivity. Rash, muscle pain, itching, and fever should be reported immediately to a physician or nurse.

Brown Recluse Spiders

There are 19 species of recluse spiders. The brown recluse *(Loxosceles reclusa)* can be identified by a characteristic fiddle or violin shape on the thorax. The spider is small, light to dark brown, and has six sets of legs. It prefers indoor or outdoor shelter and often lives in drawers, closets, attics, sheds, and other enclosed areas.

The female brown recluse has a more potent bite than the male. The spider often bites when its victim is asleep. Common sites are the buttocks, thighs, and feet, usually because the victim sat on or near the spider. The initial bite may go unnoticed, with pain developing 2 to 8 hours after the bite. Brown recluse venom is coagulotoxic; it disperses rapidly into the dermis and may stay biologically active in the tissue for up to 12 days. Skin manifestations are very unpredictable, possibly because of the small amount of venom injected, or because the individual developed humoral immunity from previous bites.

The bite site may show a tiny puncture surrounded by any or all of the following: erythema, wheal, edema, blister, purpura, cyanosis, or induration. A gray-blue halo often develops around the puncture site. Within several days the center may erode, harden, and develop a necrotic, crater-like ulceration (Figure 7-1). The center of the ulcer may become depressed, with sharply demarcated edges. Initial improvement may be followed by episodes of recurring erosion for several weeks. The ulceration may take weeks to heal and require plastic surgery for closure. Surgical intervention should be delayed until no additional tissue necrosis is evident.

Systemic reactions to a brown recluse bite also vary. Fever, chills, weakness, malaise, arthralgia, nausea, vomiting, diarrhea, and petechiae may occur up to a week after the bite. More severe symptoms may include anaphylactic reactions, hemolysis, deep vein thrombosis, paralysis, renal failure, pulmonary edema, atrial fibrillation, and shock.

HYMENOPTERA

The order Hymenoptera includes honeybees, yellow jackets, paper wasps, hornets, and ants. These insects usually sting because their normal habitat has been accidentally or intentionally disturbed. The stings generally are immediately and intensely painful for anywhere from 10 to 15 seconds up to several hours. Hypersensitive individuals or those with several stings are at most risk for serious complications. Most hymenopterans inflict individual stings, executed in one motion by a stinger that injects formic acid and proteins. The stinger, which is an adaptation of the ovipositor, has species-specific types of barbs. The barbs anchor the stinger to the skin, tearing the stinger and venom sac from the insect, which consequently dies. The unhappy recipient of the stinger may need help in removing it properly. The stinger may be pinched with tweezers or forceps where it protrudes from the skin and pulled free. A blunt instrument or fingernail may be scraped along the skin from the entry site toward the end of the stinger to flick the stinger from the skin. Quick action is important, because the venom sac continues to contract even after being pulled from the bee. The protruding stinger should not be grasped, because this will push the remaining venom into the skin. The sting produces a red papule, which becomes urticarial and edematous.

> Patients known to be hypersensitive to Hymenoptera venom may need to keep emergency equipment available at all times. When teaching the patient how to use a self-injecting epinephrine pen, be sure the patient can demonstrate self-injection.

Bees, Wasps, and Hornets

People can best avoid painful encounters with bumblebees, honeybees, yellow jackets, paper wasps, and hornets by becoming familiar with the insects' habitats and behavior. All hymenopterans discussed here have a hard exoskeleton and three pairs of legs. All have specialized mouthparts, and all have wings, except for ants.

The bumblebee is the largest of this group of hymenopterans. Along with the honeybee, it plays an important role in the pollination of fruits and flowers.

Bees tend to be rather gentle if left undisturbed. However, a new, more aggressive strain is making its way across the United States. During the 1950s, researchers in Brazil tried to develop a bee that would be a better pollinator. African queen bees were used in the experiments, because they develop quicker, fly faster, and produce more offspring in the same time span as honeybees. Breeding the African bees to honeybees produced offspring that were very aggressive, like the African parent.

The Africanized honeybees crossed the Mexican border in 1990 and are now making their way north. They cannot be distinguished from the more sedate honeybee and therefore are more dangerous if encountered. A disturbed honeybee will pursue its enemy for 50 yards—the Africanized honeybee will continue the chase for a quarter of a mile, inflicting numerous stings.

Bees raised in commercial hives, as well as those found in the woods, are less easily agitated when the skies are sunny and the weather calm, especially if there is an abundance of flowers. Clothing that has bright colors or a rough texture tends to attract bees. When a bee becomes agitated and stings, it releases a chemical called a pheromone, which alerts others of its kind; this can result in a swarm of stinging bees. The smoke cannisters used by beekeepers block the bees' ability to sense this pheromone, preventing swarming even if one or two bees sting.

A person who works in a fruit orchard can reduce the chance of being stung by yellow jackets by taking advantage of these insects' natural attraction to decaying fruit. A bucket of decaying fruit placed away from the fruit trees may serve as a decoy. Wearing mosquito netting and long sleeves while picking fruit or pursuing other outdoor activities may offer some protection. On picnics, food should be kept covered to reduce the attraction to wasps.

All flying hymenopterans become more aggressive if their hive or nest is approached, or if a person makes jarring or striking motions. If a nest must be eliminated, the job should be delayed until all members have returned at nightfall. Insect bombs contain chemicals that interrupt the insects' breathing mechanism, causing paralysis.

Honeybees occasionally find their way into a house and build a hive. They can be moved by a professional beekeeper, which eliminates the risk to the family and allows the bees to continue their vital work of pollination.

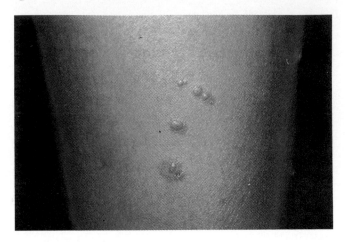

FIGURE 7-2
Erythema chronicum migrans (ECM) in Lyme disease. (Courtesy Dermatology Department, University of Texas Southwestern Medical School, Dallas, Texas.)

Local skin reactions to a bee, wasp, or hornet sting can be minimized by applying cold or ice compresses and elevating the affected part, if possible. Applying meat tenderizer to the sting has not been scientifically proven to provide any relief, because the papain cannot penetrate the skin to the depth of cellular involvement.

Imported Fire Ants

Ants come in many varieties. They generally are 2 to 5 mm long and vary in color from red through black. The most feared member of this group is a fairly recent import to the United States.

During the early part of this century, two species of this particularly vicious ant were accidentally introduced from South America into the southern states. The two species of imported fire ant (IFA), *Solenopsis invicta* and *Solenopsis richteri*, have migrated into surrounding states, moving both north and west, and entomologists predict that they eventually will spread to as much as 25% of the land area of the states.

Like the three domestic species, which are less aggressive, the imported fire ant lives in colonies. As many as 200,000 ants may live in a mound, with one queen. Their mounds have side tunnels that may extend 80 feet from the center. Like bees, the ant aggressively defends its colony, swarming on anything unlucky enough to disturb the mound.

The imported fire ant inflicts its sting in two steps. First it bites, thereby attaching itself to its victim; then it rotates its body to position the abdominal stinger for one or more stings. The injected venom of the imported fire ant has two components. About 95% of the venom is an alkaloid that contains piperidines, which are responsible for the intense reaction to the sting.

The protein portion contains four parts, which are responsible for the antigen response in allergic individuals. The bite may cause both local and systemic reactions. The initial response is an immediate flare followed by development of a wheal up to 10 mm. Then a vesicle containing clear fluid develops. The injected venom attracts neutrophils, and the vesicle becomes cloudy over the next several hours. This pustule is surrounded by a bright red halo (Figure 7-2). The piperidines cause cellular necrosis within 30 minutes of the sting and spread into the local connective tissue over the next several days. The sterile pustule lasts more than a week before rupturing and forming an eschar. The resulting scar may remain hypertrophic.

Generalized reactions may range from mild nausea, malaise, and fever over the first 24 to 48 hours, to anaphylactic shock. About 1% of IFA envenomations result in systemic allergic reaction within 30 to 45 minutes. Common symptoms include flushing, urticaria, pruritus, angioedema, wheezing, dysphagia, nausea, vomiting, diarrhea, abdominal cramping, and syncope.

Local reactions can be treated by applying ice or alcohol to the site and elevating the limb to reduce edema. Although the pustule is sterile, scratching may introduce bacteria into the opening. Cleansing the skin with soap and water or antiseptic reduces the incidence of secondary infection.

When a person is identified as reacting systemically to IFA stings, he or she should be referred for skin testing and possibly immunotherapy. Apparently some cross-reactivity exists between IFA venom and that of other hymenopterans.

BLOODSUCKING INSECTS

Fleas

Fleas are wingless, bloodsucking insects with three pairs of legs. They can jump distances far out of proportion to their size. Most flea species are adapted to a particular host. *Pulex irritans* prefers humans, but the rat flea, cat flea, and dog flea accept human blood if their host animal is not available. Fleas have a life cycle of about 6 weeks. Their eggs may lie dormant in the pupal state for as long as a year if left undisturbed. Just walking onto the carpet in a closed house may result in sudden release from the pupal stage to jumping insect.

Fleas are attracted by movement and will jump onto a human for feeding. Because they do not like bright light, they crawl underneath clothing, feeding as they move upward until stopped by constricting clothing—hence the often-described "breakfast, lunch, dinner, and snack" clusters of erythematous papules. Bites are most often noted around the ankles, where they produce reddish papules or wheals that may progress to a blister. Local application of cold compresses; lotions that contain menthol, phenol, or camphor; or local anesthetics may help reduce the itching.

A three-pronged eradication program is the best defense against fleas in the home. The pet, the flooring, and the yard must be treated at the same time to eradicate the eggs and prevent reintroduction of adult fleas. Simply removing the pet from the area during treatment is not helpful, because the fleas will feed on humans and are readily reintroduced to the house when the pet returns. Because fleas can serve as vectors for plague, typhus, tapeworms, and filariasis, they should not be allowed to multiply.

Mosquitos

Earth has more than 4,000 different types of mosquitos, and most areas of the globe have one or more species. The male generally feeds on nectar, but the female is attracted to humans by their body heat, the lactic acid in their sweat, and the carbon dioxide they exhale.

The female mosquito punctures the skin to ingest a blood meal. Several antigens have been identified in the mosquito's salivary venom, which accounts for the intense pruritus. If the person has not been previously sensitized, the lesion appears as a small, urticarial papule. Itching develops within 10 minutes of the bite and lasts as long as a week.

The mosquito is a vector for several diseases, including malaria and forms of encephalitis. If the victim is bitten numerous times, toxicity may result, producing disorientation and delirium in the absence of vector diseases.

Diethyltoluamide (DEET) is an effective repellent but must be reapplied every 2 to 3 hours. Bathing in a tub of water to which 1 or 2 teaspoons of chlorine bleach has been added also produces a repellent effect. Numerous home remedies have been proposed, and some perhaps have some benefit as a repellent. Eating foods high in serotonin (e.g., bananas and peanuts) produces natural odors that attract the insect.

As with fleas, local treatment may ease the itch of mosquito bites. If the person has numerous bites or the itching is severe, oral antihistamines may be needed. Taking diphenhydramine hydrochloride (Benadryl) or hydroxyzine (Atarax) before exposure to mosquitos may prophylactically reduce the local bite reaction.

Ticks

Tick bites can cause two very serious vector diseases: Rocky Mountain spotted fever (RMSF) and Lyme disease. Both diseases are spread by deer ticks during the blood meal the female requires to propagate.

The two genera of ticks that spread these diseases, *Ixodes* species and *Dermacentor* species, have three stages of development: larva, nymph, and adult. Ticks have only three blood meals during their lives: just before molting from larva to nymph; with the molt from nymph to adult; and finally, for females, as an adult to aid in the production of hundreds of eggs. The full cycle takes about 2 years. Although all stages of *Ixodes* species feed on humans, only the adult *Dermacentor* tick does so.

Rocky Mountain spotted fever was identified in the early twentieth century. It is caused by the intracellular bacterium *Rickettsia rickettsii*, which is transferred during the blood meal of *Dermacentor andersoni* or *D. variabilis*.

Approximately 1,000 cases of RMSF are reported annually in the United States. Most infections are acquired between April and September, although the disease can occur year-round.

The usual incubation period is 4 to 7 days. The initial symptoms may include fever, malaise, a severe frontal headache, myalgia, and a maculopapular rash that appears within a week of the tick bite. This rash, usually the hallmark of the disease, may not develop or may occur late in the disease. The rash generally appears as macules on the wrists and ankles and spreads centripetally to the trunk, where it becomes more defined with papular, petechial, or purpuric features. The soles and palms often are involved; the face usually is spared.

RMSF produces a multisystem effect. Gastrointestinal symptoms (nausea, vomiting, diarrhea, abdominal pain) often occur early in the disease. Pulmonary manifestations may occur during all phases and may include cough, dyspnea, and pulmonary edema. Neurologic, renal, and cardiac involvement may produce a confusing array of symptoms.

Early diagnosis and treatment with appropriate antibiotics dramatically reduce the mortality associated with RMSF. Death from the disease generally stems from disseminated intravascular coagulation, caused by the rickettsia-induced vasculitis.

The cutaneous and neurologic symptoms of a peculiar disease, later known as Lyme disease, were first described in Europe in 1909. A study of a cluster of children from Lyme, Connecticut, all diagnosed with juvenile rheumatoid arthritis and having had tick bites, led to the description and naming of the disease in 1975. The spirochete *Borrelia burgdorferi* was identified as the cause of Lyme disease in 1982. This established the eastern deer tick, *Ixodes dammini*, and its western cousin, *Ixodes pacificus*, as the vectors for Lyme disease. About 9,600 cases of Lyme disease were reported in the United States in 1992.

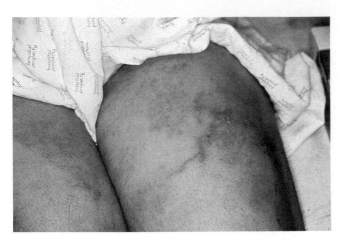

FIGURE 7-3
Multiple bites of the imported fire ant. (Courtesy Dermatology Department, University of Texas Southwestern Medical School, Dallas, Texas.)

Ixodes ticks can live as long as 3 years. The eggs hatch into six-legged larvae, known as seed ticks, which are about the size of a pinhead. The tick lives in the woods and on grasses, feeding from passing animals or humans. Bites are common in children, because they play in endemic areas. Unlike *Dermacentor* ticks, *Ixodes* ticks can transmit disease to humans in any stage of development. Because of the *Ixodes'* small size, its bite may go unnoticed.

The tick comes into contact with human skin as people walk through grass and brush. The tick moves about the body seeking a crevice or tight area, where it attaches to feed. It uses its barbed hypostoma mouthpart to penetrate the skin and secretes a cementlike substance to secure its attachment. Often crawling onto the scalp or attaching to any area where its movement is restricted, the tick feeds until engorged before falling off the victim. If noticed before this release, the tick is very difficult to remove. There are numerous folk remedies for removing ticks; many achieve only limited success, and most increase the danger of expressing organisms from the tick into the host.

For the preferred method for removing a tick, the nurse wears gloves and uses forceps or tweezers. The tick is firmly pinched as close to the skin is possible, to avoid expressing the contents of the digestive tract into the victim. Steady traction is applied to the tick without twisting. With patience, the tick will release its hold. The site should be cleaned with antiseptic and the tick disposed of in alcohol or flushed intact.

When *B. burgdorferi* is introduced into the body, about half of victims show a skin reaction in 3 to 20 days. Lyme disease does not have a linear presentation, making diagnosis difficult. Initially a small erythematous papule may appear, which grows in annular fash-

ion to as large as 50 cm in diameter with central clearing. This almost diagnostic marker, erythema chronicum migrans (ECM), develops a firm border that may be bluish red and up to 1 cm wide. The rash may extend in concentric circles and appear distant to the initial bite. Additional secondary lesions may appear over the next several days (Figure 7-3). These lesions tend to be less pronounced and migrate less. The rash usually resolves within 3 weeks. More than half of infected persons develop flulike symptoms that last about 1 week.

If the disease is not treated with appropriate antibiotics during this first phase, more than three fourths of untreated patients develop additional rashes or cardiac or neurologic involvement. Over a period of months to years, untreated patients may develop arthralgia and arthritis.

The skin manifestations of Lyme disease generally are not bothersome to the patient. They may reappear in later stages of the disease but tend to resolve with antibiotic therapy.

Preventing tick bites is the best defense against these vector diseases. Using caution in endemic areas, wearing appropriate clothing, and using insect repellents have some success. Most important, the body should be examined for ticks after being outdoors. The scalp, pubic area, axillary hair, and anatomic crevices should be inspected, because the tick spends some time on the body before attaching to feed. Ticks that have fed for less than 24 hours are thought to have a low incidence of disease transmission. A person who removes a tick should watch for any signs of rash or illness and call a physician if they occur.

Chiggers

Chiggers are six-legged, reddish mites about 0.25 mm long, barely visible to the human eye. They live in the woods and on grain and grasses.

Chiggers serve as vectors for several diseases, including rickettsial typhus, viral encephalitis, and *Pasteurella* plague.

Although chiggers can be found in northern areas of the United States, they are more prominent in warmer regions. Chiggers depend on passing animals or humans for a blood meal. Children playing in the grass or lying in hay are ready victims.

Like ticks, once on the skin of an unsuspecting host, the chigger moves to an area where it is constricted by skinfolds or clothing before seeking a blood meal. Strings of bites under socks or along belt lines are common. The mite uses an enzymatic, venomous, digestive saliva to dissolve epidermal cells as it drills into the skin (contrary to popular belief, chiggers do not burrow under the skin). Within hours an intense pruritus develops at each puncture site. The initial papule may extend to wheals, and the victim often excoriates the skin, causing secondary infection, including impetigo. Vesicles, pustules, and ecchymoses may develop. All exhibit severe pruritus.

Scratching may be so intense that the victim is unable to sleep. Applying ice or heat may interrupt the itch cycle. Ice water compresses or cautious use of heat from a hair dryer also may provide some relief. Topical cortisone sprays and oral antihistamines may help reduce the pruritus. The patient or family must be cautioned to watch for signs of secondary infection.

Many folk remedies have been offered to alleviate the maddening itch of chigger bites; camphor, phenol, alcohol, and clear fingernail polish are just a few. Although these generally are not harmful, prevention is probably the best cure. Children should be told to avoid playing in grassy areas known to be endemic for chiggers. A repellent such as permethrin, DEET, 6-12 Plus, or flowers of sulfur should be used when camping or picnicking. Play areas should be sprayed cautiously with malathion and allowed to dry before children are permitted in the area.

Bedbugs

Bedbugs are six-legged, reddish brown, flattened ovoid, bloodsucking insects about 0.5 cm long. They live in crevices and cracks, behind baseboards and wallpaper, and in furniture, including beds. They emerge at night, perhaps only once or twice a year, seeking a blood meal. They use their two stylets, which are designed to pierce the skin, to feed. The bedbug remains attached about 10 minutes while it ingests dissolved epidermal tissue and blood. The bite, which rarely disturbs the sleeping victim, leaves two small red marks. Within a few minutes the site develops pruritic red papules, which progress to wheals, vesicles, or hemorrhagic bullae. Although some individuals appear immune to the bites, others may develop asthma, arthralgia, and papular urticaria. Anaphylactic reactions have been reported.

Treatment for the lesion is symptomatic, and preventing secondary infections is important. Thorough cleaning and vacuuming, followed by use of environmental insecticides, will rid an area of bedbugs.

Although now very rare in the United States, bedbugs can be vectors for *Leishmania* (Oriental sore, Chagas' disease, and kala-azar) and *Rickettsia* (relapsing fever).

COMPLICATIONS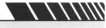

Anaphylactic reactions in susceptible individuals can produce serious complications or death. These reactions may be caused by the envenomation or from use of antivenins. Secondary bacterial infections may occur at the site of the envenomation. Local tissue necrosis, requiring surgical repair, may occur with the bite of the brown recluse spider. Individuals who have been infected with *B. burgdorferi* from the bite of a deer tick may develop cardiac complications secondary to conduction defect. This may require use of a pacemaker.

DIAGNOSTIC STUDIES AND FINDINGS

Diagnostic Test	Findings
Arterial blood gases (scorpion sting, anaphylaxis)	pH below 7.3 (infants) or 7.34 (adults); increased P_{CO_2}, decreased P_{O_2} on room air; all of these signs may be secondary to hypersalivation and obstruction of the airway
White blood count (black widow bite)	Leukocytosis possible
Complete blood count (brown recluse bite)	Hemoglobinemia and thrombocytopenia possible with systemic symptoms; pancytopenia possible after administration of dapsone; eosinophilia in type I reactions
Reticulocyte count (brown recluse bite)	May be elevated due to hemolysis
Venom-specific IgE antibodies	Elevated in approximately 80% of patients with positive results on venom skin test
Creatine phosphokinase (black widow bite)	May be elevated with cardiac muscle damage
Enzyme-linked immunosorbent assay (Lyme disease)	Four to 6 weeks after bite: positive for antibodies to spirochete
Bacterial cultures (all)	May indicate secondary bacterial infection from scratching or with tissue necrosis; joint aspirate positive for spirochete in late Lyme disease
Urinalysis (brown recluse bite)	Hemoglobinuria possible

MEDICAL MANAGEMENT

GENERAL MANAGEMENT

All victims of envenomation should be observed for complications. A very young or debilitated individual is more at risk for serious outcome. The volume of venom injected is also an indicator of outcome; the more venom injected, the more severe the reaction. Most insect bites resolve with minimal intervention. If pruritus is a problem, alternating hot and cold compresses may control the itch. The patient's fingernails should be kept short, especially on young children, to reduce the chance of secondary infection through scratching. If a stinger is present, it must be removed without squeezing to avoid injecting additional venom. Scraping with a blunt edge from the puncture site toward the exposed stinger or grasping the stinger with tweezers at the entry site before extracting minimizes venom introduction. Ticks are removed by grasping the head with tweezers or forceps as close to the skin as possible. Steady, gentle pulling is applied until the tick lets go. Care should be taken to avoid direct contact with the tick, to prevent introduction of vector diseases.

DRUG THERAPY

Scorpion, black widow, brown recluse: Appropriate antivenin may be used with all three types of envenomation. Although not without risk, use of antivenin shortens the duration of symptoms. Goat serum antivenin, used for scorpion stings, resolves the neurologic, respiratory, and cardiovascular symptoms within 1 to 3 hours. Equine antivenin, used for black widow bites, relieves symptoms within 30 minutes. The antivenin may be mixed with aqueous lidocaine and injected into the anterolateral thigh muscle of infants and children. Parenteral opioids, with or without concurrent use of benzodiazepines, also reduce symptoms of cramping and pain in this group. Although use of parenteral calcium gluconate is reported in the literature, Clark and colleagues (1992) report that an erroneous credibility may have been given to this drug because of the pattern of pain, which has been noted to "wax and wane." If tissue necrosis occurs with the bite of the brown recluse, oral dapsone (100 mg/day for 14 days) is administered. Concurrent use of prednisone (100 mg/day for 3 days) may prevent hemolysis and disseminated intravascular coagulation.

Hymenoptera stings and bites: Bronchodilators may be necessary for severe allergic reactions. Epinephrine 1:1,000 is injected subcutaneously, or aminophylline is given intravenously for bronchospasm. Oral antihistamines such as diphenhydramine (Benadryl) (25 to 50 mg PO qid) relieve pruritus. Antiinfective agents such as Bacitracin or Neosporin may be applied to scratched sites to reduce local infection.

When anaphylaxis occurs, parenteral epinephrine, oral diphenhydramine (Benadryl), and dexamethasone may be used to reduce the potentially fatal reaction. Oxygen is administered, and preparations should be made to support the airway.

Rocky Mountain spotted fever: Antibiotics are administered for 5 to 7 days. Doxycycline (100 mg bid), tetracycline hydrochloride (500 mg qid), and intravenous chloramphenicol sodium succinate (50 to 75 mg/kg/day divided into four doses) are the antibiotics of choice. Children are given appropriate weight-related dosages; tetracycline is not used during tooth development.

Lyme disease: Oral antibiotics administered early in the disease include doxycycline (100 mg bid) or amoxicillin (250 to 500 mg tid for 21 days). If the disease has progressed to late stage before diagnosis, parenteral antibiotics are indicated. Ceftriaxone or penicillin may be given for 10 to 21 days.

1 ASSESS

ASSESSMENT	OBSERVATIONS
Current health	Very young or elderly and debilitated patients may have more severe symptoms; patients with chronic disease or diabetes may be more at risk of poor outcome. Any patient with history of asthma or hypersensitivity reactions must be carefully evaluated before use of antivenin is considered.
Skin	Typical lesion (see Table 7-1), flushing, pruritus
Respiratory	Dyspnea, wheezing, shortness of breath, decreased oxygenation, cyanosis
Discomfort	May complain of discomfort at puncture site (immediate in some bites but can be delayed up to 8 hours with brown recluse bite); feeling of doom with anaphylactic response
Pain	Pain at site of envenomation (scorpion, brown recluse)
Gastrointestinal	Nausea, vomiting, diarrhea, abdominal cramping
Musculoskeletal	Peripheral motor jerking (scorpion); muscle pain, severe abdominal cramps, chest or back pain (black widow); arthralgia, weakness
Cardiovascular	Tachycardia, hypertension (scorpion); hypotension, shock
Neurologic	Confusion

2 DIAGNOSE

DIAGNOSIS	SUBJECTIVE FINDINGS	OBJECTIVE FINDINGS
Impaired skin integrity related to envenomation/bite	Reports being bitten or stung	Skin lesion, wound, local edema, erythema; identification of causative agent
High risk for alteration in respiratory function related to allergic response or excessive secretions (scorpion sting)	Reports being unable to breathe, or allergy to insect venom	Restlessness, agitation, wheezing, dyspnea, drooling, loss of control over oral secretions, cyanosis, abnormal breath sounds, difficulty speaking
Pain related to local or systemic tissue response	Reports pain at site or "all over"	Autonomic response; changes in BP, pulse, and respirations; tissue edema or necrosis, erythema
High risk for secondary infection related to disruption of skin barrier	Reports increasing pain, swelling, and "pus" at wound site	Elevated WBC, prolonged presence of erythema, increasing wound size, exudate

3 PLAN

Patient goals

1. All skin lesions will clear.
2. Patient will maintain a clear airway.
3. Patient will be free of pain and discomfort.
4. Patient will not develop a secondary infection.

4 IMPLEMENT

NURSING DIAGNOSIS	NURSING INTERVENTIONS	RATIONALE
Impaired skin integrity related to envenomation/bite	Provide wound care as ordered for brown recluse bite (e.g., moist to damp dressings if ulceration is present).	Dressings and medications provide a moist environment to promote epidermal regrowth.
	Watch for increase in erythema and signs of infection.	Normal skin flora may contaminate disrupted skin.
	Measure skin lesion and record its appearance daily.	Brown recluse venoms may cause spreading necrosis for up to 21 days; surgical repair is not indicated until no further extension is evident.
High risk for alteration in respiratory function related to allergic response or excessive secretions (scorpion sting)	Administer antivenin as ordered.	To decrease body's response to antigen.
	Prepare for suctioning and support of respirations.	Volume of secretions may impair ability to coordinate closure of the glottis, permitting oral secretions to enter the lungs.
	Administer bronchodilators as ordered.	To promote dilation of tracheobronchial tree.
	Keep patient in high Fowler's position.	To improve lung expansion and prevent aspiration.
Pain related to local or systemic tissue response	Assess degree of pain, and administer medications ordered (this may include IV or IM opioids for a black widow bite).	Degree of pain may indicate severity of envenomation; opioids block venom's effects on CNS.
	Provide cold compresses and ice as indicated.	To reduce edema, suppress local reaction, slow absorption of venom, and decrease itching (which reduces scratch response).
High risk for secondary infection related to disruption of skin barrier	Ensure meticulous hand washing by patient and staff.	Intact skin acts as a barrier against surface bacteria; this barrier has been lost at the envenomation site.
	Encourage patient not to scratch.	Persistent trauma inhibits wound healing.
	Keep fingernails short.	Long nails promote trauma with scratching.
	Administer tetanus toxoid as ordered.	Puncture site may contain contaminants.

5 EVALUATE

PATIENT OUTCOME	DATA INDICATING THAT OUTCOME IS REACHED
Envenomation site shows progressive healing.	Necrosis has stopped, and granulation tissue is present. Wound margins show no signs of erythema or purulent exudate.
Patient has normal respiratory function.	Breath sounds are normal, and blood gases are within normal limits.
Patient has no pain or discomfort.	Patient says there is no pain or is able to participate in wound care.
Patient is free of infection.	WBC is within normal limits; there are no signs of wound or systemic infection.

PATIENT TEACHING

1. Have the patient explain and demonstrate how to treat the wound to promote complete healing.
2. Teach the patient ways to avoid encounters with venomous arachnids and insects.
3. Emphasize to the patient and family the importance of follow-up treatment for ulceration from a brown recluse bite.
4. Educate the patient about the availability of medical alert identification jewelry and emergency injection kits for sensitized individuals. Have the patient give return demonstration of the epinephrine pen, if used.
5. Teach the patient the signs of delayed reaction to antivenin, that is, rash, hives, serum sickness. This reaction may occur up to 2 weeks after administration of the antivenin.

The following are guidelines and precautions, listed by type of insect, that nurses can teach their patients. **Note:** Whenever a person is stung or bitten, watch for signs of a serious allergic (anaphylactic) reaction. If these signs occur, call a doctor immediately.

Scorpions and Spiders

1. Seek immediate medical help for stings on small children or debilitated adults.
2. If you have been treated with antivenin, watch for signs of a delayed hypersensitivity reaction (rash, hives, itching, fever, discomfort, swollen glands, or joint pain). Report these immediately to your doctor.
3. Scorpions shun the light and hide under rocks and in crevices. Teach children to stay clear of such areas when hiking or picnicking.
4. Spiders hide under rocks and boards. Check closets, attics, outdoor shelters, and stored items before working in such areas or handling such items.

Hymenoptera

1. If attacked, cover your face and head and walk to a safe area without striking at the insects.
2. Seek immediate emergency care for anyone who has had a previous reaction to a bee or wasp sting, or when the sting is in the mouth or on the face.
3. If you have atopic dermatitis or some other allergic condition, ask your doctor or nurse whether you should carry a self-injecting epinephrine pen.
4. To remove a stinger properly: Pinch the stinger with a tweezers where it protrudes from the skin (do not grasp the stinger with your fingers, because this will push the remaining venom into the skin). Gently pull the stinger free. A blunt instrument or fingernail may be scraped along the skin from the entry site toward the end of the stinger to flick it from the skin.
5. If local reaction to a sting is mild, ice compresses may relieve the discomfort.
6. Be alert when working or playing in areas bees or wasps are likely to inhabit, so as not to disturb a nest or hive.
7. Teach children to wear shoes when clove is blooming, because bees love clover, and also because many varieties of wasps nest in the ground.

Continued.

8. Wear a helmet and gloves while biking or riding a motorcycle.
9. Wasps are attracted to fruit and decaying food. Cover picnic containers, keep garbage cans tightly closed, and place decoy fruit away from picking areas to reduce encounters.
10. Clean pet feeding areas regularly to avoid attracting insects.
11. Ask a local beekeeper for help if bees build a hive in your attic or some other inappropriate site.

Ticks

1. To remove a tick properly: With tweezers, grasp the tick firmly as close to the skin as possible. Exerting gentle, steady pressure, pull on the tick without twisting it. With patience, the tick will let go. Clean the area with an antiseptic (e.g., Betadine).
2. Inspect children and pets for ticks after outdoor activity; pay special attention to crevices and tight areas (e.g., belt line, scalp, armpits).
3. When hiking, wear long pants tucked into socks and sturdy shoes or boots. Long-sleeved shirts with close-fitting cuffs keep ticks off the arms.
4. Teach small children to walk in the center of paths when hiking to keep clear of grasses and bushes, where ticks cling.
5. Routinely inspect pets for ticks.
6. If someone has been bitten by a tick, watch for signs of Lyme disease. If these signs develop, see a doctor.

Ants

1. If attacked by fire ants, take quick action to get the ants off, especially if a large number of ants are involved.
2. Be ready to obtain emergency care quickly if the victim has allergies or a large number of bites and stings.
3. To treat uncomplicated bites and stings: apply cold compresses or lotions containing phenol.
4. Inspect play areas regularly for signs of loose dirt or sand, which may indicate an ant mound. Poking a stick into such an area may expose the mound. Treat mounds as needed. Do not leave young children unattended at outdoor play.
5. Do not walk through grassy areas at night without a good flashlight.
6. Use caution when gardening or mowing. New mounds may be more obvious after rainy weather.
7. When using chemicals to control ants, follow the instructions on the label carefully.

Fleas

1. Cold compresses may reduce the itching caused by flea bites.
2. Vacuum or wash pet bedding and rugs or carpets frequently.
3. Use flea collars properly on pets.
4. Regularly eradicate fleas from pets and from the house and yard.

Mosquitos

1. Avoid strong perfumes and hair sprays.
2. Use insect repellents; reapply after swimming or exercise.
3. Use screens and netting to keep mosquitos out of houses, tents, and other areas.
4. Mosquitos breed in small pools of stagnant water. Keep the yard free of old tires, cans, and debris, which can collect water.

Infestations with Ectoparasites

The two most common ectoparasites, mites (scabies) and lice (pediculosis), account for considerable embarrassment and itching among the world's population. Human scabies infestations are caused by the human itch mite, *Sarcoptes scabiei*. Two species of lice can infest humans: the pubic louse, *Phthirus pubis*, often referred to as the crab louse, and *Pediculus humanus*, which has two subspecies, the body louse (*P. humanus corporis*) and the head louse (*P. humanus capitis*) Table 7-2 gives the common skin manifestations of mite and lice infestations.

SCABIES (MITES)

Itch mites have been documented since biblical times. There was no treatment for the mite until the eighteenth and nineteenth centuries. Although insecticides were introduced in the 1940s, scabies mites continue to infect an estimated 300 million people each year worldwide. The pest has no respect for social class or economic status.

The scabies mite is transferred to a new host by close contact with another individual. Once on the human host, the female mite is impregnated by the male, which then dies. Males do not burrow into the host. Although the mite can infest other mammals, it is not transmitted from pets to humans. The animal mite can feed on humans but cannot burrow or reproduce on them.

The impregnated female penetrates the skin of the host by producing a secretion that lyses the stratum corneum. This process takes about 45 minutes. The mite does not chew into the stratum corneum; rather, she pushes her way through the corneocytes, propelled by the hind legs, always against the outward flow of cells. The motion is always forward because the mite does not turn in the burrow. Burrowing into the live stratum granulosum, she feeds on intracellular, lymph-like fluid. Because this epidermal layer has no capillaries, the mite probably is not responsible for transmitting blood-borne diseases.

The mature female mite, which is approximately 0.5 mm in diameter, continuously extends her burrow, laying one or two eggs each day during her 30-day life span. The embryo hatches in 3 to 10 days and develops into a six-legged larval stage. The larva sheds its covering twice before emerging as an eight-legged nymph, which matures into the adult mite. Both the larva and nymph can survive and mature outside the burrow. They also can be transferred during this time and can start the infestation on another unsuspecting host. Only about 10% of the developing mites survive to maturation in an immunocompetent host.

The developing burrow resembles a straight or S-shaped ridge or threadlike area about 5 to 20 mm long. A prominent dot may be visible at the end; this is actually the scabies mite. Vesicles and papules may be present. The most common burrow sites are the interdigital web spaces, the ulnar portion of the wrist, the axillae, back, areolae of the nipples, buttocks, and genitalia. Adults rarely show involvement above the neck. Children and infants, on the other hand, often have

---

Table 7-2

COMMON SKIN MANIFESTATIONS OF ECTOPARASITES

Ectoparasite	Skin manifestation
Scabies mite	Irregular, linear, gray-brown or pearly burrows less than 1 mm wide, often with a spot at the end; more prominent in the web spaces of the hands, on the flexor surfaces of the wrists, in the axillary folds, and on the buttocks; vesicles and papules may be present; in children, nodular lesions may be present on the upper back, chest, and genitals and in the axillary folds; disseminated papular eruption or crusted exfoliative areas with fissures may be seen in immunocompromised individuals
Lice	Small, erythematous papules and wheals, often with nits attached to hair shaft; cervical adenopathy may indicate severe involvement on the head and often is accompanied by purulent dermatitis, with matting of the hair; louse generally is visible on close observation

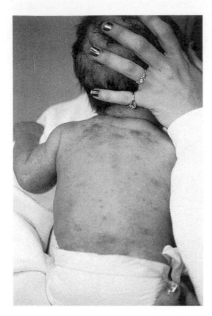

FIGURE 7-4
Erythematous papules and burrows of scabies mite in an infant. (Courtesy Dermatology Department, University of Texas Southwestern Medical School, Dallas, Texas.)

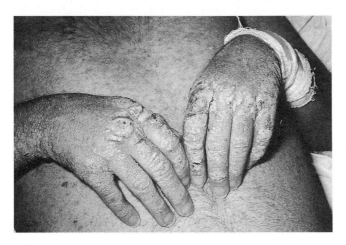

FIGURE 7-5
Disseminated papular eruption with hyperkeratotic lesions with fissures on the hands of a patient with AIDS. (Courtesy Joseph Knipper, Parkland Memorial Hospital, Dallas, Texas.)

burrows on almost any body surface (Figure 7-4).

The saliva, body secretions, and feces of the mite produce antigens, which dissolve in the cellular fluid that enters the burrow. The soluble antigen diffuses into the dermis, where it stimulates an inflammatory and immune response. The resulting infiltrate contains mononuclear T cells, some macrophages, and B cells. This process occurs over 4 to 6 weeks. During this latent period, there is no pruritus and the mite is free to multiply. As the immune response develops, the indi-

vidual begins to itch, instigating an itch-scratch-itch cycle. The allergic reaction kills a large proportion of the mites, which makes finding the live mite more difficult, especially when large numbers of mites may also have been scratched off the body. On subsequent infestation, this allergic response develops within 24 hours.

If the body fails to produce the cell-mediated response, as in immunocompromised individuals, the patient may become infested with hundreds of thousands of mites instead of the dozen or so found in immunocompetent patients. Instead of a relatively few burrows following the typical distribution, a disseminated papular eruption may occur. Hundreds of burrows may appear on almost any area of the body. Hyperkeratosis develops on the flexor surfaces, often with evidence of fissuring (Figure 7-5). Multiple tunnels often are noted on biopsy specimens. Because of the lack of immune response, the typical itch cycle, which brings most individuals to diagnosis, fails to develop. Infestation with the mite does not confer future immunity.

When members of the same family or contacts have a similar history of itching—especially when family members of various ages have a rash—scabies should be suspected. Individuals with any itching rash who work in day care centers, hospitals, shelters for the homeless, or institutions where large numbers of individuals are housed also should be suspected of having scabies. Until proven otherwise, any pruritic rash should be considered scabies.

PEDICULOSIS (LICE)

Like mites, lice are found worldwide. Although they may be found in all socioeconomic strata, overcrowding and lack of attention to personal hygiene promote their spread. Outbreaks are common in closely quartered individuals such as in schools, hospitals, military camps, and institutions.

Lice are wingless insects that need human blood to survive. The human louse is well adapted to various areas of the human anatomy. The head louse (*P. humanus capitis*) has claws that can anchor it on an average-diameter scalp hair. There it attaches its oviposit (nit), which is less than 1 mm long. The head louse is seen most frequently in girls and women of all ages, without regard to hair length. The presentation may be one of itching scalp or pruritic red papules above the shoulders. These papules result when the louse anchors its mouth to the skin, preparing to feed and inject saliva into the wound. The saliva, which prevents the blood from clotting, causes the allergic reaction. Blood is sucked into the digestive system, and fecal droppings

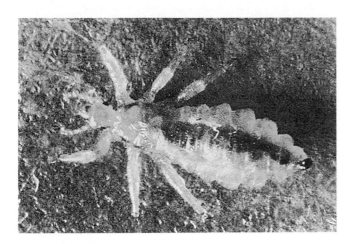

FIGURE 7-6
Pediculus corporis, or body louse. (Courtesy Dermatology Department, University of Texas Southwestern Medical School, Dallas, Texas.)

are deposited on the skin. The droppings appear as dark red spots and are seen more predominantly on the neck and shoulders. Cervical adenopathy and purulent dermatitis sometimes develop, because lice tend to concentrate in the area behind the ears and on the occiput.

Head lice seldom infest blacks but are widespread among Caucasians, American Indians, and Orientals. The shape of the hair and frequent use of oils and pomades by blacks may prevent gluing of the nit to the hair shaft.

Occasionally nits may be mistaken for dandruff. To verify that a fleck is a nit, the nurse can grasp the fleck between the fingers and try to slide the particle off the hair. If it pulls free readily, it is not the oviposit of a louse.

The claws of the pubic louse *(Phthirus pubis)* are adapted to the average diameter of pubic hair. Because hair in the axillae, beard, eyebrows, and eyelashes is similar, the pubic louse may also be found in these areas. The ova are attached to the hair at the skin line. Pubic lice also may produce gray-blue macules over the trunk and thighs. Excoriation is less likely than with body or head lice.

The body louse *(P. humanus corporis)* (Figure 7-6) lays its eggs on fabric fibers or in the seams of clothing. Its primary lesion is an urticarial papule. If infestation is prolonged, the skin becomes dry and scaly and areas of hyperpigmentation may develop, especially on the back.

All three types of lice undergo five stages of development: the egg stage (nit), three nymphal stages, and the adult stage. An adult louse can produce eight to 10 eggs a day, which are cemented to the hair shaft at the hairline or, in the case of body lice, to clothing fibers. Egg casings are firmly attached by a cementlike substance. Body heat hatches the egg in 5 to 10 days. The emerging nymph takes in air and expels it through the anus. This compressed air at the base of the egg case causes the top to pop off, expelling the nymph. The nymph goes through three molts over the next 8 or 9 days, taking frequent blood meals from the host. Lice mate within hours of reaching adulthood.

Lice can survive off the host for 10 to 30 days, depending on the temperature and humidity. Because of their dependence on the host's blood, lice generally leave a host only for another host. Pubic lice have been reported to infest dogs and then been retransmitted to humans. Lice are transmitted by person-to-person contact or the sharing of personal items such as combs, brushes, towels, and clothing.

COMPLICATIONS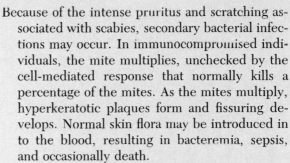

Because of the intense pruritus and scratching associated with scabies, secondary bacterial infections may occur. In immunocompromised individuals, the mite multiplies, unchecked by the cell-mediated response that normally kills a percentage of the mites. As the mites multiply, hyperkeratotic plaques form and fissuring develops. Normal skin flora may be introduced into the blood, resulting in bacteremia, sepsis, and occasionally death.

Lice infestation may be the source of keratoconjunctivitis, photophobia, and secondary pyoderma, caused by *P. humanus capitis.* Other complications include eczematization, pyodermas, nodular granulomas, urticaria, acarophobia, and delusions of parasitosis. *P. humanus corporis* serves as a vector for epidemic typhus fever *(Rickettsia prowazekii),* relapsing fever *(Borrelia recurrentis),* and trench fever *(Rickettsia quintana).*

DIFFERENTIAL DIAGNOSIS

Other skin disorders may have to be ruled out during the investigation for the cause of a pruritic rash. Atopic dermatitis, neurodermatitis, contact dermatitis, dermatitis herpetiformis, lichen planus, or psoriasis may be possible causes of skin lesions common to scabies. A similar rash present in several family members, occurring about the same time, should cause the suspicion for scabies to be heightened.

DIAGNOSTIC STUDIES AND FINDINGS

Diagnostic Test	Findings
Physical examination	Typical lesion (see Table 7-2).
Microscopic examination	*Scabies:* Scabies mite or parts (see below).
	Pediculosis: Louse, or oviposit glued to hair shaft or clothing fibers.
Mineral oil scraping (scabies)	The suspected area is covered with mineral oil to permit easier visualization. A burrow that has not been scratched or secondarily infected is likely to provide a higher yield of mites, eggs, or fecal pellets (scybala). A scalpel blade is held at right angle to the burrow, and sufficient scrapings from the epidermis are transferred to a microscope slide. A drop of mineral oil or 10% potassium hydroxide (KOH) is applied, and the scraping is viewed under lower power. The presence of the mite or parts, eggs, or scybala is diagnostic of scabies.
Burrow ink test (BIT) (scabies)	A blue or black ink pen, or felt-tipped, fine point, nonpermanent marker is used to cover the suspected burrow. The ink is allowed to penetrate the skin for several minutes before it is removed with an alcohol pad. Ink that has penetrated the burrow will remain, marking the burrow for scraping and microscopic evaluation (i.e., mineral oil scraping).
Tetracycline fluorescence technique (scabies)	Liquid tetracycline is applied to a suspicious burrow area and allowed to dry for several minutes before being removed with an alcohol pad. The area is then illuminated with a Wood's lamp. A yellow-green fluorescence will occur over burrows, marking potential areas for scraping (i.e., mineral oil scraping).
Biopsy (scabies)	Although seldom indicated, a biopsy may help in the diagnosis of crusted scabies. The biopsy shows multiple channels and tunnels in the epidermis with the presence of many mites and their egg casings and scybala. When nodular scabies is suspected, the biopsy is used to confirm the perivascular T lymphocytes and histiocytes caused by a hypersensitivity reaction. These generally occur in the intertriginous areas and on the genitalia.
IgE (scabies)	Elevated (itching may not occur in immunosuppressed or anergic individuals, who may not produce or liberate histamine).
IgA (scabies)	Decreased in crusted scabies.
Wood's light (pediculosis)	Hair infested by lice is lusterless and will fluoresce under ultraviolet light.
Complete blood count	Eosinophilia noted with crusted scabies.

MEDICAL MANAGEMENT

GENERAL MANAGEMENT

The goals of treatment are to remove the mites or lice, eliminate the itch, identify and treat any secondary infections, and provide emotional support for the patient and contacts. To prevent reinfestation, the environment, including fomites, must be treated to rid it of mites and lice.

DRUG THERAPY: SCABIES

Treatment for scabies requires the use of an insecticide by the patient and all close contacts. Insecticides may include:

5% Permethrin cream (Elimite): *Adults and children:* Massage into the skin from the head to the soles and leave for 8 to 14 hours, then wash off thoroughly; include scalp in infants; more cosmetically acceptable, although more expensive.

Benzene hexachloride-gamma (1% Lindane, Kwell): Apply as above. Because there is some evidence of neurotoxicity with infants and small children, do not use in pregnant or lactating women. Teach parents that itching may persist, but that they should not use the product repeatedly, because this increases absorption of the insecticide. For adults, one application of 30 ml usually is sufficient. For infants, the application time is shortened to 2 hours. Infants should be held to prevent introduction of the insecticide into the mouth. Repeat the treatment after 7 days if indicated.

Crotamiton (Eurax): Apply for 2 to 5 consecutive nights; bathe 24 hours after the last application. Should not be used by pregnant or lactating women.

Benzyl benzoate 25% (Ascabiol): Used for treatment only below the neck. Apply for 3 consecutive nights, then wash off thoroughly 24 hours after the last application. For children, dilute one half; for infants, dilute to one-third strength. May cause stinging and contact dermatitis.

Sulfur preparations: 5% to 10% mixtures with petrolatum may be used in pregnant and lactating women. Use caution to prevent oral contact during nursing. The mixture is applied at bedtime for 5 nights; it is very smelly and may stain bed linen.

The World Health Organization treats large populations for both lice and scabies using a preparation containing benzyl benzoate, DDT, Benzocaine, and polysorbate 80 (NBIN).

If the individual is immunocompromised, a very aggressive approach must be taken. Use of multiple agents must be considered, and careful attention must be given to reducing hyperkeratotic areas to aid in application to the mites. Keratolytics may be necessary. The fingernails tend to harbor many mites as well, and applications must include this area. Applications of permethrin and lindane may be alternated.

Topical steroids: In low to medium strength, these can be applied to lesions to reduce the pruritus that may persist for 1 to 2 months. Oral corticosteroids may be necessary for severe pruritus. Pruritic nodules may require intralesional injection of dilute corticosteroids using a suspension of triamcinolone in a 4 mg/ml strength.

Antibiotics: Either oral or systemic forms may be needed to treat secondary infections.

DRUG THERAPY: PEDICULOSIS

1% Lindane shampoo (Kwell): Apply to hair and leave in no longer than 10 minutes; rinse. This may be repeated the next day, but caution must be used because lindane may be neurotoxic, especially to children. Another treatment in 10 days will ensure that all ova have been killed. A nit comb may be used to dislodge the nit.

Continued.

MEDICAL MANAGEMENT—cont'd

1% Permethrin (Nix):   Wash the hair, rinse, and towel dry. Apply permethrin, leave on for 10 minutes, then rinse off. This is somewhat more effective than lindane and provides better ovicidal action. Although this kills the nits, some schools require their removal before children can be readmitted. If the nits are not removed, many will remain attached to the hair shaft. Any nits found farther than 0.5 cm from the skin line are dead ova or empty casings.

Pyrethrine (RID):   Apply liquid to infested area of skin, scalp, and hair. Leave in for 10 minutes, then rinse. Follow with shampoo, and wash the skin with soap and water. Treatment may be repeated once after 24 hours. This synthetic pyrethrin is less effective than other pediculicides. Lice and nits must be removed with a nit comb. Its greatest advantage is its availability as an over-the-counter product. If the patient is hypersensitive to chrysanthemums, warn him or her not to use this product, because it is chemically related to that plant and may cause hypersensitivity reactions.

0.5% Malathion lotion: Must be left on the scalp for 8 to 12 hours (has an unpleasant sulfur odor). More effective than lindane and has good ovicidal activity. Caution patients that the base is 78% alcohol, and thus the hair is flammable until completely dry.

Petrolatum: Apply to lashes twice a day, then remove lice and nits by hand. No pediculicide should be used around the eyes.

0.25% Physostigmine (Eserine):   An ophthalmic ointment applied daily to the eyelashes until clear of lice and nits.

ENVIRONMENTAL TREATMENT

Mites: Clothing, bedding, and other intimate articles should be machine washed in the hot water cycle. Because mites live as long as 96 hours if the temperature and humidity are ideal, furniture, flooring, and other nonwashable areas must be quarantined for that length of time or sprayed with insecticide. Some authorities report live mites in household dust from homes where the occupant has been continuously absent for periods exceeding 96 hours. A quarantine of 4 weeks is suggested if thorough cleaning is not possible.

Lice: All personal items such as clothing and bedding must be washed in hot water. With body lice, the extra precaution of ironing the seams of clothing should be recommended. Hats, scarves, hair ornaments, combs, and brushes must also be cleared of lice and their eggs. Although lice can live only about 10 days off the host, the eggs may hatch up for up to 30 days if kept at about body temperature.

PSYCHOLOGICAL SUPPORT

Scabies: Patients may have a severe psychological response. Delusions of parasitosis may require more intense psychological support and therapy. Reassuring the patient that continued itching does not indicate treatment failure helps to obtain compliance with treatment and reduces anxiety.

Lice: Many common expressions help account for the negative response to pediculosis, such as "lousy," "nit picking," "going over things with a fine-toothed comb," "cooties." Itching takes time to subside after treatment, much as with scabies. Many schools do not permit students to return to class with nits on the hair, even though all the egg casings may be empty or contain killed ova. Vinegar solutions have been recommended to dissolve the cement that attaches the nit to the hair shaft, but research does not support this claim. Nits can be removed by meticulously combing through each section of hair with a fine-toothed comb. It is not necessary to cut the hair unless the patient cannot cooperate with combing. A commercially available cream rinse can be used to aid in nit removal.

1 ASSESS

ASSESSMENT	OBSERVATIONS
General	Withdrawn or anxious, scratching, hair without luster, swollen lymph nodes, evidence of nits in hair, lice on skin in distribution related to type
Social history	Close contact with others; parent and infant or sexual partner with skin lesions or pruritus
General complaint	Intense pruritus and scratching, except for immunocompromised patients; sensation of something crawling on the skin
Skin	Typical lesion (see Table 7-2), excoriation, secondary infection, areas of hyperpigmentation, maculae

2 DIAGNOSE

NURSING DIAGNOSIS	SUBJECTIVE FINDINGS	OBJECTIVE FINDINGS
Impaired skin integrity related to mechanical factors	Reports itching that worsens at night	Typical skin lesions, linear scratch marks, open bullae
High risk for secondary infection related to loss of skin barrier	Complaints of having to scratch constantly	Swollen lymph nodes, evidence of secondary skin lesions, elevated WBC
Potential for transmission of ectoparasites related to lack of knowledge of mode of transmission or fear of disclosure of infestation	Expresses fear of others knowing about infestation; shows casual attitude during instruction	History of previous infestations; undue concern about or lack of interest in treatment plan
Social isolation related to stigma of diagnosis	Expresses fear of loneliness	Agitation, concerned or anguished facial expression, decreased contact with family, asks about return to school or work

3 PLAN

Patient goals

1. All lesions will heal.
2. Patient will not develop a secondary infection.
3. Patient will be free of ectoparasites.
4. Patient's family and contacts will remain free of ectoparasites.
5. Patient will have a positive self-image.

→ > >

4 IMPLEMENT

NURSING DIAGNOSIS	NURSING INTERVENTIONS	RATIONALE
Impaired skin integrity related to mechanical factors	Assess all areas of the skin and hair to detect any burrows (scabies) or lice and eggs (nits).	Proper identification of infested areas is vital to adequate treatment.
	Instruct patient in proper use of insecticide.	Overuse of insecticide may cause further skin disruption.
	Caution patient to avoid excessive or prolonged use of topical steroids.	Topical steroids cause epidermal thinning, resulting in greater susceptibility to further injury; wound healing may be delayed.
High risk for secondary infection related to loss of skin barrier	Treat infestation.	Presence of mites or lice prolongs itch response.
	Use cool baths, antipruritics, and topical steroids as ordered.	To decrease itch response and reduce scratching.
	Use meticulous handwashing, and reinforce this behavior in the patient.	Surface bacteria are readily introduced into the skin with excoriation.
	Instruct parents to cut children's fingernails.	Children are less aware of scratching and often have dirt under the nails.
Potential for transmission of ectoparasites related to lack of knowledge of mode of transmission or fear of disclosure of infestation	Instruct patient and significant others in proper use of insecticides (see Medical Management).	To minimize repeat exposure.
	Identify all contacts.	Failure to identify and treat contacts is the most common cause of reinfestation.
	Isolate patient and fomites for period of treatment.	To minimize risk of reinfestation.
	Instruct patient in proper technique for environmental and fomite treatment.	To minimize reinfestation from fomites.
	Instruct patient in methods for aiding nit removal.	Medications may not be 100% effective in killing ova.
	Teach patient the signs and symptoms of new infestations.	Treatment failures are common and must be retreated.
Social isolation related to stigma of diagnosis	Encourage patient to express feelings about infestation.	To provide an opportunity for education about mode of transmission and identification of contacts; promotes acceptance.
	Reassure patient that infestation can be successfully treated.	Realistic expectations promote compliance with treatment plan and involvement of contacts.
	Provide patient with education materials for contacts, workplace, and school or institution.	To promote improved behavior to break the mode of transmission.

5   EVALUATE

PATIENT OUTCOME	DATA INDICATING THAT OUTCOME IS REACHED
All lesions have healed.	Lesions have granulated, and excoriations have resolved.
Patient has no secondary infection.	Patient has no lymphedema; WBC and vital signs are within normal limits.
Patient is free of ectoparasites.	Pruritus resolved within 1 month; there is no evidence of new burrows or lice and nits; clothing is free of ectoparasites.
Patient's family and contacts are free of ectoparasites.	No family member or personal contact of the patient has developed scabies or lice infestation.
Patient has a positive self-image.	Patient dresses appropriately for occasion and shows evidence of good personal hygiene; he or she can describe activities for educating contacts and school or workplace, as indicated.

PATIENT TEACHING

1. Instruct patient and family or significant other in the correct application of pediculicide.
2. Instruct patient and family or significant other in the appropriate handling of linens, clothes, brushes, and combs.
3. Explain to patient and family or significant other that pruritis may persist for up to 2 weeks after treatment.

CHAPTER 8

Tumors of the Skin

Tumors of the skin may be benign, premalignant, or malignant. Benign lesions generally cause only a cosmetic problem for the individual, whereas premalignant lesions must be identified early to prevent evolution into malignant forms. Benign lesions include seborrheic keratoses, acrochordons, dermatofibromas, keloids and hypertrophic scars, keratoacanthomas, and epidermal cysts. Actinic keratoses are the most common premalignant lesion; malignant lesions include basal cell carcinoma, squamous cell carcinoma, malignant melanoma, and cutaneous T-cell lymphoma.

Benign and Premalignant Lesions

PATHOPHYSIOLOGY

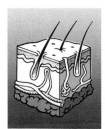

Seborrheic keratoses are common, benign growths that originate in the epidermis. Their cause is unknown, but they have no malignant potential. It is important to distinguish seborrheic keratoses from other potentially malignant lesions. Seborrheic keratoses appear in areas of the body exposed to sunlight and have a "stuck on" appearance. They generally are asymptomatic (but may produce itching, particularly in the elderly) and are easily and quickly removed.

Skin tags, or **acrochordons,** are common skin lesions found mainly in the axilla, on the neck, and in the inguinal area. They are brown or skin-colored excrescences attached by a short stalk.

Dermatofibromas are common, benign, asymptomatic (to slightly pruritic) lesions that can be seen on any part of the body. They are more prevelant in women and have a predisposition for the anterior surface of the lower legs. The tumor is thought to be caused by a fibrous reaction to viral infection or a reaction to an insect bite or trauma. Dermatofibromas are slightly raised, scaly, hard growths that are slightly pinkish brown in color. Attempts to compress and elevate the lesion will cause it to retract beneath the skin's surface. Individuals with systemic lupus erythematosus may have multiple dermatofibromas.

Keloids and **hypertrophic scars** appear secondary to injury or surgery in individuals who are predisposed to the condition. Keloids extend beyond the site of injury and do not regress spontaneously. Hypertrophic scars, in contrast, stay confined to the wound site and generally regress over time.

Keratoacanthoma is a relatively common, benign, epithelial tumor. It may be viral in origin, and the tumor generally is seen in the sixth decade of life. The tumor is a smooth, dome-shaped, erythematous papule that resembles molluscum contagiosum. Keratoacanthoma generally manifests as a solitary lesion, but multiple lesions occasionally may occur. Spontaneous remission with scarring is common.

Epidermal (sebaceous) cysts manifest primarily on the face, back, base of the ears, or chest, but they may be found on any area of the body that has sebaceous glands. The cysts are palpable and movable and may

range in size from a few millimeters to several centimeters. Small cysts have a blackhead at the skin's surface ("giant comedones"); larger cysts may be closed on the surface.

Actinic keratosis (AK) is a common premalignant lesion. These lesions are seen on sun-exposed areas of the body, because they are caused by long-term exposure to sunlight. The number of lesions increases with age, and light-skinned individuals have a higher risk of developing them. They initially manifest as an area of increased vascularity with a rough surface. With time a yellow, adherent crust forms. If induration, inflammation, and oozing occur, a biopsy should be performed to rule out malignancy.

COMPLICATIONS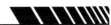

Seborrheic keratosis
Leser-Trélat sign (may indicate internal malignancy)
Keloid/hypertrophic scar, keratoacanthoma, acrochordon
Cosmetic impairment
Epidermal (sebaceous) cyst
Pain
Secondary infection
Actinic keratosis
Evolution into malignancy

DIAGNOSTIC STUDIES AND FINDINGS

Diagnostic Test	Findings
Skin biopsy	Inflammation

MEDICAL MANAGEMENT

DRUG THERAPY

Keloid/hypertrophic scar

Corticosteroids: Intralesional injections at least once every 4 weeks.

Keratoacanthoma

5-Fluorouracil (5-FU) or corticosteroids injected intralesionally.

Adrenocorticosteroids applied topically.

Oral isotretinoin and oral etretinate when multiple lesions are present.

Continued.

MEDICAL MANAGEMENT—cont'd

DRUG THERAPY

Topical 5-fluorouracil (Efudex) applied in rapid growth phase; pretreatment of lesions on the forearms, hands, or legs with salicylic acid (Keralyt) or urea cream (Carmol 20) to enhance penetration of 5-FU.

Actinic keratosis

Topical medications: Tretinoin (Retin-A) alone or in combination with 5-FU (tretinoin enhances effectiveness of 5-FU).

OTHER MEDICAL MANAGEMENT

Cryosurgery

Seborrheic keratoses, actinic keratoses

Curettage

Seborrheic keratoses

Curettage and desiccation

Actinic keratoses

Surgery

Acrochordon, keloids, epidermal cysts

Compression

Hypertrophic scars

GENERAL MANAGEMENT

Patients with actinic keratosis should use sunscreens and avoid chronic exposure to sunlight.

1   ASSESS

ASSESSMENT	OBSERVATIONS
General health	Usually good
Skin and mucous membranes	Characteristic lesion

2 DIAGNOSE

NURSING DIAGNOSIS	SUBJECTIVE FINDINGS	OBJECTIVE FINDINGS
Impaired skin integrity related to presence of lesions	Reports finding lesions	Lesions present
High risk for infection related to impaired skin integrity	Reports symptoms indicative of secondary infection	Signs of cutaneous infection present
Body image disturbance related to presence of skin lesions	Reports difficulty with social interaction	Defining characteristics of body image disturbance

3 PLAN

Patient goals

1. Patient's skin integrity will be restored and maintained.
2. Patient will be free of infection.

3. Patient's body image will be restored and maintained.

4 IMPLEMENT

NURSING DIAGNOSIS	NURSING INTERVENTIONS	RATIONALE
Impaired skin integrity related to presence of lesions	Assess skin lesions, including distribution and signs of progression.	To allow early intervention and to protect skin's barrier function.
High risk for infection related to impaired skin integrity	Assess skin lesions for signs of infection.	To aid early intervention and treatment.
Body image disturbance related to presence of skin lesions	Assess patient's current perceptions and feelings.	To identify distortions and to assist patient with negative feelings.

5 EVALUATE

PATIENT OUTCOME	DATA INDICATING THAT OUTCOME IS REACHED
Skin integrity has been restored.	Skin lesions have been treated successfully.

→ > >

PATIENT OUTCOME	DATA INDICATING THAT OUTCOME IS REACHED
No infection is evident.	Lesions are not secondarily infected.
Patient has positive body image.	Patient's reactions to body image are positive.

PATIENT TEACHING ■■■■■■■■■■■■■■■■■■■■■■■■■■■■■■■■■■■■■■

1. Teach the patient the signs of progression, particularly for lesions that are premalignant.
2. Emphasize to the patient the importance of using sunscreens and avoiding overexposure or prolonged exposure to the sun.
3. Describe benign lesions to the patient to allay any fears.
4. Instruct the patient in the use of topical medications as indicated.

Skin cancer is the most common malignancy found in humans. An estimated 600,000 cases are discovered each year. Most involve the highly curable basal cell and squamous cell carcinomas. Malignant melanoma, the most serious skin cancer, is diagnosed in about 32,000 people annually, and the incidence is increasing by 4% per year. The increasing incidence of all types of skin cancer is believed to arise from a widespread change in life-style, with greater exposure of successive generations to sunlight—specifically, ultraviolet radiation.

Other, less common but clinically significant skin cancers include Bowen's disease (squamous cell carcinoma in situ), Kaposi's sarcoma, lymphangiosarcoma, dermatofibrosarcoma protuberans, leiomyosarcoma, and mycosis fungoides.

Basal Cell and Squamous Cell Carcinomas

EPIDEMIOLOGY

Basal cell and squamous cell cancers are more common among people with lightly pigmented skin and those at latitudes near the equator. Basal cell carcinoma is more common in men than in women and occurs more often in people over 40 years of age. Squamous cell carcinoma also is more common in men, and the average age of onset is 60 years. Other risk factors are excessive exposure to the sun and occupational exposure to coal, tar, pitch, creosote, arsenic compounds, and radium.

The sections on skin cancers are reprinted with the kind permission of Anne E. Belcher, Ph.D., R.N., author of *Cancer Nursing*.

Blacks, because of their darker pigmentation, are at low risk of developing these skin cancers.

Prevention and detection focus on decreasing exposure to the sun and finding the cancer early through skin self-assessment (see Patient Teaching Guide.) Simply protecting the cutaneous surfaces of the skin from excessive exposure to the sun would significantly reduce the current high incidence of skin cancer. General guidelines for such protection are outlined in the box on page 121.

GUIDELINES FOR PROTECTING THE SKIN AGAINST EXCESSIVE EXPOSURE TO THE SUN

- Avoid intense sunlight between 10 AM and 3 PM, when ultraviolet rays are the strongest.
- Plan such outdoor activities as walking, gardening, and other hobbies for early morning or late afternoon.
- Wear protective clothing such as hats and long-sleeved shirts.
- Use a sunscreen with a sun protection factor (SPF) of 15 or higher. The sunscreen should be applied 15 to 30 minutes before going out into the sunlight and every 2 to 3 hours during exposure (it may need to be applied more often because of heat, humidity, and sweating). Sunscreen should be applied liberally to the head and neck, with special attention to the nose, rims of the ears, cheeks, and forehead.

PATHOPHYSIOLOGY

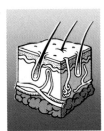

A **basal cell carcinoma** often appears as a single, small, firm, dome-shaped, flesh-colored nodule with raised edges and pearly white borders. Small, red, focal lesions (telangiectatic vessels) are often prominent and can be seen through the thin epidermis. The lesion may resemble a pimple that has not healed, with an ulcerated, bleeding center. The most common form, noduloulcerative cancer, frequently occurs on the face, especially on the cheeks, forehead, eyelids, nasolabial folds, and rims of the ears. Invasion usually is local, although metastatic disease does occur in rare cases. Left untreated, the tumor will invade such vital structures as blood vessels, lymph nodes, nerve sheaths, cartilage, bone, lungs, and the dura mater. The histologic appearance of the tumor is that of small, undifferentiated basal cells with minimum nuclear atypia. Recurrence indicates that initial treatment did not completely eradicate the tumor; however, 90% to 95% of patients are considered cured after surgery or radiation therapy.

A **squamous cell carcinoma** is a scaly, slightly elevated lesion with or without a cutaneous horn. This tumor frequently occurs on the hands and forearms, as well as on the head and neck (especially the ears, lower lip, scalp, and upper face). It is found most often in sun-damaged skin previously affected by actinic keratoses, which are erythematous, scaly lesions found especially on the face, shoulders, and dorsa of the hands. With complete tumor eradication, the prognosis is excellent. Tumors more difficult to treat are those arising in an old, unstable thermal burn scar (Marjolin's ulcer); a chronically ulcerated area at the site of a chronic sinus tract (such as that caused by osteomyelitis); or a site of previous radiation damage. Squamous cell carcinoma can metastasize, with 2% to 3% of tumors spreading to regional lymph nodes or to the lungs. Primary tumors of the lip metastasize at a rate greater than 10%. The cure rate for this type of cancer is 75% to 80% when it is treated with surgery or radiation therapy.

SIGNS AND SYMPTOMS

The clinical characteristics of superficial basal cell cancer include barely elevated, moderately firm plaques, usually with crusted and erythematous centers and raised, threadlike, pearly borders. Noduloulcerative basal cell cancer is characterized by moderately firm, elevated lesions with umbilicated, ulcerated centers and raised, waxy or pearly borders.

The appearance of squamous cell carcinoma varies. It may look like an elevated nodular mass; a punched-out, ulcerated lesion; or a fungating mass. Unlike basal cell carcinomas, these lesions are opaque.

SURGERY

Excisional surgery is the treatment of choice in 90% of basal cell cancers, including large tumors or those with poorly defined margins on the cheeks, forehead, trunk, and legs. Along with the lesion, a 3 mm margin is removed. Excision may also be indicated when metastatic spread is present. With squamous cell carcinoma, the margin should be slightly larger. It is also important to examine the regional lymph nodes in individuals with evidence of nodal involvement because of the greater likelihood of metastases with this cancer. When immediate coverage of the surgical wound is required, a free full-thickness skin graft is used.

Cryosurgery (the destruction of tissue by freezing) is used only in small-to-large nodular and superficial basal cell carcinomas. Electrodesiccation and curettage (the application of heat to destroy cancerous tissue) is used with small-to-medium nodular and superficial basal cell carcinomas with well-defined margins. This procedure may be performed using electrocautery or a carbon dioxide laser.

Mohs micrographic surgery is the removal of the tumor layer by layer until all margins are free of tumor, as verified by microscopic examination. This is the treatment of choice in recurrent basal cell lesions or those without well-defined margins. This procedure is also indicated when the basal cell carcinoma occurs in a cosmetic or functional area such as the eyelid or nose.

COMPLICATIONS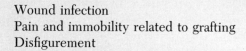

Wound infection
Pain and immobility related to grafting
Disfigurement

Preoperative Care

In addition to the usual preparation for surgery, the patient must be informed and reassured about the healing phases of the surgical wound and the plans for cosmetic surgery, such as grafting or later reconstruction.

Postoperative Care

Postoperative care focuses on keeping the surgical wound clean while observing for signs and symptoms of infection. If skin grafting is required, the nurse must help the patient keep the grafted area immobile to prevent stress on the edges of the wound. The graft site must also be kept clean and free of clots. Patients often have pain at the donor site and may need analgesics.

Disfigurement, real or perceived, requires reassurance and planning for reconstructive surgery when possible. Patients often find comfort in speaking with a plastic surgeon or a specialist in nonsurgical reconstructive procedures, such as individually prepared makeup and clothing.

RADIATION THERAPY

External beam therapy may be the treatment of choice for elderly or debilitated individuals who cannot tolerate surgery. One of the benefits of radiation therapy is tissue conservation, especially when treating lesions on the nose, eyelid, or lips. Extensive tumors may require a combination of preoperative and postoperative radiation, and surgery. Treatment failures, which usually are seen within 1 year of primary intervention, are best treated by surgery, since the skin and subcutaneous tissues will be poorly vascularized as a result of the earlier radiation therapy.

CHEMOTHERAPY

Topical 5-FU is recommended for treating premalignant actinic keratosis. Systemic retinoids have produced response rates greater than 70% in individuals with advanced squamous cell carcinoma; topical and systemic retinoids have shown some activity against basal cell carcinoma. 5-FU may be used in nevoid basal cell carcinoma syndrome but is contraindicated in other types, because it destroys the surface tumor without affecting deeper malignant cells.

Biologic response modifiers, especially interferon-alpha (IFN-α), have produced a response rate as high as 75% in recurrent or advanced local, regional, or metastatic basal cell carcinoma.

NURSING CARE

See pages 126 and 127.

DIAGNOSTIC STUDIES AND FINDINGS

Diagnostic Test	Findings
Punch, incisional, or total excisional biopsy	Malignant cells

MEDICAL MANAGEMENT

SURGERY

Excisional surgery

Cryosurgery

Electrodesiccation and curettage

Mohs micrographic surgery

RADIATION THERAPY

External beam radiation

CHEMOTHERAPY

Topical 5-fluorouracil (5-FU)

Biologic response modifiers

Malignant melanoma

Malignant melanoma is a more serious problem than other skin cancers, because it can spread quickly and insidiously, thus becoming life threatening at an earlier stage of development.

EPIDEMIOLOGY

Malignant melanoma is much more common in whites. When it does occur in dark-skinned people, the most common sites are the palms, soles, nail beds, fingers, toes, and mucous membranes. Melanoma may occur in individuals in their teens, twenties, and thirties, although the highest incidence is in those over 60 years of age. The incidence is equal in men and women; the upper back is the most common site in men, whereas the back and lower extremities are the most common sites in women.

Exposure to the sun and geographic latitude are important environmental factors. The risk of melanoma is increased for fair-skinned individuals who have intense, intermittent exposure to the sun, especially during childhood and adolescence. Countries with areas of high solar exposure (i.e., those close to the equator) have the highest incidence of melanoma.

People who burn easily and do not tan well are at greater risk of developing melanoma, as are those with intermittent heavy sun exposure. A personal or family history of dysplastic nevus syndrome, congenital nevi, or melanoma also increases the risk.

The key to diagnosing malignant melanoma is early detection. Monthly skin self-examination is essential, especially for those at high risk (see Patient Teaching Guide). The early warning signs of melanoma are identified in the acronym ABCD (see box on p. 124).

The key prognostic factor in malignant melanoma is the thickness of the lesion. Individuals with lesions less than 0.76 mm thick have a survival rate nearing 100%, whereas those with lesions 3 mm thick or thicker have survival rates of less than 50%.

Even though more people are using more effective sunscreens, the incidence of melanoma will continue to

---

ABCD RULE FOR EARLY DETECTION OF MELANOMA

A = Asymmetry

Most true moles tend to be symmetric. Melanomas tend to be asymmetric (one half does not match the other).

B = Border

Most true moles have a clear-cut border. Melanomas tend to have a notched, scalloped, or indistinct border.

C = Color

True moles may be dark or light, but they usually are uniform in color. Early melanomas have an uneven or variegated color (may range from various hues of tan and brown to black, with red and white intermingled).

D = Diameter

Once they have the A, B, and C characteristics, most melanomas are larger than 6 mm in diameter. Moles tend to be smaller. A sudden or progressive increase in the size of a mole should be reported.

---

rise in the years ahead, because there is a delay of 10 to 20 years from the time damage is inflicted by ultraviolet radiation until the cancer appears.

PATHOPHYSIOLOGY

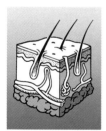 Malignant melanomas arise from three distinct types of moles, or nevi: common acquired nevi, dysplastic nevi, and congenital melanocytic nevi. The most common pigmented lesion is the common acquired nevus, which is not present at birth. Nevus production begins in childhood and tapers off at about 35 to 40 years of age. Most adults have about 20 to 40 nevi on their bodies. Common acquired nevi usually are small and uniform in color, surface, symmetry, and regularity of borders. The risk of this type of nevus developing into a melanoma is small.

Dysplastic nevi are considered precursors of melanoma, as well as markers of those at risk for melanoma. Dysplastic nevus syndrome usually becomes apparent during young adulthood, with the individual having more than 100 nevi on the body. Dysplastic nevi are larger than common acquired nevi and have irregular borders and variegated colors. They can occur anywhere on the body but are found more often on the trunk, back, breasts, buttocks, genitals, and scalp. Those with dysplastic nevi who have two or more first-degree relatives with melanoma have almost a 100% chance of developing melanoma, whereas people with sporadic dysplastic nevus syndrome have a 5% to 25% greater risk of developing melanoma than does the general population.

Congenital melanocytic nevi are raised, dark brown to black, oval or round macules that may have coarse hairs. They are present at birth and usually are small (under 1.5 cm) or medium-sized (1.5 to 19.9 cm). People with congenital nevi larger than 3 to 5 cm are thought to be at greatest risk for developing melanoma, although those with small and medium-sized nevi may have a risk as high as 22 times that of the general population.

The four distinct forms of malignant melanoma, in order of decreasing incidence, are:

Superficial spreading melanoma (70%), which occurs anywhere on the body surface. The lesion has a haphazard combination of colors and an irregular shape. It occurs more often in women 40 to 50 years of age. Common sites are the lower extremities and back.

Nodular melanoma (15%), which also occurs anywhere on the body surface. It occurs twice as often in men 50 to 60 years of age. Common sites are the head, neck, and trunk.

Lentigo maligna melanoma (5% to 10%), which occurs on exposed surfaces, especially the face, lower legs, and hands. It usually undergoes many color changes.

Acral lentiginous melanoma (less than 10%), which tends to occur on the palms, soles, nail beds, fingers, toes, and mucous membranes. It is the most common type of melanoma in blacks, Orientals, and Hispanics.

Malignant melanoma may spread to any organ or remote viscera, although common sites are the skin (intracutaneous or subcutaneous metastasis), bones, brain, liver, and lungs.

All melanomas except the nodular type have an initial radial growth phase (spreading outward from a common center) that may last longer than 10 years, during which time the melanoma cells remain confined to the epidermis. The tumor expands horizontally with only a slight increase in depth. During the vertical phase, der-

---

mal penetration occurs, and the melanoma cells invade the dermis and subcutaneous tissue. The tumor may then metastasize by vascular or lymphatic spread, with rapid movement of melanoma cells to other parts of the body. This accounts for the high mortality rate of malignant melanoma. When these tumors progress into the dermis or subcutaneous fat, "leaking" pigment or "satellite" nodules may appear around the periphery. Nodular malignant melanomas usually are convex and are palpable because of the tumor's growth elevation above the level of the epidermis.

SIGNS AND SYMPTOMS

The signs of melanoma include any unusual skin condition: scaliness, oozing, and/or bleeding of a nevus or other pigmented lesion; spread of the pigment beyond the normal border; a change in sensation, itchiness, tenderness, or pain; and development of a new nodule (see the box at left).

SURGERY

Wide excision of the primary lesion is the treatment of choice. The surgeon makes an excision of at least 2 cm around a lesion less than 1.5 mm thick; for lesions thicker than 1.5 mm, the margin of 5 cm includes the underlying fascia. Surgery may also be used for palliation if metastatic disease is present.

Regional lymph node dissection is somewhat controversial, with some surgeons recommending the procedure only if there is a significant possibility of node involvement without evidence of metastatic disease. If this exploration is done, postoperative lymphedema can be minimized by elevating the limb above the level of the heart (see the section on basal cell and squamous cell carcinomas for other aspects of preparation and postoperative care).

RADIATION THERAPY

Because melanoma tends to be radioresistant, radiation therapy is not recommended as primary treatment. It is useful for alleviating the signs and symptoms of metastatic disease to the bones, brain, and gastrointestinal tract.

CHEMOTHERAPY

Drugs with some value against melanoma are dacarbazine, nitrosoureas, cisplatin, and methotrexate. Hyperthermic regional perfusions may be used to administer such drugs so that large doses can be delivered to the extremity affected by the malignant melanoma with minimum systemic toxicity. This procedure often is combined with wide local excision and regional lymph node dissection.

Biologic response modifiers such as interferon and interleukin are being investigated for their therapeutic value. Hormonal therapy with agents such as tamoxifen and diethylstilbestrol is also under study.

DIAGNOSTIC STUDIES AND FINDINGS

Diagnostic Test	Findings
Excisional biopsy and measurement of maximum thickness of tumor	Malignant cells

---

MEDICAL MANAGEMENT

SURGERY

Wide excision

Regional lymph node dissection

RADIATION THERAPY

External beam radiation

CHEMOTHERAPY

Dacarbazine (DTIC), nitrosoureas (BCNU), cisplatin, and methotrexate

Biologic response modifiers: Interferon, interleukin

Hormonal therapy: Tamoxifen, diethylstilbestrol (DES)

---

1   ASSESS

ASSESSMENT	OBSERVATIONS
Skin	Scaliness, oozing, and/or bleeding of a nevus or other pigmented lesion; spread of pigment beyond normal border; change in sensation, itchiness, tenderness, or pain
Psychosocial	Fear

2   DIAGNOSE

NURSING DIAGNOSIS	SUBJECTIVE FINDINGS	OBJECTIVE FINDINGS
Impaired skin integrity related to presence of lesion	Complains of change in sensation, itchiness, tenderness, or pain	Scaliness, oozing, or bleeding; spread of pigment beyond normal border
Fear related to cancer, its treatment, and prognosis	Expresses fear of disease, treatment, and possibility of disfigurement and death	Appears sad, withdrawn, angry, and depressed
Knowledge deficit	Relates lack of knowledge regarding diagnosis	Unable to verbalize pertinent information about diagnosis, treatment, or outcomes

3 PLAN

Patient goals

1. Patient's skin will be free of infection or ulceration.
2. Patient will be less fearful about the diagnosis, treatment, and prognosis.

4 IMPLEMENT

NURSING DIAGNOSIS	NURSING INTERVENTIONS	RATIONALE
Impaired skin integrity related to presence of lesion	Observe lesion or lesions for change in shape, size, and color and for bleeding.	To detect progressive disease.
Fear related to cancer, its treatment, and prognosis	Assess presence and quality of support system.	To determine need for other sources of support.
	Listen to and accept expression of anger, sadness, and helplessness.	To foster expression of strong emotions.
	Encourage patient to identify fears, obtain needed information, generate alternative solutions, and focus on actions to be taken.	To support coping and problem solving.
Knowledge deficit	See Patient Teaching.	

5 EVALUATE

PATIENT OUTCOME	DATA INDICATING THAT OUTCOME IS REACHED
Patient's skin has healed.	Skin integrity is maintained without evidence of infection or ulceration.
Patient shows progress in lessening fear.	Patient talks about diagnosis and treatment options and has realistic plans for reconstructive procedures.

PATIENT TEACHING

1. Explain to the patient the need for regular physical examinations and regular skin self-assessment (see Patient Teaching Guide, page 177).
2. Encourage the patient to protect her skin from the sun by using sunscreens and protective clothing and by limiting exposure.
3. Instruct the patient and family to notify the health care provider if there are changes in the skin or other signs and symptoms indicating recurrent or metastatic disease.

Cutaneous T-Cell Lymphoma

Cutaneous T-cell lymphoma (CTCL) is a category of lymphomatous neoplasia of helper/inducer T cells that have an affinity for the skin. It can progress to involve lymph nodes, peripheral blood, and viscera. Mycosis fungoides and Sézary syndrome are the most common manifestations of CTCL.

PATHOPHYSIOLOGY

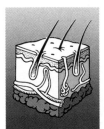

Mycosis fungoides (MF) is a rare T-cell lymphoma that originates in the skin. It generally first appears in the fifth or sixth decade of life. The course is unpredictable, depending on the presentation. Three distinct presentations have been identified—patch, plaque, and tumor. Tumor presentation has the worst prognosis, with a survival period of 3 years or less.

The *patch phase* often may be misdiagnosed as psoriasis or eczema because of its clinical presentation. Clinically it manifests as an erythematous, scaly, eczematous-like eruption, or as an atrophic, mottled, telangiectatic eruption that is diagnosed as parapsoriasis or poikiloderma vasculare atrophicans. Persistent, nonspecific, flat, erythematous areas that remain fixed are typical of MF, as are the sharply demarcated margins. This phase, which is called the premycotic phase, may persist for months or years. Cutaneous lesions of MF do not respond to topical corticosteroids, as do the lesions of eczema or atopic dermatitis. Poor response to steroids should lead to further investigation of the diagnosis.

Poikiloderma vasculare atrophicans appears on the abdomen, buttock, and thigh. It manifests as telangiectasia, mottled pigmentation, and fine wrinkling and atrophy ("cigarette paper" skin).

The *plaque stage* generally is the second phase in the evolution of the disease process. Clinically lesions manifest as dusky red to brown, sometimes scaly, elevated areas of skin. Plaques may appear as round, oval, arciform, or serpiginous, involving isolated areas or generalized. Central clearing may be seen on occasion. Intense pruritus is a characteristic sign of this phase. The plaque stage may persist for an indefinite period, with some regression, no change, or evolution into nodules and tumors.

Presentation of tumor has a very poor prognosis. The tumors may develop from preexisting plaques or from uninvolved skin. Pruritus may decrease with the appearance of tumors. Tumors and plaques may necrose and develop central ulceration. Lymphadenopathy is detectable, and with visceral involvement, deep lymphadenopathy develops. Visceral metastasis is seen in the spleen, lungs, or gastrointestinal tract.

Sézary syndrome has been called the leukemic form of MF. It consists of erythroderma, leukemia, and large peripheral lymphadenopathy. The cause of this syndrome is unknown. The clinical presentation (generalized erythema with scaling and thickening of the palms and soles) is similar to that of atopic dermatitis, psoriasis, or a severe drug reaction; therefore, misdiagnosis may occur. If the cutaneous lesions do not respond to conventional treatment or if the history is not consistent with the diagnosis, Sézary syndrome should be suspected.

COMPLICATIONS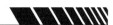

Metastasis to viscera
Secondary infection (with necrosis and ulceration of plaques or tumors)
Pruritus

DIAGNOSTIC STUDIES AND FINDINGS

Diagnostic Test	Findings
Skin biopsy	
MF	Perivascular lymphocytic infiltrate; thickens epidermis; infiltrates of lymphocytes, eosinophils, and plasma cells
Sézary syndrome	Resemble findings seen in MF
Hematologic studies	
Sézary syndrome	Sézary cells in peripheral blood
Lymph node biopsy	
Sézary syndrome	Monoclonal antibody and T-cell receptor testing in erythrodermics shows common T-cell receptors for visceral malignancy

MEDICAL MANAGEMENT

DRUG THERAPY

Corticosteroids: Used topically in stable, localized, nonplaque disease.

Chemotherapy: Topical nitrogen mustard, topical carmustine, psoralen with UVA (PUVA).

OTHER MEDICAL THERAPY

Radiation: Electron beam with or without chemotherapy used for tumors and erythroderma.

Extracorporeal photopheresis: Used for tumors and erythroderma.

GENERAL MANAGEMENT

Emollients and antipruritics are used for comfort.

1 ASSESS

ASSESSMENT	OBSERVATIONS
General health	In early stages, otherwise healthy
Skin and mucous membranes	
MF	Cutaneous lesions may resemble psoriasis, atopic dermatitis, or eczema; **patch phase:** red, scaly, eczematous eruption or atrophic, mottled, telangiectatic eruption; **plaque phase:** dusky red to brown, sometimes scaly, elevated areas; **tumor:** appears on reddened or normal skin, may necrose and ulcerate
Sézary syndrome	Generalized erythema with scaling and thickening of palms and soles
Hematologic	Normal except for identification of Sézary cells in peripheral blood
Neuropsychiatric	Body image disturbance; depression with associated poor prognosis in advanced stages of the disease

2 DIAGNOSE

NURSING DIAGNOSIS	SUBJECTIVE FINDINGS	OBJECTIVE FINDINGS
Impaired skin integrity related to presence of lesions	Reports itching, discomfort	Characteristic and diagnostic lesions

→ > >

NURSING DIAGNOSIS	SUBJECTIVE FINDINGS	OBJECTIVE FINDINGS
High risk for infection related to impaired skin integrity	Reports symptoms of secondary infection	Signs of cutaneous infection (redness, swelling, pus)
Body image disturbance related to presence of skin lesions	Reports difficulty with social interaction	Defining characteristics of body image disturbance
Ineffective individual coping related to prognosis	Verbalizes inability to cope	Unable to make decisions or to verbalize fears

3 PLAN

Patient goals

1. Skin integrity will be restored and maintained.
2. Patient will be free of secondary infection.

3. Patient will be able to accept body image and incorporate it into self-concept.
4. Patient will be able to develop adequate response to situation.

4 IMPLEMENT

NURSING DIAGNOSIS	NURSING INTERVENTIONS	RATIONALE
Impaired skin integrity related to presence of lesions	Assess skin, noting distribution of lesions and signs of their progression; apply medications as ordered.	To protect the skin's barrier function and to arrest further progression of disease involvement.
High risk for infection related to impaired skin integrity	Assess skin lesions for signs of infection; apply medications as ordered; teach meticulous handwashing and good hygiene to prevent secondary infection.	To aid early detection and intervention, and to promote healing and prevent secondary infection.
Body image disturbance related to presence of skin lesions	Assess patient's current perceptions and feelings; help patient express feelings about body appearance or fear of rejection by others.	To identify distortions and to assist patient with negative feelings and self-acceptance.
Ineffective individual coping related to prognosis	Assist patient in identifying needs and goals; encourage verbalization.	To enhance engagement in the coping process.

5 EVALUATE

PATIENT OUTCOME	DATA INDICATING THAT OUTCOME IS REACHED
Skin integrity has been restored and is maintained.	Skin lesions have been treated and existing lesions are healing.
No infection is evident.	Lesions are not secondarily infected; there is no redness, swelling, or pus in healing lesions.
Patient has positive body image.	Patient verbalizes acceptance of altered body image.
Patient exhibits positive coping.	Patient can verbalize feelings and has capacity to deal with feelings in a positive manner; patient engages in usual activities and relationships.

PATIENT TEACHING

1. Teach the patient about the disease and its progression.
2. Emphasize to the patient the importance of complying with the medical regimen prescribed.
3. Teach the patient how to apply topical nitrogen mustard properly.

CHAPTER 9

Hypersensitivity Reactions and Cutaneous Vasculitis

Cutaneous vasculature has unique properties that set it apart from other vasculature of the body. Thermoregulation is an important function of the skin, and the cutaneous vasculature is the primary anatomic structure that allows for temperature control. The body's thermoregulatory demands dominate the control of human cutaneous blood vessels.[68]

Many abnormalities may manifest in the skin, and the vasculature plays an important role in the various presentations. Abnormalities occur in a variety of diseases as either primary or secondary alterations. *Inflammation* is the term used to describe pharmacologic, physiologic, or immunologic processes that secondarily involve the vasculature. Erythema, erythema multiforme, Kaposi's sarcoma, stasis dermatitis, purpura, and hypersensitivity vasculitides are some of the manifestations seen in the skin.

Cutaneous vasculature develops from mesoderm components during the fourth month of fetal life. As blood flow is established with the organization of the pumping heart, the capillary network differentiates into arteries, veins, and capillaries. During the fifth month, arteries, arterioles, venules, and veins are organized. The transparent skin of the neonate is bright red because of this dense network of capillaries.

Vasculature is served by two types of major arteries, musculocutaneous arteries (supplying skin and muscle), and cutaneous arteries (supplying only the skin). Most changes in the vasculature develop over a long period, but changes may occur within a few days, as with psoriasis.

Nutritional and thermoregulatory functions are the two major functions of the cutaneous vasculature. Damage to the vasculature leads to reduced blood flow to tissue and a decrease in the delivery of nutrients, which eventually lead to tissue death and necrosis, as seen in pressure necrosis. To accomplish thermoregulation, the blood passes through shunts in various levels within the superficial dermis, which allows for optimum dissipation of heat.

Neural and hormonal factors mediate vasodilation and vasoconstriction of the vessels. Cutaneous blood vessels are extremely sensitive to circulating norepinephrine and epinephrine and extremes of temperature. In periods of circulatory stress, sympathetic vasoconstrictor innervation enables the vasculature to respond by shifting blood from the skin to other areas where it is required.

Erythema does not always indicate an increase in cutaneous blood flow. The redness is secondary to an increase in the visible mass of erythrocytes in the superficial cutaneous vasculature. Erythema occurs secondary to primary changes in the skin, to an increase in the superficial vascular capacitance, and/or to a change in the optical properties of the skin. When the skin is hot and arterial blood flow is brisk, the skin color usually is bright red. When the skin is cold and blood flow is sluggish, the dark, reduced hemoglobin combines with other cutaneous components to produce a bluish hue. When the cutaneous vasculature is constricted, the skin has a pale white appearance, which is caused by hormonal or pharmacologic agents that produce vasoconstriction or by local edema that constricts vessels.

Hypersensitivity Reactions

PATHOPHYSIOLOGY

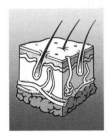

Erythema is a primitive, nonspecific cutaneous response to many noxious stimuli or diseases. It is considered part of the spectrum of response that includes urticaria, vasculitis, ischemia, and necrosis. Erythema may be localized or generalized and may manifest in such disorders as exfoliative erythroderma, psoriasis, dermatitis/eczema, febrile states, and topical corticosteroid atrophy. Generalized erythema causes the greatest concern because of the systemic effect this condition may have. With generalized erythema (i.e., exfoliative erythroderma), a substantial proportion of the cardiac output can be directed to the skin. This may lead to high-output cardiac failure and an increase in the basal metabolic rate; it also may leave the body unable to maintain a normal temperature because of thermoregulatory disturbance. A thorough, careful history and physical examination, as well as attention to distribution of the lesions, are of prime importance in the differential diagnosis of erythema.

Erythema multiforme (EM) is a relatively common, acute inflammatory disorder that often recurs. It is a self-limiting, episodic illness. The lesions erupt in less than a week and resolve over 1 to 2 weeks. The entire episode should last less than 4 weeks. However, healing may take up to 6 weeks in very severe cases. EM may be caused by one of several factors, such as infectious agents, drugs, connective tissue disease, physical irritants, x-ray therapy, pregnancy, skin diseases, and internal malignancy. In many cases no cause is found. The formation of immune complexes and their subsequent deposition in the cutaneous microvasculature have been indicated as the pathogenesis of EM.

Clinically, EM manifests with a characteristic lesion, inflammation with concentric zones of color. These lesions are commonly referred to as "bull's eye" (target) or "iris" lesions. A lesion begins as a round, erythematous papule and evolves into the characteristic lesion described above. Early in this process, the papule may be surrounded by an area of blanching and may resemble an insect bite. As the lesions evolve, the centers may become dusky or show necrosis. The central color may be opaque yellow, white, or gray, and accumulation of fluid leads to the formation of blisters, which break easily. Postinflammatory hyperpigmentation is not uncommon, but scarring from resolving lesions is. EM is classified into two categories, erythema multiforme minor (EM minor) and erythema multiforme major (EM major).

Erythema multiforme minor is the most common form of the disease. The lesions generally are distributed symmetrically and usually are found on the extremities, showing a predilection for the extensor surfaces. Sites of recent physical trauma (including sunburn) explain the isomorphic phenomenon and photodistribution seen in many cases. Superficial erosions may be seen on the mucosal surfaces and may precede, follow, or occur simultaneously with the skin involvement. Serious complications (e.g., involvement of organ systems other than the skin and mucosa) are rare in EM minor. Complications generally associated with EM minor include itching and burning of the skin, swelling and tenseness of the hands and feet, and pain with oral erosions, leading to difficulty maintaining food and fluid intake.[28]

A more severe form of the reactive process is *ery-*

Examples of erythema multiforme in white skin and black skin are shown in Color Plates 40 and 41 on p. xix.

thema multiforme major. Clinical manifestations include extensive erosions on two or more mucosal surfaces (generally the eyes and mouth), along with skin lesions. In very severe cases any mucosal surface may be involved. The complications associated with EM major are serious and may be systemic. They are fever, myalgia, prostration, damage to the eye (keratitis, conjunctival scarring, uveitis, permanent visual impairment), upper airway erosions, pneumonia, esophagitis, esophageal stricture, and hepatitis. Vesiculobullous erythema multiforme involving the mouth, eyes, and genitals is called *Stevens-Johnson syndrome.* This disorder, which occurs predominantly in children and young adults, is preceded by symptoms of upper respiratory infection. Cutaneous lesions develop suddenly in 1 to 14 days after prodrome. Prodromal symptoms include fever, headache, and sore throat. Mucous membrane lesions, including stomatitis and conjunctivitis, and pruritus occur 1 to 2 days before the onset of cutaneous lesions. Hemorrhagic crusting is characteristic of the lesions. Pulmonary involvement may be seen, evidenced by a harsh, hacking cough and patchy changes on the chest x-ray. The disease is self-limiting, and the prognosis is good if adequate supportive measures are taken.

TEN is illustrated in Color Plates 18 and 19 on p. xv. If the mucous membrane disease of Stevens-Johnson syndrome progresses to include confluent, cutaneous lesions, the result is the most severe form of EM major, *toxic epidermal necrolysis* (necrosis of extensive areas of skin). In toxic epidermal necrolysis (TEN), the patient may develop the complications associated with severe burns, electrolyte imbalance, and sepsis. EM major can be fatal if it evolves into toxic epidermal necrolysis. Death may ensue if the patient develops secondary complications such as overwhelming sepsis in denuded skin or the lungs.

Cutaneous features include a diffuse, hot erythema that becomes painful within a few hours. Nikolsky's sign (ready separation of the epidermal layers with only fingertip pressure) is positive in the erythematous skin and indicates that a life-threatening event is evolving.

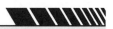

```
 ┌─────────────────────────────────┐
 │  DRUGS REPORTED TO CAUSE        │
 │  ERYTHEMA MULTIFORME MAJOR      │
 ├─────────────────────────────────┤
 │  Sulfonamides                   │
 │  Sulfonamide derivatives        │
 │  Phenylbutazone                 │
 │  Penicillins                    │
 └─────────────────────────────────┘
```

Early in the development of TEN, the mucosal surfaces show inflammation, blistering, and erosions. Purulent conjunctivitis is a constant feature. Respiratory failure is a complication that may evolve with involvement of the pulmonary mucosa. Septicemia and fluid-electrolyte imbalance also may evolve as TEN progresses.

Drugs are the primary cause of EM major and often cause extensive disease. The box above lists drugs that have been documented to lead to EM.

COMPLICATIONS

Stevens-Johnson syndrome
  Fever
  Decreased intake of food and fluids
  Blindness secondary to corneal ulcerations
  Pruritus
  Secondary infection
Toxic epidermal necrolysis
  Sepsis
  Decreased intake of food and fluids
  Chronic photophobia
  Chronic decreased visual acuity
  Blindness
  Bronchopneumonia
  Respiratory failure
  Fluid-electrolyte imbalance
  Leukopenia
  Renal involvement (hematuria, proteinuria)

DIAGNOSTIC STUDIES AND FINDINGS

Diagnostic Test	Findings
Skin biopsy	Granular IgG and C3 deposits in blood vessels
Complete blood count	Leukopenia—in TEN unknown cause; may be due to toxins from absorbed silver sulfadiazine or immune complexes
Urinalysis	Hematuria, proteinuria seen in TEN with renal involvement
Serum creatinine	May be elevated

MEDICAL MANAGEMENT

DRUG THERAPY

Systemic corticosteroids: Used in Stevens-Johnson syndrome for 1 week or until no new lesions are seen; used in the early phase of TEN, but withdrawn during healing phase to minimize infections and complications. Overall, use of systemic corticosteroids in both Stevens-Johnson syndrome and TEN remains controversial.

Antihistamines: Used to control pruritus in Stevens-Johnson syndrome.

Topical corticosteroids: Used on papules and plaques; should never be applied to eroded areas.

Oral lidocaine hydrochloride (viscous Xylocaine): Frequent rinsing may relieve symptoms caused by oral lesions.

Systemic antibiotics: Based on causative organism, to treat secondary infections.

OTHER MEDICAL MANAGEMENT

Burow's compresses: Cool compresses are applied to blisters and erosions of Stevens-Johnson syndrome.

Porcine xenografts: Prevent pain and provide temporary barrier function to decrease risk of infection; provide scaffolding for reepithelialization.

Plasmapheresis: Some studies have shown enhanced healing.

Hyperbaric oxygen: Some studies have shown enhanced healing.

GENERAL MANAGEMENT

Adequate fluid and food intake are maintained; airway is maintained (tracheostomy may be indicated); pain relief measures are used.

---

1 ASSESS

ASSESSMENT	OBSERVATIONS
Current health	Prodromal symptoms: mild EM (itching, fever, cutaneous lesions); more severe forms (malaise, fever, symptoms of upper respiratory infection [headache, sore throat], stomatitis, conjunctivitis, prostration, and pruritus)
Skin and mucous membranes	*EM minor:* Papular eruptions, target/iris lesions, coalescing to produce small plaques with rim of edema (lesions are symmetric; superficial erosions may be seen on mucosal surfaces) *EM major:* Extensive erosions on two or more mucosal surfaces (including the eyes); skin lesions as in EM minor that become bullous; erythema involving large areas of skin surface
Neuropsychiatric	Body image disturbance; depression may be evident with life-threatening disease

→ > >

ASSESSMENT	OBSERVATIONS
Hematologic	Leukopenia possible in TEN; elevated WBC in secondary infection
Cardiovascular	High-output cardiac failure in TEN
Pulmonary	Bronchopneumonia possible in patients with TEN; respiratory failure secondary to mucus retention and sloughing of tracheobronchial mucosa
Renal	Hematuria, proteinuria, elevated serum creatinine

2 DIAGNOSE

NURSING DIAGNOSIS	SUBJECTIVE FINDINGS	OBJECTIVE FINDINGS
Impaired skin integrity related to hypersensitivity reaction and presence of lesions	Reports finding lesions; pruritus and burning; difficulty eating and drinking	Target or iris lesions; mucosal surfaces may show erosions
Body image disturbance related to presence of lesions	Reports difficulty accepting altered appearance	Has difficulty talking about feelings about appearance
Ineffective thermoregulation related to diffuse erythema in TEN	Reports chills and difficulty staying comfortable	Fluctuations in body temperature evident
Altered oral mucous membranes related to presence of lesions	Reports inability to tolerate food and liquids due to discomfort from oral lesions	Erosions; patient may be dehydrated
Pain related to presence of lesions	Complains of pain	Exhibits guard behavior
Altered vision related to involvement of eyes	Reports photophobia, decreased visual acuity	Signs of involvement in mucous membranes

3 PLAN

Patient goals

1. Skin's integrity and barrier function will be restored.
2. Patient will accept body image change as a temporary change and exhibit adequate coping mechanisms.
3. Patient will maintain normal body temperature.
4. Patient will have an intact oral mucosa and increased fluid and food intake.
5. Patient's pain will be relieved.
6. Patient's vision will be protected.

4 IMPLEMENT

NURSING DIAGNOSIS	NURSING INTERVENTIONS	RATIONALE
Impaired skin integrity related to hypersensitivity reaction and presence of lesions	Apply wet dressings and topical medications.	To provide temporary barrier and give some relief from discomfort.
Body image disturbance related to presence of lesions	Assess patient's current perceptions and feelings about disease.	To identify distortions and give direction toward positive outcome.
Ineffective thermoregulation related to diffuse erythema in TEN	Adjust environmental temperature; adjust clothing and covers as needed; use warm, wet wraps to help decrease erythema and conserve body heat; monitor serum pH and glucose.	To provide comfort; decreased pH level indicates presence of acidosis due to increased oxygen demands to generate heat; decreased blood glucose is due to increased use of carbohydrate stores to generate heat.
Altered oral mucous membranes related to presence of lesions	Establish an oral care regimen.	To provide comfort and enhance oral intake.
Pain related to presence of lesions	Assess degree of pain, and administer appropriate medication.	To assess adequacy of pain medication in providing relief.
Altered vision related to involvement of eyes	Apply medications as ordered; assess condition of lesions and reactions to light.	To protect the eyes from infection and to preserve the integrity of the mucous membranes.

5 EVALUATE

PATIENT OUTCOME	DATA INDICATING THAT OUTCOME IS REACHED
Skin's integrity and barrier function have been restored.	Lesions have healed; skin's barrier function has been restored.
Patient shows a positive body image.	Patient expresses positive feelings and acceptance of disease process.
Patient's body temperature is normal.	Body temperature remains normal with no fluctuations; patient reports being comfortable.
Patient's oral mucosa has healed.	Oral lesions are no longer evident; oral intake has improved.
Patient has achieved maximum comfort.	Pain medication requirements have decreased.

PATIENT OUTCOME	DATA INDICATING THAT OUTCOME IS REACHED
Patient's vision is normal.	Patient no longer complains of photophobia; ophthalmologic examination reveals normal vision.

PATIENT TEACHING

1. Teach the patient about the evolution of the disease and the possible complications.
2. Explain the treatment regimen.
3. Explain the need for adequate intake of food and fluids.
4. Explain the need for good oral hygiene.

Cutaneous Vasculitis

Inflammation of the vessel wall, which is called *vasculitis* or *angiitis*, may be set off by deposition of immune complexes. Cutaneous vasculitic diseases are classified by the type of inflammatory cell seen within the vessel wall (i.e., neutrophils, lymphocytes, or histiocytes) and by the size and type of blood vessel involved. The small vessel diseases affect arterioles, capillaries, or venules; these are leukocytoclastic vasculitis and Henoch-Schönlein purpura (HSP). The large vessel diseases are polyarteritis nodosa, cutaneous periarteritis nodosa, and allergic granulomatosis. Vasculitic diseases may be confined to the skin or may involve other organs.

PATHOPHYSIOLOGY

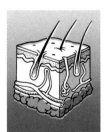 **Small vessel vasculitis** (necrotizing vasculitis) is most commonly seen in the skin and rarely affects other organ systems. In the rare cases in which another organ system is involved, it is most commonly the kidney. Signs of vasculitis include urticaria, palpable purpura, nodules, bullae, and possibly ulcers. The urticaria is characterized by minimal inflammation and necrosis of the vessel. Palpable purpura is a nonblanchable, red, slightly elevated lesion caused by exudation and hemorrhage from damaged vessels. If the vessel wall inflammation and necrosis are severe, nodules, bullae, or ulcers may manifest. Deposition of immune complexes

secondary to hypersensitivity to chemicals, drugs, microorganisms, and endogenous antigens is seen in vasculitis. An inflammatory response and release of leukocytes are initiated in the walls of the small vessels, leading to release of lysosomal enzymes, damage to the vessel walls, and extravasation of erythrocytes.[25]

Leukocytoclastic vasculitis is the most common type of small vessel vasculitis. It generally is limited to the skin, but it may involve other organs. Histologically, the disease is characterized by fibroid necrosis of small dermal vessels, with associated leukocytoclasis, swelling of endothelial cells, and extravasation of red blood cells. Fever, malaise, myalgia, and joint pain are prodromal symptoms. The lesions are asymptomatic and initially appear as localized areas of cutaneous hemorrhage. As the lesions progress, they become palpable (palpable purpura) because of the leakage of blood from the damaged vessels. The lesions may coalesce, leading to formation of nodular or urticarial lesions. If inflammation becomes severe, necrosis may occur and ulceration may result. The lower extremities most commonly are affected, although any dependent area of the body can be affected. Pruritus may accompany the small lesions; the larger purpura, nodules, ulcers, and bullae may be painful. The lesions can last from 1 to 4 weeks.

Viral infection or a drug reaction can lead to vasculitis. Recurrent vasculitis is most commonly due to systemic disease (e.g., systemic lupus erythematosus or rheumatoid arthritis). Systemic conditions associated with leukocytoclastic vasculitis are listed in Table 9-1.

Table 9-1

ORGAN SYSTEMS AFFECTED BY SYSTEMIC LEUKOCYTOCLASTIC VASCULITIS

Organ system	Manifestations
Kidneys	Microscopic hematuria and proteinuria
Nervous system	Peripheral neuropathy, hypoesthesia or paresthesia
Gastrointestinal tract	Abdominal pain, nausea, vomiting, diarrhea, melena
Lungs	Pulmonary vasculitis, cough, shortness of breath, hemoptysis
Joints	Pain, erythema
Heart	Myocardial angiitis, arrhythmias, congestive heart failure

The box at right lists possible causes of leukocytoclastic vasculitis.

Anaphylactoid purpura, known as **Henoch-Schön-lein purpura (HSP)**, is a cutaneous manifestation seen in children. It is a benign, self-limiting disease. The characteristic lesions, palpable purpura, commonly are found on the legs and buttocks, although they also may be seen on the ears, face, and arms. Systemic findings include abdominal pain, gastrointestinal bleeding, arthralgia, and hematuria. The disease is thought to be caused by entrapment of IgA-containing immune complexes in blood vessel walls in the skin, kidneys, and gastrointestinal tract. These immune complexes are thought to be released in response to an infectious process or drugs.[25]

Polyarteritis nodosa occurs in adults (generally those over 50 years of age) and is relatively rare. Chronic infection, drugs, or acute streptococcal infection may be the cause. The arteries are involved, leading to formation and possible rupture of aneurysms. Segmental lesions may occur, leading to occlusion and distal infarction. Cutaneously, the disease is manifested by recurring, subcutaneous nodules that appear in groups along the course of an artery, generally on the lower leg. The lesions may necrose, leaving a small, punched-out ulceration on the nodule. Two other forms of polyarteritis nodosa may be seen, cutaneous periarteritis nodosa and allergic granulomatosis. Cutaneous periarteritis nodosa is limited to the skin and has no systemic manifestations. The clinical lesions form a red, blanchable, livedo pattern on the legs that may develop into the recognizable nodules of periarteritis. Asthma, peripheral eosinophilia, and fever characterize allergic granulomatosis. The systemic symptoms and cutaneous signs are the same as those seen in polyarteritis nodosa.

POSSIBLE CAUSES OF LEUKOCYTOCLASTIC VASCULITIS

Drugs

Penicillins, thiazides, aspirin, phenothiazines, sulfonamides, iodides

Infections

Streptococcal upper respiratory infection (URI); *Escherichia coli* urinary tract infection (UTI)

Connective tissue disease

Malignant neoplasms

Other systemic illnesses

COMPLICATIONS

Systemic

Microscopic hematuria	Diarrhea
Proteinuria	Melena
Peripheral neuropathy	Pulmonary vasculitis
Hypoesthesia	Hemoptysis
Paresthesia	Joint pain
Abdominal pain	Myocardial angiitis
Nausea	Arrhythmias
Vomiting	Congestive heart failure

DIAGNOSTIC STUDIES AND FINDINGS

Diagnostic Test	Findings
Skin biopsy	Infiltrate of mononuclear cells and neutrophils; fibrinoid necrosis of blood vessel walls
Throat culture	Streptococcal infection
Erythrocyte sedimentation rate	Elevated
Serum complement	May be depressed
Angiography	Aneurysmal dilation
Renal biopsy	*Large vessel disease:* Focal segmental necrotizing glomerulitis; *Henoch-Schönlein purpura:* minimal involvement to diffuse mesangial proliferation
Other blood tests	No diagnostic relevance in Henoch-Schönlein purpura

MEDICAL MANAGEMENT

DRUG THERAPY

Systemic corticosteroids: Short courses of prednisone.

Colchicine: Effective in chronic cutaneous leukocytoclastic vasculitis.

Dapsone: Used with only cutaneous involvement.

Azathioprine: Used for recalcitrant disease.

Cyclophosphamide: Used with multiple organ involvement.

Plasmapheresis: Used in severe manifestations of Henoch-Schönlein purpura to remove IgA immune complexes.

OTHER MEDICAL MANAGEMENT

Identify and remove offending antigen.

GENERAL MANAGEMENT

Supportive measures to relieve pruritus and pain.

1 ASSESS

ASSESSMENT	OBSERVATIONS
Current health	May appear healthy; may exhibit symptoms of congestive heart failure, nephritis, UTI, or URI
Skin and mucous membranes	Palpable purpura, urticaria, nodules, bullae, ulceration, and ecchymoses, generally on lower extremities

ASSESSMENT	OBSERVATIONS
Musculoskeletal	Joint pain: arthralgia involving ankles, knees, and dorsum of hands and feet
Gastrointestinal	Colicky abdominal pain, vomiting, gastrointestinal bleeding, diarrhea
Hematologic	Elevated erythrocyte sedimentation rate, low complement levels
Cardiovascular	Myocardial angiitis, arrhythmias, congestive heart failure
Pulmonary	Nodular or diffuse infiltrates on x-ray, cough, shortness of breath, hemoptysis
Renal	Microscopic hematuria, proteinuria
Nervous system	Peripheral neuropathy, hypoesthesia or paresthesia

2 DIAGNOSE

NURSING DIAGNOSIS	SUBJECTIVE FINDINGS	OBJECTIVE FINDINGS
Impaired skin integrity related to presence of lesions	Reports finding skin lesions	Palpable purpura, nodules, ecchymoses, ulcers; may have bullae
Pain related to presence of lesions; systemic involvement	Reports discomfort	Guarding behavior

3 PLAN

Patient goals
1. Skin's integrity and barrier function will be restored.   2. Patient's pain will be relieved.

4 IMPLEMENT

NURSING DIAGNOSIS	NURSING INTERVENTIONS	RATIONALE
Impaired skin integrity related to presence of lesions	Assess skin; keep lesions clean, and monitor for signs of infection.	To facilitate early intervention if lesions progress to ulceration; to detect infection or secondary infection.
Pain related to presence of lesions; systemic involvement	Administer drugs as needed for pain; monitor reaction to pain medication.	To relieve pain and adjust medication as required.

→ › ›

5 EVALUATE

PATIENT OUTCOME	DATA INDICATING THAT OUTCOME IS REACHED
Skin's integrity and barrier function have been restored.	Lesions have healed; barrier function is restored.
Patient has achieved maximum comfort.	Pain medication requirements have decreased.

PATIENT TEACHING

1. Teach the patient about the evolution of the disease and the possible complications.

2. Explain the treatment regimen.

CHAPTER 10

Acne and Rosacea

Acne is an inflammatory disorder of the pilosebaceous unit of the skin. It manifests with eruptions of papules or pustules, caused when oil delivered to the skin's surface meets with resistance. **Rosacea** (acne rosacea, or adult acne) is a fairly common inflammatory condition that affects the blood vessels in the central part of the face. It may resemble and be associated with acne, appearing as a rosy red pustular eruption without comedones.

PATHOPHYSIOLOGY

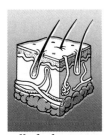 *Acne* originates in the sebaceous follicle and characteristically first occurs during adolescence with the onset of puberty, although it may be seen up to the seventh decade. The exact cause of acne is unknown, but it is believed to be caused by a complex of interrelated factors, called the pentagon of acne pathology (Figure 10-1). The five factors are genetic predisposition, androgens, abnormal intrafollicular keratinization, sebaceous follicles and sebum, and *Propionibacterium acnes.*

Acne occurs in all races but is more common among Caucasians. The onset most often occurs at puberty with the production of testosterone and the activation of the sebaceous glands. The severity of acne during adolescence varies; up to 30% of teenagers have acne severe enough to require medical treatment.

Sebaceous glands empty into hair follicles rather than directly onto the skin's surface. Any disruption in the epithelial lining of the follicle effectively blocks sebum from emptying normally. Sebum collects in the hair follicle, which is blocked by a proteinaceous plug. *P. acnes* (normal flora) exerts a lipolytic effect on the trapped sebum, causing the release of free fatty acids and other lipids. Free fatty acids have an inflammatory effect and become potential irritants, which when released into the dermis cause cysts to form. The box on page 145 lists the factors involved in the development of acne.

Factors such as stress, the environment, drugs, greasy cosmetics, and mechanical irritants may contribute to or aggravate acne. The areas most often affected are the face, chest, back, and shoulders, because sebaceous glands are most densely clustered in these areas. The severity of the condition can range from an occasional pimple or blackhead (open comedo) to the formation of large, painful cysts. Large abscesses may develop and if not treated may result in deep scarring or pock marks.

Acne produces a spectrum of clinical lesions. The primary lesion is the comedo, either open or closed (see terminology in the box on page 145). Open comedones rarely progress to more serious lesions, because they are more resistant to rupture and may be expressed intact with only minimal pressure. Closed

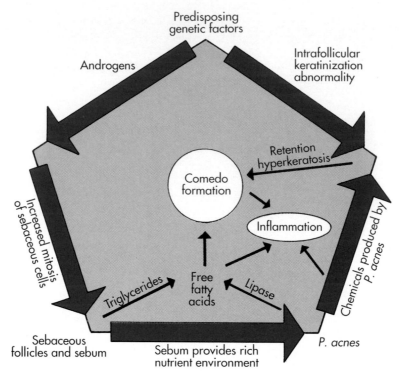

FIGURE 10-1
Pentagon of acne pathology. (From Laudano J et al: *Dermatology Nursing* 2(6):329, 1990.

CLASSIFICATIONS OF ACNE

Papulopustular

- Most common type—combination of comedones and inflammatory pustules or papules
- Severity determined by the quantity and type of lesions

Cystic

- Predominant lesion—"secondary comedones" due to multiple ruptures and reencapsulations
- Most severe form is acne conglobata
- Common sites of predilection—back, buttocks, chest
- Cysts, nodules, abscesses, and draining sinus tracts
- Severe inflammation
- Scarring

---

comedones are located deeper in the skin and are more prone to rupture, even with the slightest pressure. With rupture the contents are released into the dermis, resulting in inflammation, cyst formation, and possibly scarring. Intermediate lesions appear clinically as erythematous papules. In the spectrum of lesions they fall between noninflammatory comedones and inflamed pustules or cysts. Pustules develop purulent contents in response to inflammation. Even though these lesions contain purulent material and may look infected clinically, most often they are not secondarily infected. The contents of the pustule are leukocytes (response to inflammation) and proteolytic enzymes.

Cystic lesions are the most serious in the spectrum of acne lesions. Because they are located in the deeper structure of the skin (dermis), they can cause pain and may leave scars on healing. Extensive involvement with cystic lesions may cause systemic symptoms such as fever, malaise, and prostration. Acne is classified by the severity and type of lesions seen clinically (see the box at left).

Rosacea (adult acne or acne rosacea) is a disease that

can resemble and may be associated with acne. It primarily affects women over 30 years of age, but clinical manifestations are worse in men. It also may appear in the midteen years. The cause of the disorder is unknown. Rosacea must be distinguished from seborrheic dermatitis, contact dermatitis, lupus erythematosus, actinic damage, acne vulgaris, and perioral dermatitis.

Clinically, rosacea appears as erythema and dilated blood vessels (telangiectases), generally in the central part of the face. In the early phase the individual shows a pronounced tendency to flushing and blushing. This phase is followed by the appearance of small, inflammatory papules and pustules. Few or numerous lesions may be seen. Comedones do not develop unless rosacea is coexisting with acne vulgaris. The last phase of rosacea, more commonly seen in men, is the development of rhinophyma (pronounced enlargement of the nose). Rhinophyma is a direct result of the overgrowth of sebaceous tissue. Ocular disorders, including blepharitis, conjunctivitis, keratitis, and iritis, may occur. Numerous environmental factors, foods, drinks, chemicals, and topical preparations (see the box at lower right) have been proved to aggravate rosacea.

COMPLICATIONS

Complications of acne may include secondary infection, but they generally are due to side effects of medications used in treatment. With long-term use of tetracycline drugs various laboratory studies may be required to monitor for anemia or renal or hepatic problems. Isotretinoin may cause birth defects, headaches, fatigue, and joint aches and pains. Other complications are:

Impaired skin integrity related to lesions

Pain related to cystic lesions

Risk for secondary infection related to compromised integument

Altered body image secondary to acne lesions/scarring

Risk of adverse side effects from therapy

DIAGNOSTIC STUDIES AND FINDINGS

Acne and rosacea are diagnosed by direct observation of cutaneous manifestations. However, certain laboratory studies may be done before therapy is started (see Medical Management).

FACTORS INVOLVED IN THE DEVELOPMENT OF ACNE

Androgens

Testosterone (secreted after puberty) and dihydrotestosterone stimulate development of sebaceous glands and initiation of sebum production.

Intrafollicular keratinization abnormality

Defects in the keratinization of the epithelial lining of the pilosebaceous follicle block egress of sebum, leading to "plugging."

Propionibacterium acnes (part of skin's normal flora)

Exert lipolytic effect on stagnant sebum; release free fatty acids; cause inflammation when they escape from the pilosebaceous follicle into the dermis

---

TERMINOLOGY USED IN ACNE

Comedo (Comedones): basic lesion; two types—open (blackhead), closed (whitehead)

Erythematous Papules: intermediate lesions between noninflammatory comedones and purulent inflammation of pustules and cysts

Pustules (Pimples): inflamed lesions containing pus

Cysts: seen in the most severe cases; deeper lesions and with inflammation can cause pain and scarring; extensive involvement can lead to systemic symptoms (fever, malaise, and prostration)

AGGRAVATING FACTORS IN ACNE ROSACEA

Alcohol

Hot drinks of any kind

Spicy food

External irritants

Extremes of heat or cold

MEDICAL MANAGEMENT

Acne can be treated with systemic or topical drugs. However, because treatment is more effective in preventing new lesions than in clearing current ones, rapid improvement should not be expected. The goal of acne therapy is to interrupt the degeneration of the pilosebaceous unit by affecting one or more of the underlying causes of lesion formation. A stepwise approach to therapy should be taken, starting with the least potent therapy first. Each type of treatment should be given a sufficient trial before it is abandoned for newer, more potent therapy. Treatment must also be tailored to the location of the acne lesions. For example, lesions on the back and chest are more resistant than those on the face.

GENERAL MANAGEMENT

Patients are given a regimen that involves routine cleansing and instructions for applying topical medications. Instructions and warnings are given for administration of parenteral medications. Emotional support and encouragement are crucial to the treatment of acne in patients of any age.

SURGERY

Surgical treatment of acne involves incision and drainage of pustules and cysts to reduce the risk of scarring. Extraction of open or closed comedones removes the lesions but does nothing to prevent recurrence.

Other types of surgery, such as scar revision, scar excision, and dermabrasion (as well as collagen injections), are done to improve the patient's appearance after the acne has cleared.

DRUG THERAPY

Numerous medications, both topical and parenteral, are available for treating acne. Most of the topical drugs come in the form of gels, creams, and lotions. Topical preparations unblock the pilosebaceous units, thus removing the sebum. Benzoyl peroxide is the most commonly used topical medication. It acts as an antibacterial agent through the release of hydrogen peroxide and as a keratolytic producing desquamation; it may reduce the secretion of sebum and possibly the size of the sebaceous gland. The action of releasing hydrogen peroxide can reduce 84% of the aerobic bacteria and 98% of the anaerobic bacteria on the skin after 14 days of treatment. This also decreases the concentration of free fatty acids on the skin by 50% to 60%. The keratolytic effect helps reduce plugging of the pilosebaceous unit. Benzoyl peroxide preparations are most effective on mild acne, which consists primarily of comedones and few pustules.

Retinoic acid (tretinoin) increases cell turnover in the pilosebaceous unit. This leads to a decrease in the cohesion between keratinized cells, thus decreasing follicular plugging. Retinoic acid has been found beneficial in all forms of acne.

Many antibiotics are used to treat acne. The most useful are tetracycline, erythromycin, and clindamycin, because they reach therapeutic level in the pilosebaceous follicle. These preparations are available in topical forms, which have proved successful in treatment without causing the side effects commonly seen with the parenteral forms. Treatment with topical antibiotics may take longer than treatment with systemic forms, but the reduced risk of toxicity is worth the prolonged treatment course. Systemic antibiotics are used when the severity of the disease warrants. Tetracyclines are the most commonly used systemic drug.

Systemic steroids (prednisone) are used to treat acne, particularly the nodulocystic form, if the disorder proves resistant to conventional topical and systemic antibiotics. Steroids may be injected into the lesions of nodulocystic acne. Intralesional therapy supplements other forms of treatment and gives prompt relief from large painful cysts.

Other systemic drugs used to treat severe acne include oral contraceptives and oral retinoids (isotretinoin). Oral contraceptives and antiandrogens are effective in reducing the production of sebum in females who have not responded to other forms of therapy. Estrogen therapy can reduce the size of the sebaceous glands and decrease production of androgens by the ovaries. Oral retinoids are reserved for extremely severe, recalcitrant cases of cystic acne. Retinoids are related to vitamin A, and their mechanism of action is not clearly defined, but studies have shown they have a direct effect on the proliferation and differentiation of epithelial cells. This action results in suppression of sebaceous gland activity and has an antiinflammatory effect. Isotretinoin is used in severe, recalcitrant cystic acne because of its ability to reduce the size of sebaceous glands, thus reduc-

MEDICAL MANAGEMENT—cont'd

ing the synthesis of sebum. Even though these effects are temporary, patients may continue to improve after the effects have worn off. Because of the potential serious side effects of oral retinoid therapy, patients must be selected carefully according to criteria published by the pharmaceutical company.

Once it has been determined that drug therapy is necessary, certain laboratory studies may be ordered before treatment is begun. A complete blood count (CBC) to check for anemia may be done before systemic antibiotics are begun and may be repeated at regular intervals for long-term therapy. Serum androgen levels may be checked in females to determine whether the acne will respond to hormonal therapy (oral contraceptives).

With isotretinoin (Accutane) therapy, a pregnancy test, triglyceride level, CBC, and liver function studies must be done before treatment is started. The pregnancy test result must be negative. The triglyceride level must be within normal limits before treatment is started; it must be checked again 2 to 3 weeks after treatment begins, and every 4 weeks thereafter. If the triglyceride level exceeds 700 to 800 mg/dl, the drug must be discontinued. The CBC should reveal no sign of anemia, and the values for the liver function studies must be within normal limits, because isotretinoin is metabolized in the liver.

OTHER MEDICAL MANAGEMENT

Numerous soaps, facial masks, and washes are available for use in the treatment of acne. Many make antibacterial or keratolytic claims. Every treatment regimen should be tailored to meet the specific needs of the individual based on the severity of the disease and the individual's ability to comply with therapy.

1 ASSESS

ASSESSMENT	OBSERVATIONS
Medical history	Family history of acne or individual history of oily skin
Current health status	May complain of increasing oiliness; women may complain of irregular menstrual periods and hirsutism
Skin	Oily, erythematous skin with comedones, papules, pustules, or cysts; assess for evidence of picking or squeezing; assess personal hygiene habits and use of cosmetics
Pain	Involved areas may be sore to touch (frequently more painful in males)
Drugs	Obtain a complete drug history, including both topical and systemic drugs being used for any reason

2   DIAGNOSE

NURSING DIAGNOSIS	SUBJECTIVE FINDINGS	OBJECTIVE FINDINGS
Impaired skin integrity and high risk for infection related to skin lesions and compromised integument	Reports presence of lesions	Acne lesions Pustules, open and closed comedones; evidence of picking, manipulation, and secondary infection
Pain (discomfort) related to lesions	Complains of pain in involved areas	Shows signs of pain or discomfort with manipulation of lesions or surrounding area
Body image disturbance related to secondary lesions	Expresses concern about appearance	Shows embarrassment about skin; avoids direct eye contact; uses heavy makeup to camouflage lesions
Knowledge deficit related to disease and treatment	Does not understand cause of acne	Repeats common misconceptions about cause of acne and its treatment

3   PLAN

Patient goals

1. The barrier function of the skin will be restored.
2. The patient will be free of pain and discomfort caused by acne lesions.
3. The patient will maintain a positive body image.
4. The patient will have no infection.
5. The patient will understand the disease and its treatment.

4   IMPLEMENT

NURSING DIAGNOSIS	NURSING INTERVENTIONS	RATIONALE
Impaired skin integrity and high risk for infection related to skin lesions and compromised integument	Assess for inflammatory process.	Treatment may need to be adjusted based on degree of severity.
	Plan schedule for treatment regimen.	Patients tend to comply better if regimen is acceptable to life-style.
	Encourage patient to seek medical attention with onset of lesions.	Early treatment may prevent secondary infection and complications.
	Discourage picking and squeezing of lesions.	Manipulation increases the risk of infection.

NURSING DIAGNOSIS	NURSING INTERVENTIONS	RATIONALE
	Apply hot packs to cystic lesions.	To promote circulation and suppuration.
	Identify and eliminate predisposing or aggravating factors.	To reduce flare-ups.
Pain (discomfort) related to lesions	Discourage manipulation of lesions.	Manipulation may increase discomfort and cause secondary infection, which contributes to discomfort.
	Use warm, moist compresses.	To speed healing by increasing circulation and suppuration.
	Encourage patient to adhere to treatment regimen.	Compliance promotes healing.
Body image disturbance related to secondary lesions	Encourage patient to discuss feelings about appearance.	Verbalization allows for assistance with coping and development of realistic self-evaluation.
	Inform patient of availability of noncomedogenic agents for camouflage.	To allow patient to maintain normalcy during flare-ups.
Knowledge deficit related to disease and treatment	Dispel myths about causes of acne.	Accurate information allows better understanding and acceptance.
	Teach patient how to follow treatment regimen.	To be effective, treatment must be understood.

5   EVALUATE

PATIENT OUTCOME	DATA INDICATING THAT OUTCOME IS REACHED
Skin's barrier function has been restored.	Lesions have healed or are in an advanced stage of healing.
Patient is free of pain.	Patient reports that pain is gone.
Patient's body image has improved.	Patient makes positive statements about appearance.
Patient has no infection.	There are no signs of secondary infection.
Patient understands course of disease and treatment required.	Patient can describe disease process and understands the need to comply with treatment regimen.

PATIENT TEACHING

1. Provide information about acne to dispel any misconceptions.
2. Set up a realistic treatment schedule, and explain the approximate length of treatment required before improvement is seen.
3. Stress the importance of complying with the medication regimen and of adhering strictly to follow-up visits with the physician.
4. Explain the complications possible with the therapy being used.
5. Discuss ways to avoid factors known to exacerbate the disease.
6. Discuss the importance of avoiding sun exposure when using certain drugs, especially retinoic acid or antibiotics.
7. Instruct the patient in local care of lesions, including the need to avoid picking or squeezing.
8. Instruct female patients in the appropriate type of cosmetics to use to avoid exacerbation; instruct male patients in the use of tinted topical medications that can help camouflage lesions.

CHAPTER 11

Dermatologic Treatments

Only a small percentage of patients with a skin disease are seriously ill. Admission to the hospital usually is a matter of complicated or frequent treatments; thus quality nursing care is vital to these patients, both in providing the care immediately required and in teaching them how to perform treatments properly at home.

Unsightly, slowly healing lesions may make the patient feel "untouchable." The patient may have been around people who fear the skin disease is contagious or dirty. The nurse must show acceptance of these patients and allow them time to ventilate their feelings. The nurse should care for the patient's skin without showing distaste or a reluctance to touch.

Many dermatologic conditions are associated with pruritus. Constant itching interferes with rest and prompts scratching, which may lead to secondary infection. Therefore, relieving pruritus is vital. The patient should be kept in a cool environment, and topical and antipruritic agents should be administered as ordered. The patient's fingernails should be kept short, and diversional activities should be offered. At bedtime, an additional or higher dose of an antipruritic drug or a sedative may be necessary to provide sufficient relief for sleep. A warm bedtime bath, followed by application of a topical medication, may help. If pruritus increases after a topical agent is applied, it should be removed. Foods that may cause flushing, such as condiments, coffee, and alcohol, should be avoided, because vasodilation is associated with increased pruritus.

The nurse should always handle the patient gently, because some dermatologic diseases, such as herpes zoster, are painful. Good handwashing and clean technique (sterile technique usually is not required) are necessary to prevent infection.

Because the skin acts as protective insulation against the environment, a breakdown in normal cutaneous integrity may result in loss of body heat, predisposition to infection, and loss of protein-containing fluids. Thus the patient must be kept warm and hydrated. Rest and good nutrition also are essential and must be encouraged.

These measures apply to most patients with skin diseases. Specific therapies are dictated by the disease or the patient's general condition, or both.

APPLICATION TECHNIQUES FOR TOPICAL MEDICATIONS

Nurses responsible for either direct patient care or patient education should become familiar with the various classes of topical medication and the proper application technique for each. These types of preparations are defined in Table 11-1. Each preparation may be nonmedicated or may incorporate drugs (e.g., steroids, antibacterials, antifungals, and antipruritics). Table 11-2 provides a guide for choosing the proper type of topical

Table 11-1

TOPICAL MEDICATIONS

Class/content	Purposes	Disadvantages	Inert examples
Cream Oil-in-water emulsion; water content 60% or more	Ease of application Ease of removal Lubrication Deliver medication	Removed by perspiration Low penetration of medication	Dermatology Formula Nutraderm
Ointment Water-in-oil emulsions; water content 40% or less	Marked lubrication Maintains a layer of medication on skin Delivers medication with enhanced penetration	Greasy sensation May stain clothing May inflame hair follicles	Aquaphor Eucerin Nivea Petrolatum Lanolin
Gel Semisolid mixture; between cream and ointment in content; often contains alcohol	Ease of application Greaseless layer of medication	May cause burning on eroded skin	
Powder Finely ground solid particles	Absorbs moisture, thereby promoting drying Decreases skin friction Delivers medication best in intertriginous areas	Wears off easily	Talcum Bentonite Cornstarch Zinc oxide
Lotion Powder suspended in liquid (water, alcohol, oil)	Cooling effect on evaporation May absorb moisture, promoting dryness Delivers medication as uniform residual film Useful in hairy areas	Wears off easily Can overdry skin	Ken Lubriderm WIBI Cetaphil
Solution Powder dissolved in liquid medium	Similar to lotion Useful in hairy areas	Similar to lotion	Vehicle-N C-solve
Aerosol Spray Lotion delivered by airborne propellant	Similar to lotion but even more drying Useful in hairy areas	Similar to lotion	
Paste Powder mixed in ointment; 50% or more powder content	Leaves a protective coating while delivering medication	Low rate of penetration Messy to use	Zinc oxide paste (Lassar's)

Table 11-2

CHOOSING TOPICAL VEHICLES

Description of skin condition	Example	Topical vehicle of choice
Red, hot	Exfoliative erythroderma	Dermatologic wet dressing
Red, irritated, sore, oozing	Contact dermatitis	Lotions or sprays
Acute, red, wet skin; not painful to touch	Atopic eczema	Creams, gels
Chronic, scaly skin with redness	Seborrheic dermatitis	Creams, gels
Thick, hyperkeratotic skin	Psoriasis	Ointments

medication based on the skin condition. The location also affects this decision, as noted in Table 11-1.

The object of topical therapy is to lubricate or medicate the skin, or both. Applying the topical drug gives the nurse the opportunity to examine the patient's skin regularly and to assess the response to treatment.

SUPPLIES

Ordered topical medication
Drapes, if needed
Gloves
Tongue blade
Paint brush or gauze

NURSING CARE

The following are some general principles that guide the use of topical agents:

1. Review orders, checking site(s) and frequency of application.
2. Assemble necessary medication(s).
3. Ensure the patient's privacy, and drape properly.
4. Make sure intended application site is clean and dry. If topicals become "caked," remove before applying additional treatments. Creams can usually be removed with water-soaked cheesecloth or by gently bathing with tap water. Ointment bases are more difficult to remove. Cheesecloth dampened with cottonseed or mineral oil usually removes caked-on ointments or pastes.
5. **For creams, ointments, and pastes:**
   - Apply a small amount (approximately ½ inch from tube) of ointment or cream to your hands and rub

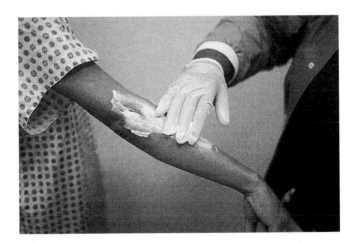

FIGURE 11-1
Applying topical cream. (Note the clinician's gloved hand.)

briskly. Hands should have a thin sheen of medication.
   - With long, downward strokes of the palms, apply medication to the affected area (Figure 11-1). Be systematic to be certain that all areas are covered. Skin should be lubricated but should not feel greasy. Only a thickness of 100 μm is needed for effective treatment. Excess medication will only rub off on clothing or linen. Do not rub up and down with medication.

- Pastes may be applied with a tongue depressor, because they have a thick, semisolid consistency.
6. **For lotions and solutions:**
   - Shake the lotion or solution well.
   - Pour a small amount into your hands.
   - For lotions with water or alcohol base, pat onto the skin. Use a brush or gauze only if the mixture is too thin to control. Do not use cotton, because it can filter out the suspended medication and can stick to the skin, causing inflammation.
7. **For sprays and aerosols:**
   - Shake the container well.
   - Direct toward affected area from the distance recommended in the package insert (usually 6 to 12 inches).
   - Spray in short bursts.
8. **For powders:**
   - Make sure the area is *dry* to minimize caking.
   - Apply a thin layer by gently shaking on the powder ("dusting").
   - Apply powder with gauze or powder puff if the area is difficult to reach.
9. Document on patient's records:
   - Patient teaching
   - Observation of the lesions
   - Apparent results of treatment
   - Any side effects, such as irritation, thinning, or atrophy
   - Patient acceptance (e.g., does the patient feel that the ointment is too greasy to wear under clothing)

NURSING CONSIDERATIONS

- Remember that using a large amount of medication is not better than using a small (proper) amount. Using more medication than necessary can result in a tremendous increase in expense without an increase in benefit. Excess medication may also pose an increased risk of side effects.
- Suspect allergic contact dermatitis if the patient's condition worsens in spite of adequate topical therapy. Patients may become allergic to active ingredients (e.g., neomycin), vehicle components (e.g., propylene glycol), or preservatives (e.g., paraben compounds) contained in topical preparations.
- Do not rub in topicals. Rubbing the applications can lead to folliculitis. Ointments and tar preparations predispose the patient to this complication.
- Do not apply a cover or dressing over topical medications unless this is specifically ordered or required.
- Apply all topicals downward (in the direction of hair growth) to minimize the risk of folliculitis.
- Do not use cotton balls to apply topicals.

- Do not allow a powder to cake and harden by using repeated thick applications.
- Do not apply topicals to eyelids, ears, or ear canals unless specifically ordered. When applying medication to the face, use a gloved fingertip.
- If lotions or sprays are to be used on the scalp, apply with the supplied applicator. The hair should be parted at ¼-inch intervals and the applicator directed along the parts until the scalp is systematically covered.

PATIENT EDUCATION

Teach the patient good technique by example. Review the points covered in Nursing Considerations. Have the patient practice the application in your presence to verify that he is using the correct technique.

APPLICATION OF TOPICAL CORTICOSTEROIDS

Topical corticosteroids are used to reduce inflammation, relieve pruritus, and induce remission of certain skin diseases.

SUPPLIES

Ordered topical medication
Nonsterile gloves
Paint brush or gauze

NURSING CARE

1. Review orders, checking site(s) and frequency of application.
2. Assemble necessary supplies.
3. Ensure patient's privacy.
4. Make sure application site is clean and dry.
5. **For creams, ointments, and pastes:**
   - Apply a small amount (approximately ½-inch ribbon) onto gloved hand.
   - Apply medication to the affected area, using downward strokes (apply in the direction of hair growth). Skin should be lubricated but should not feel greasy. Effective treatment is achieved with a thickness of 100 µm; excessive medication will rub off on clothing and will not be of any therapeutic benefit.
   - Pastes may be applied with a tongue blade or may be warmed in the palms of the gloved hands to assist in application.
6. **For lotions and solutions:**
   - Shake well.
   - Pour a small amount into gloved hands.

Table 11-3

POTENCY OF TOPICAL CORTICOSTEROIDS

Potency	Generic name	Trade name
Very high	Fluocinonide	Lidex, Topsyn
	Halcinonide	Halog, Halciderm
High	Betamethasone benzoate	Benisone
	Betamethasone dipropionate	Diprosone
	Betamethasone valerate	Valisone
	Diflorasone diacetate	Maxiflor, Florone
Medium	Fluocinolone acetonide 0.025%	Synalar, Synemol
	Triamcinolone 0.1%	Aristocort
	Triamcinolone acetonide 0.1%	Kenalog
	Flurandrenolide	Cordran
Low	Desonide	Tridesilon
	Hydrocortisone valerate	Westcort
Very low	Hydrocortisone	Hytone, Nutracort, Cortril, Synacort

- If the lotion has an alcohol or a water base, pat it onto the skin. Use a brush or gauze if the mixture is too thin to control coverage. Cotton should not be used, because it will filter out the suspended medication.

7. **For sprays and aerosols:**
   - Shake well.
   - Direct toward affected area from the recommended distance.
   - Spray in short bursts.

8. **For powders:**
   - Dry the affected area to minimize caking of powder.
   - Apply a thin layer of powder.
   - Apply with gauze or a powder puff if the affected area is difficult to reach.

NURSING CONSIDERATIONS

- Topical corticosteroid preparations can be roughly divided into groups according to their relative potency (Table 11-3).
- Side effects of topical steroids may include thinning of the skin (atrophy), induction of striae (especially in intertriginous sites), development of an acnelike eruption (notably on the face), appearance of dilated blood vessels (telangiectasia) and, if use is widespread, suppression of the normal pituitary-adrenal gland interaction. These side effects are more common with extensive and prolonged application and use of high-potency preparations. It is wise, therefore, to initiate or maintain therapy with the *lowest potency agent possible.*

- Combination steroid-antibiotic-antifungal creams are rarely indicated. Specific therapy for a specific diagnosis is preferable whenever possible.
- Rest periods may be necessary to prevent a diminution in drug effectiveness during long-term topical steroid therapy.
- Ointment-based preparations are generally more potent than chemically equivalent, cream-based agents. The proper use of cream, ointment, solution and lotion, spray, and powder preparations is discussed in Application Techniques for Topical Medications, beginning on page 151.
- Topical steroid preparations are expensive. Always use the least possible amount to cover a treatment site. Frequency of application should be the *lowest* consistent with sustained therapeutic results, usually one to four times daily. Four or more applications a day are *rarely* indicated during topical corticosteroid therapy.

PATIENT EDUCATION

The patient should understand the key points listed in Nursing Considerations. It is especially important to stress to the patient that overuse of topical corticosteroids can result in serious cutaneous and systemic complications. Patients should be cautioned against lending their creams to friends and relatives. Self-medication can have disastrous complications.

BALNEOTHERAPY (THERAPEUTIC BATH)

The object of balneotherapy is to cleanse the skin and improve the patient's feeling of well-being. The bath loosens and removes crust or scales and relieves itching. It facilitates delivery of topical medication to a large area. The skin is well hydrated, thereby enhancing penetration of medication.

SUPPLIES

Prescribed medication and/or soap
Bath thermometer
Tub
Towels
Washcloth (if thick scales are present)

NURSING CARE

1. Check orders for specific type of therapeutic bath to be used.
2. Explain steps and purpose of treatment to the patient.
3. Assemble necessary supplies in tub room.
4. Provide for patient's privacy.
5. Ensure adequate warmth in room.
6. Draw water at 35° to 37.8° C (95° to 100° F) (Figure 11-2). Place mat in tub because tub may be slippery.
7. Help patient into tub and position comfortably with as much of the body covered as possible.
8. Soak for a total of 20 to 30 minutes.
9. Cleanse if ordered. Instruct the patient to rub with the hand, not the washcloth, which may be too abrasive to already red, irritated skin. Psoriatic patients may use the washcloth to help remove crusts after soaking.
10. Help patient out of tub if assistance is needed.
11. Pat skin with towel until damp dry.
12. Apply ordered topical medications to damp skin.
13. Dress to prevent chilling.

Table 11-4

BALNEOTHERAPY

Type of bath	Agents	Disease	Purpose
Antibacterial	Potassium permanganate (1:32,000; 1:64,000) Acetic acid Hexachlorophene Povidone-iodine	Infected eczema Dirty ulcerations Furunculosis	Lower skin bacterial load
Colloidal	Starch and baking soda (1 cup each/tub) Aveeno Colloidal Oatmeal (1 cup/tub) Aveeno Oilated Colloidal Oatmeal	Any red, irritated, oozing condition (e.g., atopic eczema)	Relieve itching Soothe
Emollient*	Bath oils: Alpha Keri, Lubath Mineral oil	Any dry skin condition	Cleanse and hydrate the skin
Tar*	Bath oils with tar: Balnetar, Zetar, Polytar Coal tar concentrate (liquor carbonis detergens)	Scaly dermatoses (e.g., psoriasis)	Loosen scale Relieve itching Potentiate UVA/UVB light therapy

*For emollient and tar baths, add 3 to 6 capfuls of therapeutic agent per standard-size bathtub.

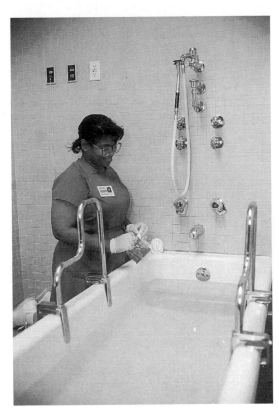

FIGURE 11-2
Preparing a therapeutic bath.

NURSING CONSIDERATIONS

- The average home bathtub holds 150 to 200 L of water.
- The type of bath that a patient is to receive should be ordered by the physician. Different diseases or skin conditions require different treatment baths. A newly admitted patient should not be bathed until orders are received!
- Hot water and soap are drying. Dry skin is more susceptible to itching, scaling, and fissuring. Therefore, even normal skin requires bathing only approximately every other day at temperatures between 35° and 37.8° C (95° and 100° F), with soap to underarms and groin only. If the skin is already dry, a 5-minute shower at the same water temperature as above using minimal soap is best.
- Using friction during bathing or drying can irritate and damage the epithelium.
- Mineral oil or cooking oil may be applied to the skin and gently rubbed off with gauze to remove accumulated topical medications.
- See Table 11-4 for types of balneotherapy.

CRYOSURGERY

Treatment with cryosurgery selectively destroys tissue through freezing, which results in cell death. Lesions commonly frozen include actinic keratoses, seborrheic keratoses, leukoplakia, molluscum contagiosum, condyloma acuminatum and, occasionally, basal cell epitheliomas or squamous cell carcinomas. Less scarring is achieved by controlling the depth of tissue destruction. For treatment of basal cell carcinomas, liquid nitrogen is applied with the aid of a thermocouple needle.

SUPPLIES

Cotton-tipped applicators
Cry-Ac (or other pressurized delivery system)
Thermocouple needles
Local anesthesia for treatment of skin cancer with liquid nitrogen and thermocouple monitoring

NURSING CARE

1. Assemble needed supplies.
2. Explain the procedure to the patient. Explain that there will be a feeling of cold and then burning pain. Instruct the patient to remain still.
3. Shield the patient's eyes or ears with gauze, as needed.
4. The physician applies liquid nitrogen.
5. Instruct the patient to expect some pain, redness, swelling, and blistering after the procedure. Blisters may be very hemorrhagic.
6. Instruct the patient that blistering will flatten and heal on its own, and he should keep the area clean by using soap and water, alcohol, or hydrogen peroxide three times daily.
7. Report extreme pain, a wide rim of redness, oozing of exudate, or fever to the physician immediately.
8. If thermocouple needles for treatment of a basal cell epithelioma are used:
   - Consult patient regarding allergies.
   - Prepare the area with alcohol or povidone-iodine solution.
   - Instruct the patient that the areas will be anesthetized. There will be a sensation of a stick and a sting.
   - Aid the physician in insertion and securing of the thermocouple needles into the base of the tumor.
   - As the physician applies liquid nitrogen, time in seconds until the tissue reaches −20° C (−4° F).
   - Record in seconds how long it takes the tissue to thaw.
   - Time the second freezing to −20° C (−4° F).
   - Instruct the patient that there will be swelling and

some discomfort. Apply ice packs and administer analgesics as ordered.

- Instruct the patient to keep the area clean with hydrogen peroxide.

NURSING CONSIDERATIONS

- Treating lesions with liquid nitrogen can give good cosmetic results with little anesthesia.
- Cryosurgery on the lips, ears, or eyelids is most painful.
- Damage to vital vessels, nerves, or tear ducts is one of the few side effects.
- Spraying liquid nitrogen with Cry-Ac (or a similar device) can result in more intense tissue destruction than using cotton-tipped applicators.
- When using thermocouple, a repeated freeze and thaw gives better destruction. Fast freezing and slow thaw gives better results.
- It takes about 3 to 6 hours for the blister to form after freezing. The blister flattens in 2 or 3 days and peels off in about 2 to 3 weeks.
- If kept clean, the cryosurgery site rarely becomes secondarily infected.

PATIENT EDUCATION

Discuss both Nursing Care and Nursing Considerations with the patient. Be certain that the patient understands the reason for freezing the lesion. The patient must be prepared for the *normal* sequelae of cryosurgery (swelling, blister formation, discomfort).

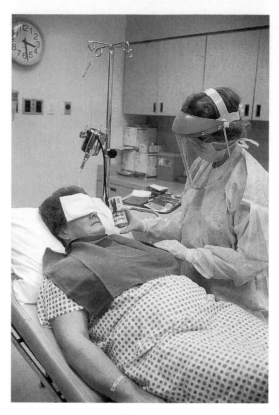

FIGURE 11-3
Patient undergoing dermabrasion of the face.

DERMABRASION

Dermabrasion is the process of planing the superficial layer of epidermis and dermis to obtain cosmetically pleasing removal of scarring or hyperplastic tissue (sufficient dermis is left to ensure reepithelization of the area planed). Dermabrasion is used to remove tattoos, to smooth out rhinophyma, or to decrease scarring from acne.

SUPPLIES

Dermabrasion apparatus
Local anesthetic
Syringe with small-gauge (27 or 30) needles
Skin preparation solution
Petrolatum gauze
Gauze pads or dressings without cotton filler
Saline irrigating solution
Gloves
Full face shields
Gowns

NURSING CARE

1. Cleanse skin as directed and drape.
2. Prepare syringe with local anesthetic. (An alternate method to provide local anesthesia is with fluoroethyl spray. Spray small areas until hard; dermabrade; move to next area and repeat procedure.) (See Figure 11-3.)
3. Physician will infiltrate and perform procedure.
4. Cover wound with petrolatum gauze.
5. Instruct the patient to expect oozing and pain. Oozing will occur for 24 hours. Crusts will form and last for about 1 week. The crust comes off, but the skin will be red for 2 to 3 months.
6. Administer analgesics as needed.
7. Keep original petrolatum dressing in place for 24 to 48 hours.
8. Apply cool saline compresses over the dressing four times a day (if ordered) for the first 2 days postoperative.
9. Assist the physician with dressing change at 24 to 48 hours.

10. After the crusts form, and until well healed, apply bland emolliating creams.
11. Cover the wound only if necessary to prevent snagging on clothing.
12. Report fear, excessive pain, swelling, or exudate to the physician immediately.
13. Face may be cleansed after 72 hours by gently applying nonmenthol shaving cream and showering, allowing the water to gently rinse the face. *Under no circumstances* should the face be rubbed or scrubbed, with or without a washcloth.

NURSING CONSIDERATIONS

- The patient may need reassurance, because results are slow to see.
- Discomfort may increase as the wound heals. Fissures may occur in the area and lead to secondary infection. Applying petrolatum helps reduce tightness and decreases the risk of fissuring.
- Observe the patient closely for infection.
- The healed skin may react abnormally to sunlight. Avoid sun exposure as much as possible, or protect skin with a sunscreen, for 3 to 4 months.
- The patient should keep the head elevated at least 45 degrees during the first 24 to 48 hours postprocedure to reduce edema.
- Saline solution for contact lenses is acceptable for wound cleansing.

PATIENT EDUCATION

Before surgery, discuss the procedure thoroughly with the patient. After surgery, review all Nursing Considerations and any specific instructions with the patient.

INTRALESIONAL CORTICOSTEROID THERAPY

The purpose of intralesional corticosteroid therapy is to achieve the prolonged, continuous antiinflammatory effects of corticosteroid therapy in a localized lesion (e.g., injecting a keloid). Intralesional therapy prevents systemic absorption.

SUPPLIES

Tuberculin syringe or pressure jets
30-gauge, ½-inch needle
Alcohol swabs
Injectable corticosteroid
Normal saline (bacteriostatic)

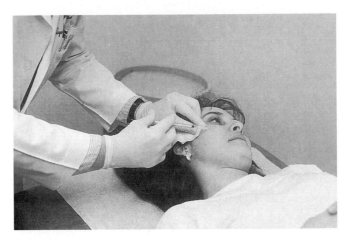

FIGURE 11-4
Clinician administering an intralesional corticosteroid injection to patient's face.

NURSING CARE

1. Prepare the intralesional corticosteroid as ordered by mixing injectable steroid with bacteriostatic normal saline. The solution may also be prepared by the physician or the pharmacist at different institutions. Dilutions of 2 mg/ml, 3 mg/ml, 5 mg/ml, or 10 mg/ml are most commonly used.
2. Explain the procedure to the patient. Explain that there will be some burning and pain. Inform the patient that it is hoped results will include decreased redness, decreased swelling, decreased size, and decreased pruritus in the localized area. If using a pressure jet, instruct the patient to expect a noise as it fires.
3. Swab the lesion with alcohol.
4. Assist the physician in injecting the lesion with the corticosteroid (Figure 11-4).
5. Apply pressure to stop any bleeding.

NURSING CONSIDERATIONS

- Watch for side effects (atrophy, hypopigmentation, infection, ulceration).
- Follow proper cleaning procedure for the pressure jets.
- Many patients believe the air jet is less painful than the tuberculin syringe. The air jet injects 0.1 ml per firing.

PATIENT EDUCATION

Explain to the patient what discomfort he may experience. Discuss what results he can expect.

OCCLUSIVE DRESSINGS

Occlusive dressings are airtight dressings that are applied over medicated skin to achieve the following results: (1) increase humidity and soften thick, dry, hyperkeratotic skin, increasing absorption of the medication; (2) increase the efficacy and decrease the expense of treatment (penetration is enhanced such that less medication is required to achieve the same goal); (3) retain moisture and prevent evaporation of the medication.

SUPPLIES

Ordered topical medication (most often corticosteroid cream)
Plastic to cover the area to be occluded:
  Saran Wrap or Handi-Wrap for arms, legs, torso, feet
  Plastic tape (Blenderm) for small patches
  Vinyl gloves for hands
  Plastic bags for hands and feet
  Plastic shower cap for scalp
  Vinyl exercise suit for total body
Paper tape to seal the edges of dressings

NURSING CARE

1. Review physician's order for occlusion. It should include the topical medication ordered, areas to be occluded, and the length of time occlusion should be in place.
2. Explain the procedure to the patient.
3. Have the patient bathe and clean the skin well between periods of occlusion.
4. Apply ordered topical medication.
5. Determine what method will cover the area effectively and comfortably. For example, occluding the hands with gloves instead of Saran Wrap allows the patient better mobility.
6. Apply the plastic, sealing edges with paper tape. Blenderm tape may be applied directly to small areas of skin for occlusion.
7. Keep the plastic in place for the ordered period of time unless the patient complains of burning, itching, stinging, or pain.

NURSING CONSIDERATIONS

- Applying occlusion over a steroid cream may increase potency of the medication 100 times.
- Occlusion helps build up a reservoir of steroid cream by hydrating the stratum corneum.
- Occlusion is very effective over lichenified (thickened) skin or thick plaques.
- Because perspiration under the plastic may lead to miliaria, folliculitis, or secondary infection, bathing between applications is important.
- Because the strength of the medication is so greatly increased under occlusion, side effects of topical steroids may appear sooner. Therefore, the nurse should observe for striae, atrophy, or thinning of the skin and report these to the physician. Occlusion is not used chronically.
- Long periods under occlusion can result in systemic absorption of the corticosteroid.
- Creams, not ointments, should be applied under occlusion. Ointments are too greasy and may result in greater risk of miliaria or folliculitis.
- A lower potency steroid may be used under occlusion, because potency is increased so greatly.
- Occlusion is not used for acute skin conditions (red, weeping, irritated). The increased humidity and heat retention may well worsen such conditions.

PATIENT EDUCATION

The patient must be cautioned not to use occlusion more often or for longer periods than ordered. (The rapid progress may encourage continued use and increase the risk of side effects.) The patient should understand the importance of bathing between applications to remove perspiration and medication and to reduce the chances of developing miliaria, infection, and folliculitis.

PINCH GRAFTING

Pinch grafting is done to promote reepithelialization and healing of an ulcer. Small pieces of skin are obtained from a healthy donor site and applied to an ulcerated area that has a clean, granulating base. Special care must be taken to prevent infection and rejection of the grafts.

SUPPLIES

Skin preparation solution ordered by physician
Shave prep kit
Skin hook
Razor blade or scalpel blade (No. 11)
Petrolatum gauze
Gauze pads

Topical antibiotic ointment
Normal saline
Local anesthetic (without epinephrine)
Syringe with 30-gauge, ½-inch needle
Elastic bandage (2 inches wide)
Gloves

NURSING CARE

1. Shave donor site (usually anterior thigh).
2. Prepare and anesthetize donor site as directed.
3. Physician obtains skin grafts by elevating donor site skin with fingers or skin hook and shaving off thin grafts with razor blade or scalpel blade. Grafts are placed into ulcer.
4. Cover both donor and recipient sites with antibiotic ointment.
5. Cover ulcer site with petrolatum gauze and then with several layers of gauze pads. Alternate regimen: Graft sites (donor and recipient) may be covered with a semipermeable adhesive, transparent plastic membrane. This remains in place for 10 to 14 days (skip steps 8 and 9 if this regimen is used).
6. Wrap recipient site loosely with elastic bandage.
7. Place patient on *strict bed rest* (usually 2 to 7 days) with recipient leg elevated.
8. Leave original dressing in place 24 to 48 hours as ordered, then remove and leave recipient site open until crusting appears.
9. Begin normal saline compresses after crusting (every 2 hours) for 4 to 7 days as ordered.
10. Fit patient for elastic stockings, to be worn for approximately 1 month after grafting.

NURSING CONSIDERATIONS

- Watch for signs of rejection (erythema, edema, purulent exudate, fever) at both the donor and recipient sites.
- Elevation of the extremity and postoperative bed rest are crucial to proper healing.
- Using a transparent dressing eliminates the need for saline compresses, but has not yet been proved superior.

PATIENT EDUCATION

Discuss the procedure with the patient before the grafting. A knowledgeable, cooperative patient will usually tolerate the postoperative restrictions. Though the ulcer may look "healed," the patient should be instructed to avoid trauma to the area, to wear elastic support stockings, and to avoid prolonged standing for at least 1 full month after grafting.

POSTOPERATIVE CARE OF DERMATOLOGIC EXCISIONS

Dermatologic excision is performed to remove or biopsy malignant or benign skin lesions for curative or cosmetic reasons. After surgery, minimal scarring is attained by preventing infection and promoting adequate skin closure.

SUPPLIES

Saline solution or tap water
Alcohol or hydrogen peroxide
Bandage or gauze pad and paper tape

NURSING CARE

1. Determine the length of time the physician wants the pressure bandage applied at the time of surgery to remain in place (usually 24 to 48 hours).
2. Instruct the patient how long to leave the bandage in place. Tell him to remove the bandage if severe swelling, erythema, or cyanosis develops above or below the dressing, and to report any of these to the physician immediately. Also instruct him to report severe pain, or bleeding that saturates the dressing.
3. The patient, nurse, or physician will remove the dressing at the specified time. Gently clean with saline solution or tap water on a gauze pad. Report wide erythema, drainage, pain, or fever. Report immediately if the wound comes open.
4. Leave the wound open unless the patient is involved in an activity in which the wound is likely to get dirty.
5. Explain postoperative care to the patient:
   - Clean two times.
   - Avoid stress to the area. Refrain from activities likely to put tension on the wound.
   - Return for removal of stitches. If Steri-Strips are applied, leave in place until they fall off.

NURSING CONSIDERATIONS

- Keep the wound clean. Leave open, because covering tightly can lead to infection.
- Instruct the patient to discontinue use of any other creams or ointments previously being used on the site.
- Pressure bandages should not be applied around a limb, because they can easily interfere with circulation and prevent healing.
- Teach the patient what symptoms to report to the physician.
- Stitches on the face are usually removed in 3 to 5 days; stitches elsewhere on the body are removed in 7 to 10 days.

PATIENT EDUCATION

The patient should be able to repeat to you the exact instructions for postoperative wound care. He should be able to state the signs and symptoms of circulatory problems or infection and should understand the need for follow-up.

PUNCH BIOPSY

The objective of punch biopsy is to obtain a small piece of tissue (2 to 8 mm) for histopathologic study. A punch biopsy may be performed to establish a diagnosis; to evaluate the efficacy of current treatment; to remove entirely a small lesion (punch excision); to search for infectious organisms; or to obtain a specimen for biochemical analysis.

SUPPLIES

Punches (reusable or disposable) of necessary diameter
Forceps, scissors, needle holder
Syringe with small-gauge (27 or 30) needles
Gauze pads, cotton-tipped applicators
Band-Aids
Shave kit (if needed)
Suture material or skin clips
Skin preparation material
10% Formalin, sterile saline, or other transport solution in container
Monsel's solution
Local anesthetic

NURSING CARE

1. Shave area if hairy.
2. Cleanse skin with appropriate solution.
3. Prepare syringe with local anesthetic and small-gauge needle.
4. Physician will infiltrate local anesthetic and use punch instrument to obtain skin plug.
5. Place tissue specimen in formalin bottle (saline if for cultures and biochemical analysis, special media for immunofluorescent studies).
6. Label specimen bottle with patient's name and identifying number.
7. Use Monsel's solution on cotton-tipped applicator to stop bleeding; alternatively, physician may suture or clip the wound closed.
8. Cover site with Band-Aid or other dressing as directed.
9. After the procedure, explain postoperative care to the patient:
   - Instruct the patient to leave the Band-Aid in place for 8 to 24 hours.
   - Remove the dressing and clean gently with saline solution or tap water twice daily.
   - Leave the site open. If necessary, keep covered for short periods. Covering is usually necessary for cosmetic reasons only.
   - Report spreading erythema or drainage.
   - If sutures are in place, dab gently with saline solution or tap water two times daily. Return as ordered for suture removal.
10. Explain that the hole made by the punch biopsy will gradually fill in and leave little scarring.
11. Stress the importance of keeping return appointments for explanation of biopsy results.

NURSING CONSIDERATIONS

- Biopsies rarely become infected if kept clean and open.
- Similar postoperative care may be used for shave or curettage biopsy sites.

PATIENT EDUCATION

Explain the procedure before it is done. This is a *minor* procedure, and steps should be taken to minimize the patient's anxiety. Ensure that signed consent is obtained when indicated by the patient's age or institutional policies. Stress the importance of postoperative care as directed. Be certain the patient understands when to return for follow-up.

THERAPEUTIC SHAMPOO

The purpose of therapeutic shampoo is to cleanse the scalp and remove accumulated scales, crusts, or medications.

SUPPLIES

Prescribed shampoo (Table 11-5)
Towels
Topical lotions, solutions, or sprays ordered for application to the scalp
Gloves

NURSING CARE

1. Gather necessary supplies.
2. Inform the patient and family of the purpose of the treatment shampoo.
3. Demonstrate the procedure so that the patient can accomplish this independently in the future, if able.
4. Wet the hair with water at 35° to 37.8° C (95° to 100° F) (Figure 11-5).

Table 11-5

THERAPEUTIC SHAMPOOS

Shampoo content	Examples
Salicylic acid/sulfur	Sebulex, Meted, Vanseb, Xseb, Ionil, P & S
Zinc pyrithione	Zincon, DHS Zinc, Danex
Other surfactants	Capitrol, PHacid
Tar	Sebutone, Vanseb-T, Xseb T, Ionil-T, Pentrax, Zetar, Polytar, T-Gel
Selenium sulfide	Selsun, Exsel

5. Apply enough shampoo to make a lather.
6. Suds, using fingertips, not nails, for 2 minutes.
7. Allow shampoo to remain on the hair for 5 minutes.
8. Rinse, and repeat the shampoo. Take care to avoid the eyes when rinsing hair.
9. Dry the hair with a towel or a hair dryer set on cool.
10. Apply topical medications as ordered. The patient should be assisted whenever possible because of the difficulty of seeing one's own scalp and applying medications evenly.

NURSING CONSIDERATIONS

- Infrequent shampooing may result in treatment failure.
- Scrubbing with fingernails may damage the scalp by forcibly removing crust or scale.
- Allowing shampoo to remain on scalp increases penetration and thus efficacy of shampoo.
- Excessive heat from an electric dryer may increase scaling and pruritus.
- If the hair becomes dry, rinsing with a solution of 2 tablespoons of white vinegar to 1 gallon of water will help.
- Shampoo with a tar base will typically be ordered for scalp conditions involving scaling (seborrheic dermatitis or psoriasis).
- A specially constructed shampoo basin may be available in day care psoriasis centers or inpatient hospital dermatology wards.

PATIENT EDUCATION

Make sure the patient understands and is able to repeat the purpose of the therapeutic shampoo and the steps in the procedure. Ensure that he is also familiar with the nursing considerations.

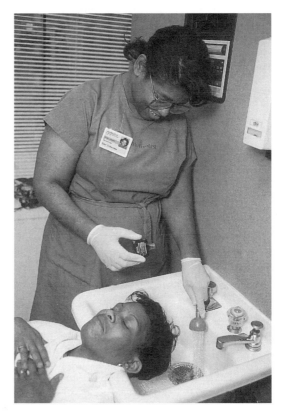

FIGURE 11-5
Patient being given a therapeutic shampoo.

SOAKS (COMPRESSES)

Soaks are applied to loosen eschar or crust, to decrease or prevent infection, to relieve itching, or to promote drying of moist areas.

SUPPLIES

Basin or tub large enough to immerse body part (if large area is to be treated)
Gauze pads—enough to cover the involved area (if small area is to be treated)
Solution ordered for soaks (Table 11-6)
Gloves

NURSING CARE

1. Obtain necessary solution.
2. Position patient comfortably; ensure privacy.
3. If area to be soaked is on an extremity:
   - Prepare ordered solution for soak at 35° C (95° F) in a basin of a size corresponding to area to be soaked.
   - Immerse area for approximately 20 minutes.
   - Remove.
   - Wipe with 4- × 4-inch gauze pad (without cotton filler) to debride, if debridement is ordered and desirable.
   - Apply a dry gauze dressing only if ordered, to prevent soilage of clothing or trauma.
   - Repeat soaks at ordered intervals (usually every 2 to 6 hours).

4. If area to be soaked is other than on hand, forearm, ankle, or foot:
   - Soak a 4- × 4-inch gauze pad (without cotton filler) in solution ordered for compresses.
   - Place plastic mat under area. This is for the protection of linen or furniture only. It is *not* used to wrap and occlude the area.
   - Apply dampened gauze to area for 10 to 40 minutes. Remove and redampen or add solution to pads using a sterile syringe approximately every 5 to 10 minutes.
   - Repeat at ordered intervals.
   - Apply dressing only if ordered. Otherwise, leave open.

NURSING CONSIDERATIONS

- Soaks are applied and *kept wet.*
- Gauze pads with cotton filler are not used for this procedure. The cotton may leave fibers in a wound, causing itching. In addition, these retain too much solution, which prevents evaporation and may cause maceration.

PATIENT EDUCATION

Go over instructions for application each time you provide care. Demonstrate the preparation of the solution and technique of application to the patient and family. If the patient does his own treatments, make frequent "spot checks" to be sure the technique is satisfactory.

Table 11-6

SOLUTIONS FOR SOAKS AND WET DRESSINGS

Solution	Purpose	Dilution
Tap water	To cool and relieve pruritus To loosen eschar and crusts	Tap water at approximately body temperature
Aluminum acetate (Domeborro, Aluwets, Burow's solution)	Same as tap water To promote drying To provide a mild antiseptic effect	Mix 1 tablet with 1 qt water (1:40) Mix 1 tablet with 1 pt water (1:20)
Potassium permanganate ($KMnO_4$)	Same as tap water To provide astringent effect To provide antimicrobial effect (especially effective against *Pseudomonas aeruginosa*)	Prepared by pharmacist at dilutions of ¼% to ½%
Normal saline	Same as tap water To provide isotonic solution to skin for cooling and antipruritic effect	0.9% saline solution
Silver nitrate ($AgNO_3$)	Astringent and antibacterial	Prepared by pharmacist at 1:1000 to 1:10,000

SUTURE REMOVAL

The object of suture removal is to provide atraumatic removal of stitches.

SUPPLIES

Suture removal kit *or*
Nontoothed forceps, scissors
Gauze
Alcohol pad

NURSING CARE

1. Check the wound to make sure that the edges appear well approximated and that there are no signs of infection (erythema, tenderness, purulent discharge).
2. Gently dab wound with alcohol to remove any crust.
3. Lift sutures slightly; cut with scissors.
4. Pull sutures out by exerting pressure *toward* the wound. *Never* remove sutures by pulling away from the wound, as this may cause dehiscence.
5. In cosmetically sensitive areas, adhesive tape strips may be placed across the wound to afford an additional week of external support.

NURSING CONSIDERATIONS

- Sutures may be removed in two separate visits if the wound appears to be incompletely healed.
- If significant infection exists, all or part of the wound may need to be opened to allow drainage.

PATIENT EDUCATION

Make sure the patient returns as directed for suture removal. After this procedure, emphasize to the patient that the wound is *not* yet totally healed. Caution the patient to favor the area, avoiding unnecessary stress or trauma, for at least 1 month.

ULTRAVIOLET LIGHT THERAPY: UVB

Ultraviolet light therapy is effective in inhibiting DNA synthesis, thereby decreasing the rapid epidermal cell turnover seen in psoriasis. UVB therapy also can produce mild erythema and desquamation, thereby reducing follicular plugging (acne).

SUPPLIES

Ultraviolet B (UVB) light source (sunlamp bulbs or units, fluorescent sunlamp bulbs FS40, or hot quartz light)
Drapes
Goggles

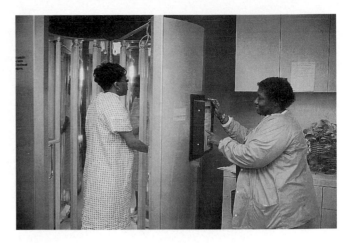

FIGURE 11-6
Patient ready to receive ultraviolet light therapy.

NURSING CARE

1. Explain to the patient the procedure, its desired effects, and possible complications.
2. Light treatment *must* be administered by a qualified person if potent hot quartz units or multibulb phototherapy boxes are used (Figure 11-6). Sunlamp units or small banks (4 to 8) of FS40 bulbs may be used at home.
3. Make sure the patient is not taking any photosensitivity medications (see the box on p. 166), because these might exaggerate the results of UVB therapy.
4. Determine the minimal erythema dose (MED) for light source to be used. This determines initial exposure time.
5. Goeckerman technique (psoriasis)
   - Patient applies a tar preparation (classically 2% to 5% crude coal tar) four times daily. More pleasant tar gels (Estar) or tar–salicylic acid gels (Baker's P & S Plus Gel) may be substituted.
   - In the morning before UVB therapy, remove tar by wiping with a towel or cheesecloth moistened with vegetable, cottonseed, or mineral oil.
   - Start UVB exposure, gradually increasing in duration, to maintain a mild sunburn effect.
   - Give a cleansing, emollient bath after therapy. Tar solutions may be added (see Balneotherapy, page 156).
   - Repeat applications of tar preparation and UVB therapy on a daily (or twice daily) basis.
   - A modified regimen involves applying topical corticosteroids during the day, with topical tar preparations applied only overnight.

COMMON PHOTOSENSITIZING DRUGS

The following drugs may interfere with UVB or UVA therapy:

Thiazide diuretics
Sulfonamides (antibiotics)
Sulfonylureas (antidiabetic)
Phenothiazines
Griseofulvins
Tetracyclines

6. Ingram technique
   - Patient has a tar bath in the morning (see Balneotherapy, page 156).
   - Start UVB exposure as in Goeckerman technique.
   - Apply anthralin paste to lesions with tongue blade or *gloved* fingertips.
   - Cover anthralin paste with dry dressing and leave in place 8 to 12 hours.
   - Repeat process daily.
   - Treat intertriginous areas with *dilute paste only* (less than ¼%).
7. Low-intensity UVB for acne
   - Position sunlamp unit at indicated distance from face or back (usually 12 inches).
   - Start therapy at 30 seconds and increase by 30 seconds at each daily treatment.
   - Maximum exposure time is about 15 minutes.
8. During all forms of UVB therapy, observe for marked erythema, blistering, or peeling as signs of overexposure. Should this occur, withhold therapy for 2 days and reinstitute at the last satisfactory level of exposure.
9. Care must be taken to protect the eyes. Gray or green polarized lenses should be worn during treatment.

NURSING CONSIDERATIONS

- The individual administering the treatments must be highly qualified. Improper administration may result in serious burns or failure of patient to progress properly.
- The intensity of the UVB rays can be affected by the source of the rays, the patient's distance from the rays, the time of exposure, or the patient's skin type.
- Disadvantages of the Goeckerman and Ingram therapies: They are messy and usually must be adminis-

tered on an inpatient basis. Treatment requires at least a 3-week stay.
- Careful attention must be given to ensure that the patient is not burned.
- Tar preparations must be applied with long, downward strokes in the direction of hair growth to help prevent folliculitis.
- Sensitivity to tar may occur. Observe for erythema, pruritus, or eczematous reaction.

PATIENT EDUCATION

Carefully discuss the procedure with the patient. Give instructions regarding proper application of topical treatments and the signs and symptoms of overexposure. Keep the patient informed of his progress.

ULTRAVIOLET LIGHT THERAPY: UVA

Administer psoralen (P) in combination with exposure to long-wave ultraviolet light (UVA). Psoralens increase sensitivity to UVA and the combination therapy decreases cell growth rate. Repeated PUVA (also called photochemotherapy) treatments usually lead to clearing of psoriasis in 10 to 20 treatments delivered over 4 to 8 weeks. PUVA therapy may also be helpful in the treatment of mycosis fungoides and atopic dermatitis.

SUPPLIES

Psoralen (usually 8-methoxypsoralen)
UVA light source
UV filtering goggles

NURSING CARE

1. Review the patient's history to make sure there are no contraindications (e.g., pregnancy; previous ionizing radiotherapy; history of arsenic ingestion; cataracts; history of skin cancer, including melanoma; immunosuppression; photosensitizing medication).
2. The physician should review potential risks with the patient. A signed statement of informed consent is recommended. Risks include cataracts, skin cancer, sunburn reaction, pigmentary abnormalities, failure of therapy.
3. Administer psoralen (8-methoxypsoralen) orally (0.5 to 0.8 mg/kg) 2 hours before phototherapy.
4. UVA exposure is determined by the amount of energy delivered. Initial dose is 0.5 joules/cm^2 to 3 joules/cm^2, depending on the patient's skin type and degree of natural pigmentation. UVA source

should be calibrated periodically to ensure proper energy output.

5. Treatment should be delivered only by a qualified, specially trained individual.

6. Shield the following areas during PUVA therapy:
   - Male genitalia
   - Depigmented skin
   - Areas of actinic damage

7. After therapy, monitor the patient for erythema or blistering. Report these symptoms of overexposure.

8. After therapy, exposed areas of the skin should be shielded from sunlight for 8 hours. UV-opaque sunglasses are advisable during all daylight exposure while treatment is in progress.

9. Patient receives therapy as ordered, usually two or three times weekly. After clearing, maintenance therapy may be required (optimum type or duration has not yet been determined).

10. Patient may require periodic blood tests, urinalysis, and ophthalmologic examination. Remind patient when it is time to undergo these diagnostic tests.

NURSING CONSIDERATIONS

- PUVA should not be administered by those unfamiliar with the subtleties of therapy and its many potential side effects
- Nausea may accompany psoralen administration.
- Although general guidelines exist, therapy must always be *individualized* and *closely monitored* by a physician.

PATIENT EDUCATION

The patient and family must be carefully informed of the risks and benefits of this therapeutic modality. Patient reliability and compliance are essential.

WET DRESSING

Wet dressings are applied to relieve inflammation, itching, and burning through evaporation. They are effective in removing scale, which allows for increased penetration of the topical medication (often corticosteroid) through dampening of the stratum corneum.

SUPPLIES

Ordered topical medication
Tap water (at body temperature)
Basin for dampening of dressings

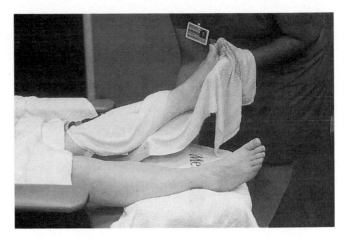

FIGURE 11-7
Applying wet dressing to patient's leg.

Dressings of approximate size to cover involved area (dressings must be clean but not necessarily sterile)
Towels, pieces of bath blanket, or other flannel wrap to wrap over the wet wraps for insulation
Safety pins or gauze ties to hold the dressings in place
Bath blankets to prevent chilling
Gloves

NURSING CARE

1. Explain the procedure to the patient.
2. Be certain that the patient's room is warm. Ensure privacy.
3. If wraps are to be applied to a large portion of the body, work with two people. It is necessary to work rapidly to prevent chilling.
4. Apply the appropriate topical medication.
5. Fill the basin with tap water approximately 35° C (95° F).
6. Soak the dressings. Squeeze out excess water. Dressings should be wet but not dripping.
7. Wrap an area with four to six layers of gauze. Immediately after wrapping, cover with a towel or a piece of flannel (Figure 11-7). Tie in place with gauze strips. Pull the bed covers over the wrapped area to insulate warmth. Start at the feet and move upward, covering as you go.
8. Leave dressings in place for approximately 3 hours. Remove and allow patient to move about and dry out before reapplying. Use the same dressings for 24 hours unless drainage is heavy.
9. If the patient must get out of bed while dressings are in place, monitor carefully for chilling. If he is to be up for more than a few minutes, remove the dressings. If the dressings are left in place without

CREATE DRESSINGS TO FIT ANY PART OF THE BODY

Face

Cut eyes, nose, and mouth openings in four to six layers of gauze burn dressings. Attach ties at the temple and chin.

Arms and legs

Use four to six layers of roller gauze. Burn dressings may also be used lengthwise on the arms or legs.

Hands

Cotton gloves may be used. The hands can also be wrapped with roller gauze.

Feet

Cotton socks or roller gauze may be used.

Total body

Combine the above dressings. The torso may be covered with large burn dressings pinned at the sides and shoulder.

adequate provision for conserving warmth, hypothermia can occur.

10. Seal soiled dressings in plastic bags before discarding.

NURSING CONSIDERATIONS

▪ The nurse should adapt the technique to the area treated. If wet dressings are ordered for one arm, for example, little heat loss will occur, and the patient can be allowed to ambulate.

▪ A damp stratum corneum absorbs steroid cream more readily. The potency of the cream may be increased 100 times by using it under a wet dressing.

▪ Creams, *not ointments*, are used under wet dressings. The water cannot readily penetrate through the ointment.

▪ Patients with red, itchy, acutely inflamed skin respond best to this treatment. Some conditions that respond well are exfoliative, erythroderma, psoriasis, and contact dermatitis.

▪ No plastic should be used over or around these dressings. The plastic prevents evaporation, leading to heat retention and maceration.

▪ Wet dressings reduce erythema by promoting vasoconstriction or decreasing vasodilation.

▪ Be certain to position the patient comfortably.

▪ Confining the patient to bed with wet dressings forces the patient to rest. This is a desirable side ef-

fect in patients with acute skin problems.

▪ At times tap water dressings alone may be ordered to cool the skin. A steroid cream or other topical medication is not always used under the dressing.

PATIENT EDUCATION

The patient and family are not usually able to do total body applications at home. The technique should be explained, however, because wet dressings may be ordered to cover a small area.

WET-TO-DRY DRESSINGS

Wet-to-dry dressings are similar to soaks. An additional major effect is tissue debridement, a technique particularly well suited to the treatment of ulcerative lesions.

SUPPLIES

Roller gauze (size is determined by area to be covered; 4-inch is commonly used)

Solution ordered for wet-to-dry dressings (see Table 11-6)

Safety pin, paper tape, or cloth strips to hold dressing in place

Gloves

NURSING CARE

1. Clean the ulcer well, using a whirlpool or soaking with ordered solution for 5 minutes and then rubbing with dry gauze pad.

2. Roll enough roller gauze to cover the ulcer twice. Leave attached to the roll.

3. Dampen this portion with ordered solution. Squeeze out excess. Roll should be damp, not dripping.

4. Fanfold the damp roller gauze over the ulcer twice. Pack into the ulcer.

5. Anchor in place with two turns of roller gauze around the limb. Do not apply too tightly, to avoid interfering with circulation.

6. Use a safety pin, tape, or gauze ties to hold in place. Do not tape to the skin, because the skin could become irritated or even denuded by the tape.

7. Leave the dressing in place for 6 to 8 hours.

8. After 6 to 8 hours, pull the dressing off. Do not dampen to loosen before removal, as this will prevent debridement. Explain to the patient that even though it may be uncomfortable to pull the dressing loose, the discomfort will be only momentary. If the patient experiences severe pain, consult the physician.

NURSING CONSIDERATIONS

- Wet-to-dry dressing means that the dressing is applied wet and *dries out* before removal. In drying, the dressing material sticks, and debridement is accomplished when the dressing is pulled off.
- Ulcers must have a clean base before granulation to allow healing; thus debridement of ulcerated or crusted lesions is essential.
- The wet-to-dry dressing must be thin enough to dry out. Otherwise, the dressing will not stick and cannot debride.
- If dressings are ordered too frequently to allow drying between applications, discuss this with the physician.
- Dry gauze pads without cotton filler are excellent for use in debridement. Wiping the ulcer base with this slightly abrasive cloth immediately after removal of the wet-to-dry dressing further removes unwanted exudate, crust, or eschar.

PATIENT EDUCATION

The patient must understand the underlying cause of the disease and the aims of treatment. Tell the patient why pulling the dry dressing off is necessary.

CHAPTER 12

Patient Teaching Guides

The responsibility for health and wellness lies with the individual and requires that the individual who strives for optimal health participate in health-promoting behaviors. Nurses can provide patients with the information they need to participate in making decisions regarding their own health care.

Written patient teaching guides can help reinforce patient teaching and encourage compliance. This chapter provides written handouts that can be photocopied and given to patients or their caregivers to take home and use for self-care.

Guides that explain measures for preventing skin cancer and avoiding acne breakouts are also included.

These teaching guides are not intended to replace direct teaching. They are to be used by the nurse to reinforce patient teaching and to encourage the patient's participation in and compliance with his or her own health care management.

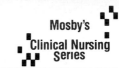
Acne

I have *some* blackheads and pimples, but not a lot. Does that still mean I have acne? What exactly is meant by "acne"?

Most people associate acne with being a teenager. It is, after all, a skin disease that commonly occurs during adolescence. At puberty hormonal activity increases, causing the oil (sebaceous) glands in the skin to become more active. These glands begin to secrete sebum, an oily substance that works its way up from the hair follicle to the skin's surface. Under normal conditions, the result is oily skin.

With acne, however, the pores of the skin (which serve as the glands' outlets) become plugged with sebum and other materials, such as pigment, dead cells, and bacteria. If the plug (comedo) remains just beneath the skin, it appears on the surface as a very small, round, whitish bump, often called a whitehead. When the comedo reaches the skin's surface, it looks like a black dot, commonly known as a blackhead. Both "blackheads" and "whiteheads" may remain in the skin for a long time. In some mild cases they are almost the only manifestation of acne. In other cases the plugged follicle may eventually burst, or the oily contents may seep into the surrounding skin. This causes inflammation. The result can be the formation of small or large, solid bumps, pus pimples, or even cavities containing a sticky fluid (cysts).

Will the acne go away?

Yes, acne usually goes away by itself eventually. In girls, it usually is at its worst from the ages of 14 to 17. In boys, it reaches its peak in the late teens. Thereafter, its severity decreases and it usually is gone by the early twenties. However, in some cases the deeper lesions may leave a small, depressed scar or a lumpy one. While the condition is active, it may alternately erupt and then improve.

I've been told that if I stop eating chocolate, my acne will clear up sooner.

Not necessarily. Although chocolate and French fries have often been named as the culprits, in truth foods seem to have little effect on the course of acne in most individuals. Of course, there are always exceptions. If you find that certain foods such as chocolate, fatty foods, or excessive amounts of milk and sweets seem to aggravate your condition, it is best to avoid them.

Does that mean that nothing affects acne? I read that makeup is bad for acne.

There are still outside influences that come into play. Probably foremost is stress. Severe or prolonged emotional tension may aggravate acne. That's why acne may often flare up before examinations or under the stress of a new experience, such as starting college. In girls, acne may also get worse shortly before menstruation because of the influence of hormonal factors.

Many cosmetics, especially some cleansing creams and moisturizers, have greasy bases that can aggravate acne. Even certain "brilliantines" used on the hair may drip onto the forehead and help cause blackheads. However, contrary to popular belief, cosmetics don't actually plug the pore or follicular opening. They apparently alter the cells of the follicle, making them more likely to stick together and form plugs or comedones. It is probably best to use as few cosmetics as possible, and when wearing cosmetics, use nonoily water-based types. (One exception might be the cosmetics used to cover acne blemishes. They are usually made of a liquid base and powder and seldom cause any harm.)

I've heard that vigorous scrubbing helps control acne.

If you feel your skin is especially greasy, wash your face *gently* two or three times a day with a mild soap. *But do not rub and scrub.* This may only make matters worse. A mature comedo is several millimeters deep. No amount of scrubbing will dislodge it, and the damage you are doing to the follicle may cause it to rupture, producing new inflammatory lesions. Other sources of friction, such as leaning on or rubbing an area of the skin affected with acne, or the pressure from helmets or tight collars, belts, or backpacks, may have similarly harmful effects.

Isn't it just an old wives' tale that pimples can't be squeezed? After all, doesn't that help get rid of them?

No, definitely not. They should be left alone. Your physician will decide what to do. In some cases he or she may drain them. This is a surgical procedure that requires experience and a special technique. But digging and squeezing with fingernails often result in scarring. In fact, more damage can be done to the skin by picking and squeezing than by the acne process itself.

What can I do to fight acne?

There are several steps you can take to help improve your acne. These include: eating a well-balanced diet; using as few cosmetics as possible; and washing your face gently several times a day with a mild soap. In addition, do *not* pick or squeeze pimples—that would probably do more harm than good. Also, be aware that *emotional stress* may cause acne to flare up. For the most part, sunshine seems to help diminish fully developed lesions and to decrease the emergence of new ones. This, together with the beneficial effects of outdoor exercise, sea bathing, and holiday relaxation, is probably the reason acne seems to improve during summer vacation. But, as a rule, individuals who tan benefit most from sunshine. Fair-skinned blonds and redheads often become worse. In addition, prolonged heat and humidity can even cause explosive outbreaks of severe cystic acne, usually called "tropical acne."

What can doctors do about acne?

Once your doctor has determined the type of acne you have, he or she will prescribe a treatment regimen suited to you. Topical medications that promote drying and peeling may be appropriate for many cases of acne. When additional control is required, your dermatologist may prescribe topical or oral antibiotics, or both. Oral antibiotics have proved to be very successful in reducing acne. Some of the newer acne therapies that are chemically related to vitamin A should be used only when other treatments, including oral antibiotics, don't work.

"Lamp treatments." These treatments are done with ultraviolet light and are sometimes used when plentiful sunlight is not available. This often causes mild peeling. If not done properly, this treatment can be dangerous to the eyes and skin.

Locally applied medications. These are usually used to reduce the skin's natural oils; they promote drying and mild peeling and help resolve acne lesions if applied diligently and in accordance with a doctor's instructions.

Antibiotics. Your doctor may prescribe either an antibiotic that is taken internally or one that is applied to the skin.

Aren't antibiotics just for infections? Does that mean acne is an infection?

No, it is not. It is not caused by the usual microbes that develop on dirty cuts or scratches. But some harmless microbes normally present in the sebaceous follicle can break down the fatty parts of the sebum into fatty acid substances that leak into the surrounding skin and cause inflammation. When your doctor suppresses these germs with antibiotics, there are fewer fatty acids and therefore fewer inflammatory acne lesions. Antibiotic therapy may be prolonged to be effective. Your doctor will make this decision. You should inform your doctor if any reactions develop.

What can I do about acne scars?

You have several choices. Scarring may disappear to a surprising extent simply with the passage of time. Dermabrasion, performed using local anesthesia, involves removing the outer layers of the skin with a rapidly rotating brush. There are other methods as well. Your doctor will recommend whether you might benefit from one of these procedures and if so, which one is best for you. It is important to understand that the success of any treatment for scars is dependent on the depth of the scar. No method can completely remove deep acne scars.

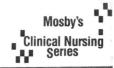
Cystic Acne

I had trouble with my complexion all through high school, but my parents always said it would go away with age. Well, it hasn't. Also, my acne is really severe. Aren't I too old for this?

You may have cystic acne—a severe and disfiguring skin disease. Although acne is considered by many to be a disease of adolescents, a person can be affected with acne into the thirties and forties. Males tend to get more severe acne than females.

How did my acne develop?

Acne develops in the oil-producing structures of the skin, called sebaceous glands, which are attached to hair follicles. During adolescence the sebaceous glands grow larger and produce more sebum (oil), especially in the face, chest, and back. Acne occurs when sebum's normal route to the skin's surface is blocked. In the case of cystic acne, the sebum builds up in the gland and mixes with dead cells. This accumulation finally ruptures the follicle wall, forming an inflamed cyst under the skin. Scarring usually results from these cysts.

When I first got acne in high school, I gave up chocolate and greasy foods. I've watched my diet for years, but it hasn't done any good.

Despite what most of us were told when were growing up, acne is not caused by a poor diet, dirt, or an oily complexion. Factors that may aggravate acne include emotional stress; fatigue; cosmetics; drugs, such as iodides and bromides; and certain foods (for certain individuals).

Can I do *anything* about my complexion?

You may benefit from a drug called isotretinoin (a common brand name is *Accutane*). Isotretinoin is used to treat severe cystic acne that has not responded to other treatments. It is important to follow the directions on the medication insert and from your doctor. Isotretinoin can have serious side effects. Call your doctor if you have any questions or develop any severe or troubling symptoms.

What do I need to know before taking isotretinoin?

If you have a family or personal history of medical conditions such as diabetes, liver disease, heart disease, or depression, please inform your doctor. Because isotretinoin is related to vitamin A, you should avoid taking vitamin supplements containing vitamin A, since they may add to the unwanted effects of the drug. Check with your doctor or pharmacist if you have any questions about vitamin supplements. Tell your doctor if you are sensitive to parabens, because they are used in the capsules. Advise your doctor if you are planning to undergo vigorous physical activity during treatment.

Blood tests will be necessary before and periodically during treatment to check your body's response to the drug. Be sure to take your medication as prescribed by your doctor. Read the prescription label on the package carefully. If there is anything you don't understand, ask your doctor or pharmacist to explain it to you.

Women patients must not take the drug until they are sure they aren't pregnant and must use effective contraception for at least 1 month before beginning and during treatment; never take this drug if you are pregnant or a nursing mother. Wait until the second or third day of your next normal menstrual period before beginning drug therapy. It is recommended that you return to your doctor every month for a pregnancy test. And if your menstrual period is delayed, stop taking isotretinoin and call your doctor.

Finally, you must continue using effective birth control for 1 month after your treatment has ended.

I've heard of isotretinoin. A friend of mine took it, and she said her complexion got worse, so she quit.

Like many patients, you may find that your acne will get worse during the early period of your treatment. Don't be alarmed; this condition usually is only temporary. However, if it does occur, please notify your doctor.

I also heard from my friend that she and a man in her office found out they were both being treated with isotretinoin, but their dosages were really different. Shouldn't there be some sort of standard dosage?

The dosage varies from patient to patient. The number of capsules you must take is determined specifically for you, by your doctor, for your particular case. Periodically during treatment your doctor may change the amount of medication you need to take. Make sure you follow the schedule you are given. If you miss a dose, do not double the next dose. If you have any questions, call your doctor. Be sure to return to your doctor as scheduled so he or she can check your progress.

What else can I expect during treatment?

During treatment you may experience some side effects, the most common of which are dry skin and lips. You may experience some redness of the eyes. Other reactions some patients have experienced are mild nosebleed, bleeding and inflammation of the gums, aches and pains, itching, rash, skin fragility, increased sensitivity to the sun, and peeling of palms and soles. These side effects usually are temporary and disappear when treatment is discontinued. If you develop any of these side effects, check with your doctor to determine if a change is needed in the amount of medication you are taking. Also, ask your doctor to recommend a lotion or cream if drying or chapping develops.

In some patients thinning of the hair has occurred. In rare cases this hair loss persisted after treatment was completed. A number of patients have also experienced decreased night vision. Because the onset can be sudden, you should be particularly careful when driving or operating any vehicle at night. If you wear contact lenses, you may find that you are less able to tolerate them during and after therapy. If you experience any visual difficulties, stop taking the medication and consult your doctor.

Are there any more serious side effects I should know about?

Yes, isotretinoin may cause some less common but more serious side effects. Be alert for any of the following: headaches, nausea, vomiting, severe stomach pain, diarrhea, rectal bleeding, blurred vision, a feeling of dryness in your eyes, mood changes, yellowing of the skin or eyes, or dark urine. If you experience any of these symptoms or other unusual or severe problems, stop taking the drug and notify your doctor immediately. These could be early signs of more serious side effects which, if left untreated, could result in permanent damage.

Finally, minimal bone changes have been detected by x-ray examination in some patients. The significance of these changes is not currently known.

What happens when I've "completed" the course of treatment? Will my acne return?

Like most patients, you may find that your skin continues to improve even after completing a course of treatment. In addition, most side effects clear up completely in a few days or a few weeks after treatment is discontinued. If your side effects persist longer than this, contact your doctor. Some patients have needed a second course of therapy for satisfactory results. If this is necessary for you, it may begin 8 or more weeks after the first course is completed.

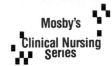
Rosacea

I thought I was getting acne, but my doctor said I have rosacea. What exactly is rosacea?

Rosacea (pronounced *rose ay shah*) is a disease that primarily affects the skin of the face. Skin affected by rosacea has one or more of the following features: a redness that looks like a blush, pimples, knobby lumps on the nose, and thin red lines caused by enlarged blood vessels.

How does it develop?

Rosacea develops slowly over time and often gradually worsens, but it can be treated. In most people the first sign is a persistent redness of the face, particularly on the cheeks and nose. This redness is caused by enlarged blood vessels under the skin of the face and looks like a blush or sunburn. The redness gradually becomes permanent and more noticeable. Facial skin may become very dry.

As the redness progresses, pimples may appear on the face. These pimples may be small, red, solid bumps (papules) or pus-filled bumps (pustules) that resemble the pimples of teenage acne. Because of this similarity, rosacea has been called "adult acne" or "acne rosacea." In rosacea, however, the pimples are not usually associated with the blackheads and whiteheads (comedones) seen in teenage acne.

Finally, small blood vessels in the skin of the face may become enlarged so that they are visible. These enlarged blood vessels look like thin red lines, and doctors call them telangiectasia.

I've always had a smattering of pimples or redness just like my dad, and it never really bothered me. But his nose often looks swollen. Is mine going to do that, too? Can I prevent that?

In some people, especially men, knobby bumps may develop on the nose. As the number of bumps increases, the nose may appear swollen. This condition is called rhinophyma. The eyes may become involved as rosacea progresses. The lids and mucous membranes can be affected. Without treatment, the course of rosacea can be progressive, with alternating periods of improvement and worsening of the condition.

Because of this gradual development, the characteristic appearance of rosacea may not be recognized in the early stages. Many people think that rosacea is a sunburn, a complexion change, or acne and do not seek treatment. This delay in seeking treatment is unfortunate, because most dermatologists believe that early treatment prevents worsening of rosacea and the formation of telangiectasia.

I admit my dad likes a beer now and then. I know drinkers tend to get rosacea, but I don't drink at all, and I still got it. Who's most likely to get rosacea, anyway?

Rosacea generally develops in adults and may affect anyone from 20 to 70 years of age. Rosacea seems to affect fair-skinned people more often than it affects people with dark skin, though it can affect all skin types. Most rosacea sufferers have a history of blushing more easily and more frequently than the average person.

Women are somewhat more likely to get rosacea than men; however, men are more likely than women to develop rhinophyma on the nose. It is unfortunate that rosacea symptoms have been associated with excessive alcohol consumption. Although alcohol usually aggravates rosacea, even people who never drink alcohol can develop the disease.

Rosacea is a long-term disorder and generally tends to worsen over time. However, in most people, the condition is cyclic—its symptoms come and go. Sudden increases in activity, called flare-ups, are common in rosacea.

So if it's not caused by alcohol, what does cause rosacea?

The cause of rosacea is unknown. Various theories have suggested that rosacea is caused by bacteria, mites, a fungus, a malfunction of connective tissue under the skin, or psychologic factors. However, none of these theories have been proven. It seems likely that there is no single cause of rosacea, and that it develops in individuals who are susceptible because of a variety of factors such as heredity, skin color, and skin structure. People who suspect that they have rosacea should consult their doctor.

I can tell by comparing my skin to my dad's that I have rosacea. Can I just treat this myself?

Self-diagnosis and treatment of conditions resembling rosacea are not recommended. Patients who self-treat rosacea using nonprescription acne medications often find that these products irritate the dry, sensitive skin of rosacea and that they often contain ingredients not appropriate for rosacea treatment.

What can a doctor do for me?

A variety of treatments are available that can decrease or eliminate the symptoms of rosacea. Some treatments may slow or even stop its progression. Medications can be used to control redness and to reduce the number of papules and pustules. Several different medications are available by prescription, including topical forms (applied to the skin) or oral forms (taken by mouth). A combination of forms can also be used. The most widely used topical medication is metronidazole, which has been proven effective. Oral antibacterial medications, such as tetracycline, are also commonly used.

I've heard that people have even had surgery for this. Is that true?

Surgery is a treatment usually reserved for correcting the nose enlargement in people with rhinophyma. Surgery with a fine electric needle or laser may also be used to eliminate enlarged blood vessels.

Short of surgery, what else besides medication can be used to help fight rosacea?

The doctor may recommend specific moisturizers, soaps, sunscreens, or other products as needed to improve the condition of the skin. Work with your doctor, too, to identify aggravating factors and avoid or reduce exposure to these factors. These include consumption of hot liquids, spicy foods, or alcohol; being exposed to extremes of heat and cold; exposure to sunlight; and stress. In general, actions that produce a facial flushing reaction or irritate facial skin should be avoided.

Proper use of a medication is very important to the success of a recommended treatment. Often, doctors prescribe two or more medications to be used at the same time. The following are some of the various types of rosacea medications: topical or oral antibacterial agents, topical steroids, special soaps or cleansers, moisturizers, and sunscreens of SPF 15 or higher. Approximately 70% to 80% of rosacea patients can expect significant improvement from oral or topical medications or a combination of both.

Is there a cure, then?

Unfortunately, there currently is no cure for rosacea; however, simple treatments can control rosacea and improve the appearance of the skin. Treatments may stop progression of the disease and, in some cases, reverse the progress. The important thing in treating rosacea is seeking medical care early and following the doctor's treatment program exactly.

How soon can I expect results from treatment?

Topical medications usually produce some improvement within 3 to 4 weeks but may take up to 2 months to show maximum improvement. Patience and faithful application of the medication as prescribed by your doctor improve the odds for successful treatment. Oral medications tend to produce results more quickly than topical medications.

The overall degree of improvement and the timing of the improvement are influenced by the stage of the disease when therapy is initiated and how well the patient follows the treatment program. Again, caution in avoiding aggravating factors is also important.

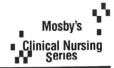

Mosby's
Clinical Nursing
Series

Preventing Skin Cancer

Can I prevent skin cancer?

To a certain extent. Although there is no sure prevention, you can significantly reduce your susceptibility by taking three simple steps: (1) ensure that you protect your skin from overexposure to the sun, both by limiting exposure and by using sunscreens; (2) get in the habit of examining your skin regularly, looking for changes in existing moles and for new "moles"; and (3) report any changes in your skin to your doctor.

However, "skin cancer" is too broad a term for a thorough discussion. Let's look at the two most prevalent types of skin cancer: basal cell carcinoma and malignant melanoma.

Basal cell carcinoma

What is basal cell carcinoma? Who's at risk for getting it?

Basal cell carcinoma is the most common type of cancer. It affects more than 400,000 Americans each year. One out of every four new cancers is a basal cell carcinoma, and one in eight Americans develops this skin cancer. The number of new cases each year has increased sharply in the past few decades. Until recently, those most often affected were older people, particularly men who had worked outdoors, but the average age of onset has steadily decreased. Anyone with a history of sun exposure can develop basal cell carcinoma, but those at highest risk have fair skin, light hair, and blue, green, or gray eyes. Those who work or spend a lot of their leisure time in the sun are particularly susceptible. Geographic location is also a factor. The closer to the equator, the higher the number of cases among fair-skinned individuals.

Although the disease is rarely seen in children, a teenager occasionally is affected. Skin specialists report that more and more people in their twenties and thirties—women especially—are being treated for this skin cancer.

What causes basal cell carcinoma?

The cause of 95% of all basal cell carcinomas is chronic overexposure to sunlight. That's why these tumors occur most frequently on exposed parts of the body—the face, ears, neck, scalp, shoulders, and back. In rare cases, however, tumors develop on nonexposed areas. In a few cases, contact with arsenic, exposure to radiation, and complications of burns, scars, vaccinations, or even tattoos are contributing factors.

What should I look for to determine whether I might have basal cell carcinoma?

Only a trained physician, usually a specialist in skin diseases, can decide for sure if that's what you have. You probably won't be able to tell just by looking. Basal cell carcinoma sometimes resembles noncancerous skin conditions such as psoriasis or eczema.

The five signs are: (1) a persistent, nonhealing, open sore that bleeds, oozes, or crusts and remains open for 3 weeks or longer; (2) a reddish patch or irritated area, usually on the chest, shoulders, or limbs, that may or may not itch or hurt; (3) a smooth growth with an elevated, rolled border and indented center; (4) a shiny bump or nodule that is pearly or translucent and that can be pink, red, white, tan, black, or brown; and (5) a scarlike area, white, yellow, or waxy, which often has poorly defined borders.

Examine your body regularly for signs of basal cell carcinoma, as often as once a month if you are at high risk. Be sure to include the scalp, backs of ears and neck, and other hard to see areas. (A full-length mirror and a handheld mirror can be very useful for the less visible parts of your body.) If you observe any one of these warning signs, other changes in your skin, or an unusual growth, see your doctor immediately.

Do I need a doctor's examination if everything looks fine to me?

The Skin Cancer Foundation recommends a total body skin examination by a qualified skin specialist, particularly for those at risk. The doctor will suggest the correct interval for follow-up visits, depending on your specific risk factors, such as skin type and history of sun exposure.

What if I am diagnosed with basal cell carcinoma? Then what?

After the doctor's examination, the diagnosis of basal cell carcinoma is confirmed with a biopsy. This procedure involves removing a small piece of tissue, which is examined in the laboratory under a microscope. If tumor cells are present, treatment—usually surgery—is required.

What can I expect from surgery?

Fortunately, there are several effective methods for eradicating basal cell carcinoma. The doctor's choice of treatment is based on the type, size, and location of the tumor and on the patient's age and general health. Treatment almost always can be performed on an outpatient basis, in the doctor's office, or at a clinic. With the various surgical techniques, a local anesthetic is used. Pain or discomfort during the procedure is minimal, and there is rarely any pain afterward. Surgery may take one of several routes: (1) excisional surgery, (2) electrosurgery, (3) cryosurgery, (4) Mohs surgery, and (5) laser surgery. Another effective treatment is radiation therapy.

In *excisional surgery,* the doctor removes the entire growth and an additional border of normal skin as a "safety margin." The tissue is sent to the laboratory to determine if all the malignant cells have been removed. *Electrocryosurgery* involves scraping the cancerous tissue from the skin with a curette (a sharp, ring-shaped instrument). An electric needle then burns a safety margin of normal skin around the tumor and at the base of the area that has been scraped. This technique is repeated several times to ensure complete removal.

In *cryosurgery,* tumor tissue is destroyed by freezing it with liquid nitrogen, without cutting the growth. This procedure may be repeated several times to ensure total destruction of malignant cells. Easy to administer, cryosurgery is the treatment of choice for patients who have bleeding disorders or an intolerance to anesthesia.

In *Mohs surgery* (microscopically controlled surgery), the physician removes very thin layers of the malignant growth, checking each layer thoroughly under a microscope. The excision is repeated as needed, until the site is tumor free. This method saves the greatest amount of healthy tissue and has the highest cure rate. It is frequently used for tumors that recur and for tumors in difficult locations (the nose, ears, and around the eyes).

In *laser surgery,* a laser beam is used to remove basal cell carcinomas surgically. To date, its role in skin cancer surgery, in relation to more conventional methods, needs to be more fully determined.

In *radiation therapy,* x-ray beams are directed at the malignant cells. Total tumor destruction generally requires a series of treatments, usually several times a week for a few weeks. Radiation therapy may be used with elderly patients or with individuals whose overall health is poor.

How easy are basal cell carcinomas to treat?

When removed promptly, basal cell carcinomas are easily treated in their early stages. The larger the tumor has grown, however, the more extensive the treatment needed. Although this skin cancer hardly ever spreads, or metastasizes, to vital organs, it can destroy surrounding tissue, sometimes causing considerable destruction and even the loss of an eye, ear, or nose.

Because all surgery involves cutting the skin, scarring is inevitable. When small skin cancers are removed, the result is usually cosmetically acceptable. After larger tumors are removed, reconstructive surgery involving a skin graft or flap may be required to cover the defect.

After the carcinoma is completely gone, what are my chances of a recurrence?

If you have one basal cell carcinoma, you have a greater chance of developing others in the years ahead. The damage your skin has already received from the sun cannot be reversed. When the first basal cell carcinoma is diagnosed, your physician may find another, or even several other tumors that you had not been aware of, on different areas of your skin.

Even though a basal cell carcinoma has been removed, another growth can develop in the same place or in a nearby area. These recurrences typically take place within the first 2 years after surgery. Basal cell carcinomas on the scalp, nose, and corners of the nose are especially troublesome. Should the cancer recur, the physician may recommend a different type of treatment the second time, because some methods (e.g., microscopically controlled surgery) are more effective than others in such cases.

Malignant melanoma

How common and how dangerous is malignant melanoma?

In the United States the incidence of malignant melanoma (cases per 100,000 people) is increasing at an alarming pace. For people born in 1930, the risk of developing malignant melanoma at some point in their lives was then one in 1,500. A baby born today has a lifetime risk of one in 135. Should this trend continue, by the year 2000 nearly one in 90 Americans will develop this form of skin cancer.

What effect does early detection have on the death rate from malignant melanoma?

Catching malignant melanoma early makes a big difference. For instance, consider this: The death rate for malignant melanoma has increased dramatically, doubling over the past 35 years. Yet in Queensland, Australia, where the first comprehensive education program on malignant melanoma was established for the medical profession and for the public, the death rate for this disease has begun to *decrease.* This decline in the death rate is especially impressive because the number of *cases* of malignant melanoma in Queensland, a very sunny part of the world, has continued to rise. This seems to prove that education and increased awareness—and thus a greater chance of early detection—can save lives.

Aren't some malignant melanomas more curable than others?

Yes. In fact, it is now possible to predict with considerable accuracy which malignant melanomas are curable and which are not. *Thickness* of the tumor is a key indicator. (With the aid of a microscope, thickness is measured from the outer surface of the skin to the deepest penetration of the tumor.) Malignant melanomas that are removed when they are less than 0.75 mm (about 1/32 of an inch) thick can be cured in virtually all cases, as long-term follow-up has repeatedly confirmed. However, progressively thicker malignant melanomas have correspondingly poorer prognoses.

Given these facts, it is essential that members of the medical profession, the allied health fields, and the general public be able to recognize early (thin) malignant melanomas, which can be so successfully treated.

Prevention seems to be the key, then. What can I do?

If you have all body surfaces examined regularly and see your doctor when you find changes in your skin, malignant melanoma can be stopped before it spreads to distant sites.

What are the key warning signs of malignant melanoma?

Any one or more of these changes occurring in a new or existing pigmented (tan, brown) area of the skin or in a mole may indicate the presence of a malignant melanoma:

- Change in size: especially sudden or continuous enlargement
- Change in color: especially multiple shades of tan, brown, dark brown, black; the mixing of red, white, and blue; or the spreading of color from the edge into the surrounding skin
- Change in shape: especially development of an irregular, notched border, which used to be regular

- Change in elevation: especially the raising of a part of a pigmented area that used to be flat or only slightly elevated
- Change in surface: especially scaliness, erosion, oozing, crusting, ulceration, or bleeding
- Change in surrounding skin: especially redness, swelling, or development of colored blemishes next to, but not part of, the pigmented area
- Change in sensation: especially itchiness, tenderness, or pain
- Change in consistency: especially softening or hardening

Really, what are my chances of developing malignant melanoma? Who's at risk?

In general, the risk of developing malignant melanoma increases as people grow older. In addition, individuals living in the Sun Belt (i.e., closer to the equator) are at greater risk. Caucasians are affected ten times more often than blacks. Beyond these general considerations, several specific factors identify individuals prone to develop this tumor. Some characteristics of people at high risk are:

- A family history of malignant melanoma
- A previous malignant melanoma
- Unusual moles (often larger than 1/4 inch, irregular in shape and multicolored),
- Fair skin, light hair, and light eye color, and a tendency to sunburn easily and tan with difficulty
- Large brown moles at birth
- A record of painful or blistering sunburns, especially when young
- Indoor occupations and outdoor recreational habits
- Considerable outdoor exposure, especially while living in sunny regions

---

THE ABCDs OF MALIGNANT MELANOMA

A = Asymmetry
B = Border (notched, scalloped, or indistinct)
C = Color (uneven, variegated—ranging from tan and brown to black to red and white)
D = Diameter (usually larger than 6 mm)

From the Skin Cancer Foundation.

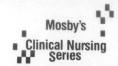

Contact Dermatitis

What is contact dermatitis?

The word "dermatitis" means inflammation of the skin. Contact dermatitis is a particular type of skin inflammation caused by contact with certain substances found in the environment. The inflammation appears as redness, swelling, itching and, at times, blistering. In severe cases the condition may cause considerable discomfort, and occasionally it can even interfere with a person's ability to work.

What substances cause contact dermatitis?

The most common cause of contact dermatitis in the United States is probably something with which you are quite familiar—the poison ivy plant (and its relatives, poison oak and poison sumac). Another very common cause is nickel, which is widely used in costume jewelry, in metal clasps on women's underclothing, and in watch bands. Some other causative substances are detergents, cleaning compounds, and cosmetics.

Contact dermatitis is extremely common. At work, at home, in the garden, and elsewhere we are exposed to innumerable chemicals, metals, plants, and other substances. There is always the possibility that some of these may cause a reaction in susceptible individuals.

How does contact dermatitis develop?

For one thing, it can develop by means of *irritation*—chemical (such as a detergent) or mechanical (such as fiberglass or wool particles). If the irritant is strong (e.g., an accidental spill of lye on your hands) a single exposure causes a violent inflammatory reaction. The skin becomes itchy, red, and swollen and often develops tiny water blisters, called "vesicles," or even large blisters. If the irritant is weak, only repeated exposure, such as repeated exposure to soaps and detergents, will show the damage. When the dermatitis develops slowly in this manner, the skin shows dull red, itchy, thickened patches, at times accompanied by blistering. If the inflammation is located on areas where the skin bends, such as the fingers, painful cracks may develop.

A second way contact dermatitis develops is by *sensitization.* This means that the first contact with the substance causes no immediate trouble. But the exposure "sensitizes," or changes, the sensitivity of the skin. Then, whenever the skin is subse-quently exposed to the same substance, even slightly, it becomes inflamed. This is called an "allergic reaction." A perfect example of this is poison ivy dermatitis.

Another uncommon but interesting mechanism in the development of contact dermatitis is what is called "photoallergy." This means that some chemicals contained in perfumes, soaps, or medications may "sensitize" the skin to the sun's rays. Afterward, when the person is exposed to sunlight, a rash develops. The types of skin reaction caused by sensitization are the same as those caused by irritants.

Who is likely to get contact dermatitis?

Actually, anybody can. But naturally, the greater a person's activity and exposure, the greater the risk of developing it. People whose daily work requires them to handle soaps, detergents, cleaning fluids, sprays, and other kinds of irritating substances are likely candidates; this sort of condition is sometimes called "industrial dermatitis."

My sister has had contact dermatitis on her face, but I always get it on my hands. Are some parts of the body more at risk than others?

Yes. The hands are most prone to developing contact dermatitis, because they get actively into everything. But the face, the feet, and the rest of the body are susceptible, too. The face is often affected by hygienic and cosmetic products such as soaps, shampoos, creams, lipsticks, hair sprays, and shaving creams. The feet may be affected by materials used to make shoes. Body rashes usually are caused by clothing, bedding, or laundry chemicals. Sometimes airborne substances may cause severe rashes involving the face and exposed parts. An example of this would be the dermatitis that develops in people sensitive to poison ivy when they are exposed to the smoke of burning poison ivy leaves.

How do I find out what causes *my* dermatitis?

In some cases the location of the rash may suggest the cause. For instance, a rash around the wrist is easily identified as caused by a watchband, and rashes in the armpits often are due to deodorants. But in most cases, identifying the cause is not that simple. Your doctor will ask you many questions about what you do and what you've handled at home and in your work. You should try to help by remembering all your activities, such as gardening, painting, using metal polishes, and touching plants, that may have caused irritation of your skin. You should mention if you've recently changed employment or recently been on vacation away from your usual environment. Confirming and sometimes even detecting the specific substance that caused the rash may require further study and patch tests.

What are patch tests?

A patch test involves applying to the skin a small amount of the material suspected of causing the rash. This patch of substance usually is placed on the healthy skin of the forearms or back, covered with a small bandage, and left on the skin for 24 to 48 hours. (If you feel intense itching or burning from the patch, it should be removed immediately.) A positive patch test shows redness, swelling, or even blistering of the small area where the substance was in contact with the skin. Never try a patch test yourself; it may cause serious trouble.

What kind of treatment can I expect, once the cause of my dermatitis has been determined?

If the cause of your rash is identified, you will, of course, be instructed to avoid further contact with it. If the specific cause cannot be found, all possible causes should be eliminated. Your treatment will depend on the degree of inflammation of the skin. Local treatment (medication you apply to the skin) may range from wet dressings to lotions, cortisone-derivative cream or ointment, or other measures. If your physician feels that increased hydration of the skin may be beneficial, he or she may also prescribe some sort of moisturizing preparation or medication with a moisturizing base. In selected cases the doctor may also prescribe or administer by injection medications such as antihistaminics or a cortisone derivative. These are aimed at reducing the itching and inflammation.

What results can I expect, once treatment is started?

If the cause of your rash is identified and you avoid further contact with the substance, appropriate treatment will stop the itching and eventually cause the rash to disappear. In the case of "one time" exposure to strong irritants or sensitizers (such as poison ivy), the skin rash probably will persist for about a week and then gradually subside. It will heal with peeling and is not likely to leave any sort of scar. Rashes stemming from repeated contact (usually of a dry, thickened appearance) tend to be more persistent. The rash heals more slowly, often leaving a patch of darker skin. This, however, eventually fades.

What else can I do to help the rash heal faster and to keep it from coming back?

First of all, don't scratch the rash. Second, follow the doctor's directions: avoid contact with the causative substance, and use the prescribed medication. Also, follow instructions regarding hygiene and protection of the affected area.

Third, try to avoid contact with *other* chemicals that may be irritants. Inflamed skin is more susceptible to irritation by other agents. And once you have had contact dermatitis, it may be wise to be extra careful with new substances. If contact with possibly troublesome substances is unavoidable, protect your hands with vinyl or plastic gloves, or use whatever other protective method your doctor recommends.

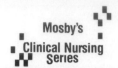
Atopic Dermatitis

What is atopic dermatitis?

The word "dermatitis" means inflammation of the skin. Atopic dermatitis is a particular type of skin inflammation that seems to occur in individuals with a family history of allergic conditions ("atopy"). The rash develops in a characteristic pattern on the body and is accompanied by itching. The condition is fairly common and is believed to occur in as many as 5% of the country's population—that's 11 million people! So you're not alone.

What causes atopic dermatitis?

The exact cause of atopic dermatitis is still unknown, but we do know that the tendency to develop atopic dermatitis is inherited, and there is an assumed allergic connection. For instance, such allergic conditions as asthma, hay fever, or hives often run in the family of a person with atopic dermatitis. Occasionally atopic dermatitis in infants is believed to be traceable to a sensitivity to milk, orange juice, or some other food. Nevertheless, exactly *how* allergy contributes is still a mystery.

My cousin claims she's had atopic dermatitis since she was an infant. Is her skin disorder the same thing as mine?

Atopic dermatitis often (but not always) starts in infancy, usually from the age of 2 to 6 months, in the form of "infantile eczema." The baby shows red, glazed blotches oozing a clear fluid. This later dries, forming superficial, itchy scabs on the face or a great part of the body, or both. In about half of the infants and toddlers with atopic dermatitis, the skin problem clears up by the age of 2 and never returns. Clearing may occur in adolescence, or the condition may persist into adulthood.

As the person grows older, the rash usually seems to shrink and become localized (limited) to certain parts of the body. It is found mainly on the bend of the elbows and knees and on the back of the hands and top of the feet. The sides of the neck and face, especially the eyelids, often are affected, and the skin becomes dry, itchy, thickened, and leathery. The more the affected person scratches, the thicker the skin gets. In general, the condition tends to improve with the passage of time; most patients, although certainly not all, are free of the eruption by age thirty.

How can I tell if I have atopic dermatitis?

Usually your family medical history, your own personal history, and a skin examination are enough to help your doctor make a diagnosis. Sometimes skin tests for specific allergies can help. Your physician probably will call the condition "atopic dermatitis," but you may hear it referred to by other names as well, such as "atopic eczema" or "generalized neurodermatitis." This simply suggests that it is an inflammation of the skin that can be affected by stress or nerves.

Nerves? What do nerves have to do with my skin?

"Nerves" or stress can make the condition worse. A flare-up of the disease can be triggered by anxiety, conflict, or stress. Some women have flare-ups just before their menstrual period; this may be due to the general stress that often precedes menstruation.

Is it true that climate can affect it, too?

Absolutely. Extreme hot or cold temperatures often make the condition worse. High humidity, as a rule, also aggravates the condition. That's why you may feel better in a warm climate like that of the southwestern United States. You may find, too, that you are sensitive to sudden changes in temperature. For instance, you may be suddenly more uncomfortable after undressing, or after leaving a bath, because both situations lead to a sudden lowering of skin temperature.

What else can affect atopic dermatitis?

Your skin may become further irritated and itchy from the use of detergents, solvents, certain ointments, or other medications. This is called "contact dermatitis." It is actually only a minor complication and can easily be controlled by your doctor.

What other complications should I watch out for?

Sometimes atopic dermatitis may become infected by bacteria, yeast (fungi), or viruses. This is called "secondary infection." Bacterial secondary infection is the most common and often occurs as the result of scratching. The rash gets angry red with pus, pimples, and scabs. If this occurs, most likely your doctor will prescribe antibiotics that will rapidly control the infection.

A more serious complication can be caused by certain viruses. The "cold sore" virus (herpes simplex) and the one used in the vaccination against smallpox may cause a severe rash with fever. If this happens, contact your doctor immediately.

Smallpox vaccinations are rarely given any longer in this country, but to avoid such a complication, you should avoid direct contact with any person who has been recently vaccinated for smallpox or any person with active cold sores.

What can I expect from treatment?

Unfortunately, there is no medication that will permanently eliminate the disease. The main objective in treating atopic dermatitis is to decrease the skin eruption and relieve the itching. Since the condition of atopic dermatitis changes from stage to stage, your doctor will note the stage of the eruption and the degree of inflammation in choosing the best medication for you.

What kind of medication?

Topical medications are the primary treatment for atopic dermatitis, including cool compresses, cortisone-derivative cream or ointment, topical antibiotics (with infection), and others. In certain stages of the condition, the skin can be excessively dry. For this reason, your doctor may also prescribe some sort of moisturizing preparation or a medication with a moisturizing base.

So there are no pills for atopic dermatitis?

Certain internal medications, called antihistamines, may help control itching. Although they are not sleeping pills, they may cause some degree of drowsiness and thus may help you sleep better at night. In selected cases, tranquilizers or other sedatives may be prescribed. On occasion, a derivative of cortisone may be prescribed for internal use. Your doctor will decide if you need it, how much you need, and how long to take the medication.

What else can I do to avoid flare-ups?

Most important is to follow your doctor's instructions about medications and general hygiene. In addition, you should avoid contact with substances you know cause itching, such as soaps, detergents, some colognes, dust, fur, wool, synthetic fabrics, or any type of scratchy clothing. In winter, wear cotton underwear or a cotton shirt or blouse under your sweater.

Bathing too frequently or with very hot water can increase dryness and itching. When you wash, do not use a scrub brush. And when you dry, dry by patting, not rubbing briskly. Try to keep the temperature and humidity in your home fairly constant, possibly using an air conditioner or vaporizers when needed. During dry winter or humid summer months, a change of environment may also be beneficial.

Don't scratch! This will only make things worse by breaking and damaging the skin; causing bleeding; producing change such as redness, scaling, and thickening; and contributing to possible infection. Perhaps the most important measure is a good mental outlook. Often, the more you worry, the worse it gets. And remember: eventually, the disease may burn itself out.

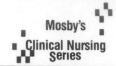
Scabies

What is scabies?

Scabies is a highly contagious skin disease caused by a mite too small to see with the naked eye. The most common symptom is a rash, which can appear anywhere on your body but usually is found on the hands, breasts, armpits, genital area, and waistline. It usually itches intensely at night.

Who is most likely to get scabies? How does it spread?

Scabies can affect men, women, and children of all ages. It is easily spread from person to person by close physical contact, such as between family members, sexual partners, and children playing at school.

How do I get rid of scabies?

A prescription skin cream of 5% permethrin can eliminate the scabies and relieve the itching as well, while the healing gets under way. The cream should be thoroughly and gently massaged into all skin surfaces from your head to the soles of your feet. Be sure that infants and elderly patients are treated for scabies on the neck, scalp, temple, and forehead. The cream should be left on overnight for 8 to 14 hours and removed the next morning by bathing and shampooing.

Do I only have to apply the cream to the rash itself?

No. It is extremely important to put permethrin on every square inch of your body; not just where the rash is. That includes applying it under your fingernails and toenails, around the nail beds, between your fingers and toes, and in the cleft of your buttocks and genital area. If you wash your hands or any other area during the treatment period, new cream must be reapplied immediately.

I'm relieved to find something that will relieve the itching, but are there any uncomfortable side effects with permethrin?

Yes, in some patients itching, mild burning, and/or stinging may occur after application. Also, keep the cream away from your eyes. If any cream accidentally gets in your eyes, flush them with water immediately.

Anything else I should know about treatment, or is using the cream enough?

To avoid getting scabies all over again, everyone affected in your family or relationships should be treated at the same time, as directed by your doctor.

In addition, as you undergo treatment, be sure to change your clothes and bed linens and have all the affected articles washed at the same time on a hot cycle or professionally dry cleaned. It is not usually necessary to clean sweaters, jackets, furniture, drapes, or rugs. And be sure to see your doctor for a follow-up examination.

How long will I still be contagious once treatment has begun?

You will not usually be contagious after one treatment if these instructions and your doctor's directions have been followed carefully. The scabies mites will be gone in a matter of days; however, the rash and itching may persist up to 4 weeks after treatment. This is rarely a sign of treatment failure and is not necessarily an indication for retreatment. If itching is excessive or if irritation persists, consult your doctor.

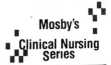
Psoriasis

What is psoriasis?

Psoriasis is a common, recurring condition in which the skin develops red patches of various sizes, covered with dry, silvery scales, which quickly progress into dry plaques. Plaques sometimes develop pustules or small elevations of skin that produce pus. Most often psoriasis affects the scalp, the trunk of the body, and the outer side of the arms and legs, especially the elbows and knees. The palms and soles may also be involved. Fortunately, the face is usually spared.

What causes psoriasis?

We don't know what causes psoriasis, but we do know something about its development. The "epidermis," or outer layer of our skin, is constantly manufacturing new cells and shedding old ones. In psoriasis, it is thought that some defect of the enzymes of the skin alters this process. Normally, the development of new cells, which grow out from the lower basal layer toward the skin's surface, takes about 28 days. In psoriasis, this process is speeded up to 4 or 5 days. Instead of shedding inconspicuously, the outer cells form scales, which remain heaped up on the skin.

My grandmother had psoriasis, and now I do. Does this mean my children will automatically get this? Do people only get it through heredity?

There are some factors that seem to determine who is most likely to get psoriasis, and possibly the most important of these is indeed heredity. Often, a person with psoriasis has a parent or grandparent who also had the condition. In terms of probability, it has been estimated that a person with one affected parent has about a 10% chance of also being affected. Having two parents with psoriasis increases the chance to about 30%.

Although the tendency to develop psoriasis is inborn, race is also an important factor. Basically, psoriasis is a disease of Caucasians. It has an incidence of 2% to 4% among the white population in the United States and an even higher incidence in Europe.

How is psoriasis diagnosed? Isn't dandruff, after all, a form of psoriasis?

The white, silvery scales of psoriasis are so distinctive that it is relatively easy to diagnose. When the scales are not evident (as often occurs in people who bathe and scrub frequently), scratching the lesions will show the typical scales. Further scratching will show bleeding pinpoints, which are also characteristic of the disease. In about a quarter of all cases, the nails may also show peculiar changes, such as pitting, thickening, and turning yellowish or opaque, with ridges and scales heaped up at the free edge. These characteristics, plus the scaly patches on the body and the family history, aid in diagnosis. In cases of doubt, a biopsy using local anesthesia can confirm suspicions.

Dandruff is not the same thing as psoriasis. Dandruff covers most of the scalp, whereas psoriasis occurs in patches, with normal scalp in between. Passing your fingers over your scalp, you cannot feel dandruff; you only see the flakes on your shoulders. But you can feel the psoriatic lump caused by heaped up scales held together by the hairs.

I have psoriasis on my scalp. Does this mean I'm going to lose my hair?

No, not at all. Some hairs may break when squeezed by the scales, but the roots, deep down in the skin, are not affected. Once your scalp is clear, the hair will grow as healthy as before.

A friend told me she had an aunt whose psoriasis was caused by "nerves," and that maybe with stress management I could get rid of it altogether. Is that true? I guess I am a little high strung sometimes.

"Nerves" don't cause psoriasis and seldom trigger the first attack. But it is true that they can aggravate and perpetuate the disease. For instance, the patches or plaques of psoriasis may clear up during a restful vacation on a sunny beach. . . only to relapse when you return to the pressures and stress of a responsible job.

Someone else told me psoriasis is caused by allergies or strep throat. Is that an old wives' tale? I don't remember ever having strep throat or allergies.

Streptococcal sore throat in children often triggers an attack of psoriasis. In addition, an adult with chronic psoriasis may develop a flare-up after a strep throat infection. This reaction develops about 2 weeks after the infection, which may indicate that it is of an allergic nature. However, this is the only evidence that allergy may play a role in psoriasis.

My psoriasis disappeared altogether during pregnancy. Does that mean hormonal changes can affect it?

Yes. We know that there is some relationship between psoriasis and hormonal changes in different stages of life, but we don't know exactly what it is. In both men and women, psoriasis develops more frequently or gets worse at puberty, and there is another smaller peak at menopause. Often the lesions improve or disappear during pregnancy, only to reappear after childbirth.

Can changing my diet improve my condition?

Currently, diet is thought to play only a small role in psoriasis. Some dermatologists like their patients to reduce their intake of greasy food. In general, obese individuals respond better to therapy if they lose weight. And some people have flare-ups following an excess of alcoholic drinks. In general, a well-balanced diet is advisable in people with psoriasis, just as it is in everyone.

My children and I spent a summer in Arizona, and my skin improved dramatically. When I came home, it flared up right away. What is the role of climate and sunlight?

Hot, humid environments tend to make bad cases of psoriasis worse. In contrast, sunlight and dry, sunny climates, as a rule, are helpful, particularly in mild cases. In fact, in temperate climates, where sunlight is not available all year, artificial ultraviolet light frequently is used in the treatment. One time-tested, effective therapy combines the application of a preparation containing coal tar with exposure to an ultraviolet lamp. Another treatment that has provided encouraging results combines a substance taken by mouth (methoxsoralen) with exposure to a special source of ultraviolet light.

I thought so. So I should sunbathe frequently?

Only if you're careful. Exposure to sunlight or artificial ultraviolet light should always be done cautiously and in moderation. The exposure should be just enough to cause a mild redness the first time, then gradually and carefully increased on subsequent occasions. Prolonged exposure to sunlight may do considerable harm, especially if you are fair skinned. A severe sunburn may actually cause the psoriasis to spread all over the sunburned areas. That's because in some people, superficial injury to the normal skin, such as sunburn, may cause a patch of psoriasis to develop at the injury site.

What is the treatment for psoriasis?

In general, the course of psoriasis is unpredict-able and irregular. Nevertheless, with treatment the plaques frequently disappear entirely, or the disease retreats to a few spots on elbows or knees. Treatment options include: opical steroids; tar and ultraviolet light; methoxsoralen and ultraviolet light; lubrication with bland emollient; and, in severe recalcitrant cases, chemotherapy or etretinate. These spots or some slight pitting on the nails may remain minimal for years. Then, under severe stress or for some other, unknown reason, the rash may again blossom over the body . . . again requiring aggressive treatment to hasten its retreat. This erratic course may go on for years, often with long periods of freedom from skin trouble.

Is it true that psoriasis is incurable?

It is not possible to make psoriasis disappear and never come back, but it is possible to make the *symptoms* disappear. Of course, individuals with a tendency to psoriasis may develop new lesions months or years later, just as those with a tendency to colds may develop another one anytime in the future.

What kind of treatment will my doctor prescribe?

Naturally, your doctor knows best what is likely to help your particular case. He or she will study your psoriasis and choose the measure or measures that seem most suitable. Routine measures may include local preparations made from coal tar or cortisone derivatives that you massage into your skin. You may even be told to cover some areas of your body or leave them uncovered. Your doctor may also inject medication into a psoriasis plaque to speed recovery.

What can I do to help get rid of psoriasis?

First and foremost, you should cooperate fully with your doctor. Set aside a certain amount of time daily for treatment. Massage the prescribed preparations into the affected skin without fail and in accordance with your doctor's directions.

Try not to scratch. Any itching will probably be minimal, and your doctor can prescribe a locally applied cream or ointment to relieve it. Avoid quick "cures," often widely advertised, and avoid situations of stress that may aggravate your condition. Finally, don't get discouraged if progress is slow. If you are more stubborn than the disease, you can control it, make it disappear or, at least, keep it to a minimum. Remember: You don't have to allow it to run your life!

Treatment of psoriasis with etretinate

What should I be especially careful of while taking this drug?

If you have a family or personal history of medical conditions such as diabetes, liver disease, heart disease, or depression, please inform your doctor. Etretinate is related to vitamin A. Therefore, you should avoid taking vitamin supplements containing vitamin A, because they may add to the unwanted effects of the drug. Check with your doctor or pharmacist if you have any questions about vitamin supplements.

You should also tell your doctor if you are sensitive to parabens, since they are used in these capsules. Call your doctor if you have any questions or experience any severe or troubling symptoms. If you are allergic to any foods or medications, let your doctor know. It could be very important. Blood tests will be necessary before and periodically during treatment to check your body's response.

If you are a woman, you must not take etretinate until you are sure you are not pregnant, and you must use an effective form of birth control for at least 1 month before beginning and during the course of therapy. It is strongly recommended that you have a pregnancy test no more than 2 weeks before beginning treatment with etretinate. Then, wait until the second or third day of your next normal menstrual period before beginning therapy. Again, never take etretinate if you are pregnant or a nursing mother.

Finally, because etretinate remains in your body for a prolonged period, you must continue using an effective form of birth control after your treatment has ended. The period of time that pregnancy must be avoided after treatment is concluded has not been determined. Consult your doctor before you stop using birth control.

What can I expect during treatment with etretinate?

Like many patients, you may find that your psoriasis worsens during the first month of treatment. Occasionally patients experience more redness or itching at first; these symptoms usually subside as treatment continues.

You may have to wait 2 or 3 months before you realize the full benefit of etretinate. In the first few weeks—perhaps before you see any healing—you may begin to have some side effects. You can expect to find peeling of the fingertips, palms, and soles; chapped lips; dry skin and nose; loss of hair; eye irritation; itching; excessive thirst; bone or joint pain; rash; fatigue; a red, scaly face; sore mouth; and fragile skin. If you develop any of these side effects, check with your doctor to determine whether the dosage of your medication needs to be changed. Also, ask your doctor to recommend an emollient if drying or chapping develops.

Most patients experience some degree of hair loss, but the condition varies among patients. The extent of hair loss that you will experience and whether your hair will return after treatment cannot be determined.

A number of patients have had a decrease in night vision. Because the onset can be sudden, you should be particularly careful when driving or operating any vehicle at night. If you wear contact lenses, you may find that you are less able to tolerate them during and after therapy. If you experience any visual difficulties, stop taking etretinate and consult your doctor.

Are there any more serious side effects I might expect?

Yes. You should be aware that etretinate may cause side effects such as headaches, nausea, vomiting, blurred vision, mood changes, yellowing of the skin or eyes and/or dark urine, a persistent feeling of dryness of the eyes, aches or pains in bones or joints, or difficulty in moving. Bone changes have been detected on x-rays in some patients taking etretinate. The significance of these changes is not currently known.

In any case, if you experience these or any other unusual or severe problems, discontinue etretinate and notify your doctor immediately. These may be the early signs of more serious side effects which, if left untreated, could result in permanent effects.

My prescribed dosage is a lot different from my neighbor's. Has my doctor given me the right amount?

The dosage of etretinate varies from patient to patient. The number of capsules you must take is determined specifically for you, by your doctor, for your particular case. Periodically during treatment your doctor may change the amount of medication you take. Make sure you follow the schedule you are given, and always take this drug with food. If you miss a dose, do not double the next dose. If you have any questions, call your doctor. Be sure to return to your doctor as scheduled. He or she will want to check your progress.

Your doctor will generally stop your treatment when your skin has sufficiently cleared. You may experience some degree of relapse within a few months after you stop your therapy. This is common. If you notice a worsening of your condition, however, contact your doctor. Subsequent courses of treatment will generally produce the same response as the first course.

CHAPTER 13

Drug Therapy for Skin Disorders

ANTIBACTERIAL AGENTS

Bacitracin (Baciguent: OTC ointment, 500 U/g)

Indications: Infection prophylaxis in minor cuts, burns, and skin abrasions. Also for treatment of superficial bacterial infections of the skin caused by susceptible organisms, primarily gram negative.

Administration: Apply to affected area one to three times daily.

Precautions/contraindications: Contraindicated in cases of prior sensitization. For external use only. Do not use in eyes or over a large area of the body. Do not use for more than 1 week unless directed by physician.

Side effects/adverse reactions: May cause allergic contact dermatitis.

Nursing considerations: Unless otherwise directed, cleanse wound before applying. Watch for allergic reaction, burning, swelling, redness, or worsening of condition. Store at room temperature. With prolonged use, watch for superinfections and overgrowth of nonsusceptible organisms, especially fungi. Notify physician if condition worsens.

Chloramphenicol (1% cream) (Chloromycetin)

Indications: Infection prophylaxis and treatment of superficial bacterial infection of the skin caused by susceptible organisms.

Administration: Apply to affected area two to four times daily.

Precautions/contraindications: Contraindicated with hypersensitivity or prior sensitization; do not use in eyes or over a large area of the body. For external use only.

Side effects/adverse reactions: Blood dyscrasia (bone marrow hypoplasia, including aplastic anemia and death); itching, burning, urticaria, vesicular, maculopapular dermatitis, and angioneurotic edema have occurred in sensitive patients.

Nursing considerations: Unless otherwise directed, cleanse wound before applying. Watch for allergic reaction, burning, swelling, redness, or worsening of condition. With prolonged use, watch for signs and symptoms of blood dyscrasias. Watch for superinfections and overgrowth of nonsusceptible organisms, especially fungi. Notify physician if condition worsens. Store at room temperature.

Chlortetracycline HCl (OTC 3% ointment) (Aureomycin)

Indications: Infection prophylaxis and treatment of superficial bacterial infection of the skin caused by susceptible organisms; pyogenic skin infections.

Administration: Apply to affected area two to four times daily.

Precautions/contraindications: Contraindicated with hypersensitivity to this drug. Pregnancy category D, lactation. May stain clothing.

Side effects/adverse reactions: Rash, urticaria, stinging, burning, dry skin, photosensitivity. Will cause tooth discoloration if used while teeth are being formed in gums; will not discolor existing teeth.

Nursing considerations: Administer enough medication to completely cover lesions. After cleansing with soap and water before each application, dry well. Store the ointment at room temperature in a dry place, in light-resistant container.

Evaluate the patient for allergic reaction: burning, stinging, swelling, redness. Evaluate the therapeutic response: decrease in size and number of lesions.

Teach patient/family:

- To watch for superimposed infections
- To use medical asepsis (hand washing) before, after each application
- To apply with glove to prevent further infection
- To avoid use of OTC creams, ointments, lotions unless directed by physician
- To avoid squeezing or poking lesions or spreading may occur
- To notify physician if condition worsens, or rash, irritation, or swelling occurs
- To avoid sunlight or ultraviolet light
- That skin may be stained

Clindamycin Phosphate (1% solution, gel) (Cleocin)

Indications: Treatment of acne vulgaris; also used to treat rosacea.

Administration: Apply a thin film to affected area twice a day.

Precautions/contraindications: Contraindicated with hypersensitivity to clindamycin or lincomycin, and with history of regional enteritis, ulcerative colitis, or antibiotic-associated colitis. For external use only.

Side effects/adverse reactions: Can cause diarrhea, bloody diarrhea, colitis, pseudomembranous colitis, and abdominal cramping; solution can cause skin dryness.

Interactions: Antagonism has occurred between clindamycin and erythromycin.

Nursing considerations: Solution has an alcohol base, which can cause burning and irritation of the eye. In case of contact with eyes or irritated skin or mucous membranes, flush with cool tap water. Use with caution around mouth. Notify physician if abdominal pain or diarrhea occurs.

Erythromycin (2% solution) (A/T/S solution, Erycette, T-stat, Eryderm 1.5% solution, Staticin)

Indications: Topical control of acne vulgaris.

Administration: Apply to affected area twice a day (AM, PM).

Precautions/contraindications: Hypersensitivity to erythromycin may develop with prolonged use; bacterial or fungal overgrowth of nonsusceptible organisms (superinfection) may occur. For external use only.

Side effects/adverse reactions: Erythema, desquamation, burning, eye irritation, dryness, oily skin.

Interactions: Antagonism has occurred between clindamycin and erythromycin. Avoid use with abrasive agents, acids, or alkaline media.

Nursing consideration: Keep away from eyes, nose, mouth, and other mucous membranes. Wash, rinse, and dry affected areas before applying.

Mafenide Acetate Cream (Sulfamylon)

Mafenide is a bacteriostatic sulfonamide active against gram-negative and gram-positive organisms. It reduces the bacterial population present in avascular tissue of second and third-degree burns. It is absorbed and rapidly metabolized to *P*-carboxybenzenesulfonamide, an inactive metabolite that is cleared through the kidneys. This metabolite has no antibacterial activity, but can inhibit carbonic anhydrase.

Indications: Adjunctive therapy for second- and third-degree burns.

Administration: Apply once or twice daily.

Precautions/contraindications: Contraindicated with hypersensitivity to any ingredients in the product. Cross-sensitivity to other sulfonamides is not known. Superinfection may result with use. Pregnancy (category C). Not recommended in women of child-bearing potential unless burned area covers more than 20% of the body surface, or benefit is greater than risk to fetus. Discontinue use during nursing. May cause metabolic acidosis as a result of carbonic anhydrase inhibition, usually compensated for by hyperventilation. Acid-base balance should be closely monitored, particularly in patients with large burns or those with pulmonary or renal dysfunction. If acidosis occurs and cannot be controlled, discontinue therapy for 24 to 48 hours while continuing fluid therapy. Use with caution in patients with acute renal failure. Use with caution in patients with sulfite sensitivity.

Side effects/adverse reactions: Pain or burning sensation on application. Rash, itching, facial edema, hives, blisters, erythema, tachypnea, or hyperventilation; decrease in arterial P_{CO_2}; metabolic acidosis.

Nursing considerations: Apply cream to debrided burn area with a sterile gloved hand, to thickness of about $\frac{1}{16}$ inch, once or twice daily. Keep burned area covered with mafenide at all times; reapply if any is removed. Dressings are not required, but if necessary, use only a thin layer. Bathe daily if possible to help debridement. Continue treatment while risk of infection exists or until the site is ready for grafting. Discontinue if allergic reactions or marked hyperventilation occurs. Cleanse with soap and water; dry well before applying unless otherwise directed. May stain skin. Monitor for superinfection. Store at room temperature.

Metronidazole (MetroGel: 0.75% gel)

Metronidazole is an antiprotozoal, antibacterial agent. When it is applied topically, and with normal usage, systemic absorption is minimal.

Indications: Topical treatment of inflammatory papules and pustules, and erythema of rosacea.

Administration: Apply and rub in a thin film twice daily.

Precautions/contraindications: Contraindicated with hypersensitivity to metronidazole, parabens, or other ingredients of the formulation. Adverse experiences reported with oral form have not been reported with gel. Use with caution in patients with evidence or history of blood dyscrasia. For external use only.

Side effects/adverse reactions: Eye irritation if applied too close to eyes; transient redness, mild dryness, burning, skin irritation.

Interactions: Less likely with topical administration, but use with caution in patients receiving anticoagulant treatment with warfarin may prolong prothrombin time.

Nursing considerations: Do not apply close to eyes. Wash area before applying. Significant therapeutic results should be noticed within 3 weeks, and improvement should continue for 6 more weeks. Cosmetics may be used after application of topical metronidazole.

Mupirocin (2% ointment) (Bactroban)

Indications: Topical treatment of impetigo caused by *Staphylococcus aureus*, beta-hemolytic streptococci, and *Staphylococcus pyogenes*.

Administration: Apply a small amount to affected area three times daily.

Precautions/contraindications: Contraindicated with hypersensitivity to any components of the product. Avoid contact with the eyes. Monitor for superinfections.

Side effects/adverse reactions: Burning, stinging or pain, itching, rash, nausea, erythema, dry skin, tenderness, swelling, contact dermatitis.

Nursing considerations: For external use only. Avoid contact with eyes. If skin reaction develops, stop therapy. Wash affected area. Contact physician if improvement is not seen in 3 to 5 days. Treated area may be covered with gauze dressing if desired.

Nitrofurazone (0.2% solution, ointment, and cream) (Furacin)

Indications: Adjunct therapy in patients with second- and third-degree burns when bacterial resistance is a real or potential problem. Also used in skin grafting when bacterial contamination may cause graft rejection or donor site infection.

Administration: Apply daily or every few days, depending on dressing technique.

Precautions/contraindications: Contraindicated with known sensitization to nitrofurazone. Use ointment with caution in patients with known or suspected renal impairment. Monitor for superinfection. Use with caution in individuals with glucose-6-phosphate dehydrogenase deficiency (G6PD).

Side effects/adverse reactions: Contact dermatitis, rash, pruritus, local edema.

Interactions: Sutilains' (Travase) enzyme activity may be impaired by nitrofurazone.

Nursing considerations: Apply directly to lesion, or place on gauze. Avoid exposing drug to direct sunlight, excessive heat, strong fluorescent lighting, and alkaline materials. Notify physician if condition worsens or if irritation occurs.

Tetracycline HCl (OTC 3% ointment, 0.22% solution) (Achromycin)

Indications: Infection prophylaxis and treatment of superficial bacterial infection of the skin caused by susceptible organisms; acne vulgaris.

Administration: Apply to affected area twice daily.

Precautions/contraindications: Contraindicated with hypersensitivity; pregnancy category D. Discontinue if redness, irritation, swelling, or pain persists. Use with caution during lactation. For external use only.

Side effects/adverse reactions: Rash, urticaria, stinging, burning, redness, swelling, photosensitivity.

Nursing considerations: Cleanse area well with soap and water, and dry before applying unless otherwise directed. Apply enough to cover entire affected area, using aseptic technique. Avoid eyes, nose, and mouth. Clothing or skin may become stained. Notify physician if condition worsens.

ANTIVIRAL AGENTS

Acyclovir (5% ointment) (Zovirax)

Indications: Management of initial episodes of herpes genitalis and in *limited*, nonthreatening mucocutaneous herpes simplex viral infections in immunocompromised patients.

Administration: Apply every 3 hours six times daily for 7 days.

Precautions/contraindications: Contraindicated with hypersensitivity to any components of the formulation.

Use with caution during lactation. Do not use in eyes. Will not prevent recurrences or transmission of the virus to others.

Side effects/adverse reactions: Mild pain, burning, stinging, pruritus, rash.

Nursing considerations: For external use only. Ointment must thoroughly cover all lesions. Use finger cot or rubber glove to apply ointment. Apply as early as possible following onset of symptoms. Notify physician if pain, burning, stinging, or rash persists or becomes pronounced.

Acyclovir Sodium (200 mg capsules; injection IV 500 mg) (Zovirax)

Indications: Mucocutaneous herpes simplex virus, herpes genitalis (HSV-1, HSV-2).

Dosage: *Herpes simplex:* Adults and children 12 years of age: IV infusion 5 mg/kg over 1 hour q8h for 5 days; children 12 years of age: IV infusion 250 mg/m^2 over 1 hour q8h for 5 days. *Genital herpes:* Adults: Oral—200 mg q4h 5 times per day during waking hours, for 5 days to 6 months, depending on whether the episode is initial, recurrent, or chronic.

Precautions/contraindications: Lactation, hepatic disease, renal disease, electrolyte imbalance, dehydration, pregnancy category C. Contraindicated in individuals with hypersensitivity to the drug and in cases of herpes zoster in an immunosuppressed individual.

Side effects/adverse reactions: Tremors, confusion, lethargy, hallucinations, convulsions, dizziness, headache; anemia, increased bleeding time, bone marrow depression, granulocytopenia, thrombocytopenia, leukopenia, megaloblastic anemia; nausea, vomiting, diarrhea, increased ALT, AST, abdominal pain, glossitis, colitis; oliguria, proteinuria, hematuria, vaginitis, moniliasis, glomerulonephritis, acute renal failure, changes in menses; rash, urticaria, pruritus, phlebitis at the IV site.

Drug interactions: Increased neurotoxicity or nephrotoxicity occurs when acyclovir is administered with aminoglycosides, amphotericin, interferon, probenecid, or methotrexate. IV acyclovir is incompatible with dobutamine, dopamine, and all protein and blood products.

Pharmacokinetics: *IV:* Activity peaks in 1 hour; the half-life is 20 minutes to 3 hours (terminal). The drug is metabolized by the liver, excreted by the kidneys as unchanged drug (95%), and crosses the placenta.

Nursing considerations: The drug should be taken when itching or pain occurs, usually before skin eruptions are present. The patient must be sure to inform any sexual partner that the patient has herpes and that the partner could become infected. The drug must be taken in equal intervals around the clock to maintain blood levels for the duration of therapy. Notify physician of bruising, bleeding, fatigue, or malaise because they may indicate blood dyscrasias. Be sure to report the occurrence of sore throat, fever, and fatigue because they could indicate superimposed infection. Make sure the patient's fluid intake is adequate (200 ml) to prevent deposit in kidneys.

ANTIFUNGAL AGENTS

Amphotericin B (Fungizone: 3% cream, ointment, or lotion)

Indications: Treatment of cutaneous and mucocutaneous mycotic infections caused by *Candida* organisms.

Administration: Apply two to four times daily (duration depends on response).

Precautions/contraindications: Contraindicated with hypersensitivity to any components.

Side effects/adverse reactions: Has only a slight sensitizing potential. May cause local irritation, particularly in moist intertriginous areas. Cream may have a drying effect.

Nursing considerations: External use only. Avoid contact with the eyes. Cleanse affected areas before applying unless otherwise directed. Apply liberally and rub in gently. Cream may cause drying and slight discoloration of skin. Lotion and ointment may stain nail lesions but not nail. Notify physician if redness, itching, or burning, particularly in skinfolds, becomes bothersome or if condition worsens. May discolor fabrics. Severe infections of the nail beds may require several months of treatment.

Ciclopirox Olamine (1% cream, lotion) (Loprox)

Indications: Treatment of tinea pedis, tinea cruris, tinea corporis, cutaneous candidiasis, and tinea versicolor.

Administration: Apply twice a day.

Precautions/contraindications: Contraindicated with hypersensitivity to any components of formulation. Avoid contact with eyes. For external use only. If sensitivity occurs, discontinue treatment.

Side effects/adverse reactions: Local irritation, pruritus, redness, pain, burning.

Nursing considerations: Cleanse skin with soap and water, and dry thoroughly before application. Gently massage cream into affected and surrounding areas unless otherwise directed. With athlete's foot, wear well-fitting, ventilated shoes, and change shoes and socks at least once a day. Use medication for full treatment time, even if symptoms have improved. Improvement usually occurs within the first week of therapy. Reevaluate if no improvement occurs after 4 weeks. Tinea versicolor usually responds after 2 weeks of treatment. Inform physician if area shows signs of increased irritation. Do not use occlusive wrappings or dressings.

Clotrimazole (OTC 1% cream, solution, lotion) (Lotrimin, Lotrimin AF, Mycelex)

Indications: Treatment of tinea pedis, tinea cruris, tinea corporis, cutaneous candidiasis due to *Candida albicans,* tinea versicolor.

Administration: Apply twice daily.

Precautions/contraindications: Contraindicated with hypersensitivity to clotrimazole or any product components. Avoid contact with eyes. If sensitivity develops, discontinue use. For external use only.

Side effects/adverse reactions: Erythema, stinging, burning, blistering, peeling, edema, pruritus.

Nursing considerations: Cleanse affected areas before applying unless otherwise directed. Rub gently into affected area and surrounding areas of skin; avoid eyes. Continue treatment for full course of therapy, even if symptoms improve. Improvement usually occurs in 1 week. If no improvement is noted after 4 weeks or if condition worsens or irritation develops, notify physician.

Econazole Nitrate (1% cream) (Spectazole)

Indications: Treatment of tinea cruris, tinea pedis, tinea corporis, cutaneous candidiasis, and tinea versicolor.

Administration: Apply once daily (for cutaneous candidiasis, use bid).

Precautions/contraindications: Contraindicated with hypersensitivity to econazole or any ingredients of product. Avoid contact with eyes. If sensitivity develops, stop use. Pregnancy category C. Do not use in first trimester of pregnancy unless essential; in second and third trimesters, use only if benefits outweigh risks. Use with caution during lactation.

Side effects/adverse reactions: Burning, itching, stinging, erythema.

Nursing considerations: For external use only; avoid contact with eyes. Cleanse area with soap and water and dry before application, unless otherwise directed. Use medication for full course of therapy, even if symptoms improve. If no improvement is noted after 2 to 4 weeks or if condition worsens or irritation develops, contact physician. Use for 2 weeks for candidiasis, tinea cruris, and tinea corporis. Use for 4 weeks with tinea pedis. Do not use occlusive dressing.

Haloprogin (1% cream, solution) (Halotex)

Haloprogin is a synthetic antifungal agent used to treat superficial fungal infections of the skin. Its mechanism of action in dermatophytes is unknown.

Indications: Topical treatment of superficial mycotic infections, including tinea pedis, tinea cruris, tinea corporis, and tinea manuum; also for treatment of tinea versicolor.

Administration: Apply liberally to affected areas twice daily for 2 to 3 weeks. Intertriginous areas may require 4 weeks of therapy.

Precautions/contraindications: Contraindicated with hypersensitivity to any components of the product. Keep out of the eyes. Use with caution during lactation.

Side effects/adverse reactions: Burning, irritation, erythema, scaling, itching.

Nursing considerations: For external use only; avoid contact with eyes. Discontinue if sensitization develops or irritation increases. Use for full course of therapy, even if symptoms have abated. If no response is noted after 4 weeks, reevaluate.

Ketoconazole (2% cream, shampoo) (Nizoral)

Indications: *Cream:* Treatment of tinea corporis, tinea cruris, tinea pedis, tinea versicolor, cutaneous candidiasis, and seborrheic dermatitis. *Shampoo:* Reduction of scaling caused by dandruff.

Administration: Apply once daily for cutaneous candidiasis, tinea corporis, tinea cruris, and tinea versicolor. Apply twice daily for seborrheic dermatitis. (For dandruff scale, see Nursing Considerations.)

Precautions/contraindications: Contraindicated with hypersensitivity to any ingredients of product. Avoid contact with eyes. Cream has sulfites, which may cause allergic-type reactions, some potentially severe.

Side effects/adverse reactions: *Cream:* Severe irritation, pruritus, stinging. *Shampoo:* Increase in normal hair loss, loss of curl from permanently waved hair, itching, irritation, mild dryness of skin.

Nursing considerations: For external use only; avoid contact with eyes. *Cream:* Apply to affected area, including immediate surrounding areas. Treat tinea cruris, tinea versicolor, and tinea corporis for 2 weeks. Treat tinea pedis for 6 weeks. In seborrheic dermatitis, apply twice daily for 4 weeks or until cleared. *Shampoo:* Wet hair, lather, and massage for 1 minute. Rinse thoroughly and repeat, leaving on scalp for 3 more minutes. Then rinse well. Shampoo twice a week for 4 weeks with at least 3 days between each shampooing. Then use as needed for control.

Miconazole Nitrate (2% cream, powder, spray) (Micatin, Monistat-Derm)

Indications: Treatment of tinea pedis, tinea cruris, tinea corporis, cutaneous candidiasis, and tinea versicolor.

Administration: Apply twice daily (AM, PM); once daily for tinea versicolor.

Precautions/contraindications: Contraindicated with hypersensitivity to any components of the product.

Side effects/adverse reactions: Irritation, burning, maceration, allergic contact dermatitis.

Nursing considerations: For external use only; avoid contact with eyes. Lotion is preferred in intertriginous areas. With cream, rub in sparingly to avoid maceration. Use for full treatment time, even if symptoms improve. Treat tinea cruris, tinea corporis, candidiasis, and tinea versicolor for 2 weeks. Treat tinea pedis for 1 month. If no improvement is noted after 1 month, reevaluate. If condition worsens or doesn't respond, or if irritation develops, discontinue and notify physician.

Naftifine (1% cream, gel) (Naftin)

Naftifine is a synthetic allylamine cream derivative with broad-spectrum antifungal activity. It appears to interfere with sterol biosynthesis, decreasing the amount of sterols (especially ergosterol), which results in corresponding accumulation of squalene in the cells. Naftifine penetrates the stratum corneum to inhibit growth of dermatophytes.

Indications: Topical treatment of tinea pedis, tinea cruris, and tinea corporis.

Administration: *Cream:* Apply once a day. *Gel:* Apply twice a day (AM, PM).

Precautions/contraindications: Contraindicated with hypersensitivity to any components of the product. Use with caution during lactation.

Side effects/adverse reactions: Burning, stinging, dryness, erythema, itching; may cause irritation.

Pharmacokinetics: After a single topical application systemic absorption was approximately 6% with the cream and 4.2% or less with the gel. Naftifine and its metabolites are excreted in the urine and feces. Its half-life is approximately 2 to 3 days.

Nursing considerations: For external use only; avoid contact with eyes, nose, mouth, and mucous membranes. Apply enough to cover affected areas and surrounding skin. Wash hands after application. Do not use occlusive dressing unless otherwise directed. If no improvement is noted after 4 weeks, reevaluate.

Nystatin (100,000 U/g cream, ointment, powder) (Mycostatin, Nilstat, Nystex)

Indications: Cutaneous or mucocutaneous mycotic infections caused by *Candida albicans* and other *Candida* species.

Administration: Apply 2 to 3 times daily (apply powder freely).

Precautions/contraindications: Pregnancy category B; use only if clearly needed. Contraindicated in patients with hypersensitivity to any component of the product.

Side effects/adverse reactions: Very well tolerated; virtually nontoxic and nonsensitizing.

Nursing considerations: For external use only; avoid contact with eyes. Apply after cleansing and drying affected area unless otherwise directed. If irritation develops, stop use and notify physician. Use until healing is complete. Cream is preferred for intertriginous areas; powder is best for very moist lesions.

SCABICIDES AND PEDICULICIDES

Crotamiton (10% cream, lotion) (Eurax)

Crotamiton is a scabicidal, antipruritic agent. Its mechanism of action is unknown.

Indications: Eradication of scabies and symptomatic treatment of pruritic skin.

Administration: Shake lotion well before using. Massage thoroughly into skin from the chin down. Second application is recommended 24 hours later. A cleansing bath should be taken 48 hours after last application. For pruritus, massage into affected areas of skin. Repeat as necessary.

Precautions/contraindications: Contraindicated with hypersensitivity to any components of the product. Do not apply to inflamed skin; raw, exposed surfaces; eyes; or mouth. If sensitivity occurs, discontinue use. Use on pregnant women only when clearly needed (category C). Avoid contact with eyes.

Side effects/adverse reactions: Itching, rash, irritation, contact dermatitis.

Nursing considerations: For external use only. Apply after patient bathes with soap and water. Cover body from chin down, including folds and creases, but not to face, eyes, mouth, lips, any mucous membranes, anus, or meatus. Change clothing and bed linens the next day and wash in hot water or dry clean. Discontinue use if irritation or sensitization occurs. Itching may continue for 4 to 6 weeks.

Lindane (Gamma benzene hexachloride) (1% cream, lotion, shampoo) (Kwell, Scabene, G-Well)

Lindane is an ectoparasticide and ovicide. It stimulates the nervous systems of arthropods, resulting in seizures or death.

Indications: Effective against pediculosis capitis (head lice) and pediculosis pubis (crab lice) and their ova. The cream and lotion are also indicated for scabies.

Administration: *Lotion:* For the treatment of crab lice and head lice. *Crab lice:* Apply enough lotion to cover hair and skin of pubic area and surrounding areas if infested. Rub in and leave for 12 hours, then wash well. Treat sexual contacts simultaneously. Retreatment is not necessary unless living lice are seen after 7 days. *Head lice:* Apply enough lotion to cover hair and affected surrounding areas. Rub in and leave on for 12 hours, then wash well. Retreatment is not necessary unless living lice are seen after 7 days. *Shampoo:* For the treatment of head lice. Apply a sufficient quantity (1 to 2 ounces) to dry hair; work thoroughly into hair and leave on 4 minutes. Add small quantities of water until a good lather forms. Rinse thoroughly and towel briskly. Nits or nit shells should be removed with tweezers or a nit comb. Retreatment is not usually necessary unless living lice are seen 7 days after treatment. *Cream and lotion:* For the treatment of scabies. If crusted lesions are present, bathe before applying. Apply a thin layer to dry skin and rub in thoroughly. About 2 ounces is sufficient for an adult. Apply from the neck down, covering body, and leave on for 8 to 12 hours. Remove by washing well. One application usually is enough.

Precautions/contraindications: Contraindicated with hypersensitivity to any component of the product. Use with caution in premature neonates and patients with known seizure disorders due to the potental for systemic absorption. Potential toxic effects are greater in patients under 10 years of age. Seizures have occurred after excessive use or ingestion of lindane. Avoid contact with eyes; flush with water immediately if this occurs. If irritation or sensitivity occurs, consult physician. Nursing mothers should consider discontinuing nursing during use of lindane. Do not use on abrasions or breaks in the skin.

Side effects/adverse reactions: CNS effects ranging from dizziness to convulsions (convulsions are usually associated with oral ingestion); eczematous eruption resulting from irritation.

Nursing considerations: For external use only; do not apply to face, lips, mouth, eyes, any mucous membranes, or meatus. Wear rubber gloves, especially if applying to more than one person. Do not apply to open cuts or external excoriations. Itching may continue for 4 to 6 weeks. Wash all clothing and bed linens. Use insecticide on rugs and upholstered furniture. Use nit comb or tweezers to remove nits and nit shells. Has no residual activity. Treat sexual contacts simultaneously.

Permethrin (5% cream, 1% liquid) (Elimite, Nix)

Permethrin is a synthetic pyrethroid that is active against lice, ticks, mites, and fleas. Permethrin is rapidly metabolized in the liver to inactive metabolites and excreted in the urine.

Indications: *Cream:* Treatment of scabies. *Liquid:* Treatment of head lice.

Administration: *Scabies:* Wash and dry thoroughly; massage cream into skin from the head to the soles of the feet (usually 30 g is enough for an adult). Leave cream on for 8 to 14 hours, then remove by washing. One application is sufficient. NOTE: Scabies rarely infests the scalp in adults, but in infants and geriatric patients, the hairline, neck, temple, and forehead may be infested. Check these areas and treat if necessary. *Head lice:* Shampoo hair, rinse thoroughly, and towel dry (do not apply conditioner). Apply enough of the liquid permethrin to saturate hair and scalp. Allow to remain on hair for 10 minutes; then rinse thoroughly with water. A single treatment is sufficient.

Precautions/contraindications: Contraindicated with hypersensitivity to any component of the product, synthetic pyrethroid, pyrethrin, or chrysanthemums, and for individuals sensitized to ragweed. Use with caution, if at all, in nursing mothers.

Side effects/adverse reactions: Pruritus, mild burning, stinging, itching, numbness, tingling, erythema, rash. May temporarily exacerbate pruritus, erythema, or edema caused by infestation.

Nursing considerations: For external use only. Avoid contact with mucous membranes (may be mildly irritating to eyes; flush with water if contact occurs). Itching may continue for 4 to 6 weeks. If irritation develops and persists, notify physician. Do not exceed prescribed dose. Has residual activity for up to 10 days. Sexual contacts should be treated simultaneously.

Pyrethrins (cream, gel, shampoo) (A-200 Pyrinate, RID, R&C, TISIT)

Pyrethrins are pediculicides used with piperonyl butoxide; the two act synergistically as a contact poison, causing death by paralysis.

Indications: Treatment of infestations of head lice, body lice, and pubic lice and their eggs.

Administration: (Administration varies with each product; consult the package insert.) *Usual regimen:* Apply enough of the product to cover or saturate hair and scalp. Leave on 10 minutes, then rinse. Reapply in 2 days if needed, but not within 24 hours.

Precautions/contraindications: Use with caution in children and infants. Use on pregnant women only when clearly needed (category C). Contraindicated with hypersensitivity to any ingredients of the product and for individuals sensitized to ragweed. Do not use on eyelashes or eyebrows. Do not use on inflamed skin or cuts and abrasions.

Side effects/adverse reactions: Skin irritation, pruritus, urticaria, eczema.

Nursing considerations: For external use only;

harmful if swallowed. Avoid contact with eyes and mucous membranes; flush with water if contact occurs. Wash or dry clean clothes and bedding to prevent reinfestation. Itching may continue for 4 to 6 weeks. If irritation or infection develops, discontinue use and contact physician. Remove nit and nit shells with fine-toothed comb. Treat sexual contacts simultaneously.

KERATOLYTICS AND CAUSTICS

Coal Tar (Fototar, Estar)

Coal tar is an antipruritic, antieczematic, keratoplastic agent. It is available in various preparations (ointment, gel, cream, lotion, soap, and bath solution) ranging in concentration from 1% to 20%.

Indications: Treatment of psoriasis, dandruff, seborrheic dermatitis, atopic dermatitis, and eczematoid dermatitis.

Administration: See package insert.

Precautions/contraindications: Contraindicated with sensitivity to any component of the product. Pregnancy category C; use only when needed. Use with caution during lactation; it is not known whether coal tar is excreted in breast milk. Do not apply to axillae, face, or mucous membrane warts.

Nursing considerations: For external use only; avoid contact with eyes, mucous membranes, genital and rectal areas, open wounds, and inflamed skin. Coal tar is photosensitizing; avoid direct sunlight and do not use a sunlamp for 72 hours after applying. Do not use with other forms of psoriasis therapy unless directed to do so. May stain clothing, bathtubs, and light-colored hair.

Podofilox (0.5% solution) (Condylox)

Podofilox is a topical antimitotic drug purified from the plant families Coniferae and Berberidaceae. It can also be chemically synthesized. Treatment results in necrosis of visible wart tissue.

Indications: Topical treatment of external genital warts.

Administration: Apply twice a day (AM, PM) for 3 consecutive days, then stop for 4 consecutive days. This 1-week cycle may be repeated up to four times until no wart tissue is visible.

Precautions/contraindications: Contraindicated with hypersensitivity to any components of the product. Pregnancy category C. Do not apply to axillae, face, or mucous membrane warts.

Side effects/adverse reactions: Burning, pain, inflammation, erosion, itching, pain with intercourse, insomnia, bleeding, dizziness, vomiting, hematuria. Burning and pain are seen more often and with more severity in women.

Nursing considerations: For external use only. Avoid contact with eyes; if contact occurs, flush with water and seek medical advice. Apply to warts with a drug-dampened, cotton-tipped applicator. Apply the minimum amount needed to cover wart. Limit treatment to ≤ 10 cm^2 of wart and to ≤ 0.5 ml of solution per day to avoid possible systemic absorption and local adverse reactions. If applying in skinfolds, separate skin and allow solution to dry before releasing folds. Carefully dispose of used applicator. Wash hands. If response is incomplete after 4 weeks, reconsider treatment. Give patient the patient information leaflet provided with product.

Salicylic Acid (cream, gel, ointment, patch, shampoo, solution) (Keralyt, Occlusal, Sal-Acid)

Salicylic acid is a keratolytic agent available at concentrations of 2% to 6%. Concentrations of 10% to 17% are used to remove warts. Plasters used to remove corns and warts contain concentrations of up to 50%. These cause desquamation of the horny wart by dissolving intercellular cement substance, thereby causing the cornified epithelium to swell, soften, and macerate.

Indications: Topical aid in removing excessive keratin in hyperkeratotic skin disorders. Also used to treat dandruff, seborrheic dermatitis, psoriasis, multiple superficial epitheliomatoses, acne, and calluses.

Administration: Apply at night. Hydrate affected area for 5 minutes to enhance drug's effects. Then apply thoroughly. Use occlusive dressing overnight, and wash product off in the morning. Apply more frequently if occlusion is not possible. Once condition has cleared, occasional use usually maintains remission.

Precautions/contraindications: Contraindicated with sensitivity to salicylic acid, in children under 2 years of age, diabetics, or individuals with impaired circulation. Do not use on moles, birthmarks, unusual warts with hair growing from them, genital warts, or warts on the face or mucous membranes. Monitor for salicylate toxicity, especially with prolonged use over large areas, in children, or in people with renal or hepatic impairment (see Side Effects/Adverse Reactions). Avoid other drugs that can cause elevated salicylate levels, such as aspirin, when given with salicylates. Pregnancy category C. With lactation, discontinue either drug or breast-feeding because of serious effects on nursing infant. Do not use on open wounds or lesions.

Side effects/adverse reactions: Local irritation, drying, salicylism (hearing loss, tinnitus, dizziness, confusion, headache, hyperventilation).

Nursing considerations: For external use only. Avoid contact with eyes and mucous membranes; if contact occurs, flush with water immediately. Do not use on the face, genitals, or on broken or inflamed skin. Wash thoroughly in the morning after treatment. Use an occlusive dressing to improve effectiveness. Monitor for side effects. Apply lotion on areas if drying occurs. Avoid contact with clothing, plastics, wood, or metal, because these might be damaged. Rinse hands well after application.

ANTINEOPLASTIC AGENT

Fluorouracil (1%, 5% cream; 1%, 2%, 5% solution) (Efudex, Fluoroplex)

Fluorouracil inhibits the synthesis of DNA and, to a lesser extent, RNA. These effects are more pronounced on rapidly growing cells, which take up fluorouracil at a faster pace. Fluorouracil is not significantly absorbed. When applied to a lesion the response occurs in stages: (1) early inflammation (erythema); (2) severe inflammation (burning, stinging, vesiculation); (3) disintegration (erosion, pain, crusting); (4) healing (some residual erythema, temporary hyperpigmentation).

Indications: Treatment of multiple actinic or solar keratoses; superficial basal cell carcinomas.

Administration: Apply twice daily to lesions. Continue use until inflammatory response reaches the erosion, necrosis, and ulceration stage. Then discontinue, usually within 2 to 6 weeks. Complete healing might take 1 to 2 months after discontinuing medication. The 5% strength is recommended only for basal cell carcinomas. Treatment is usually continued for at least 3 to 6 weeks, possibly for as long as 10 to 12 weeks.

Precautions/contraindications: Contraindicated with hypersensitivity to any component of the product. Occlusive dressings may increase inflammatory response on adjacent normal skin. Avoid prolonged exposure to sunlight because of photosensitization. Monitor for delayed hypersensitivity reactions. Pregnancy category X; do not use during pregnancy or in a woman who may become pregnant while taking this drug. Mothers should not breast-feed while taking this drug, because some systemic absorption occurs.

Side effects/adverse reactions: Pain, pruritus, hyperpigmentation, irritation, inflammation, burning, scarring, soreness, scaling, swelling, stomatitis, alopecia, irritability, insomnia, medicinal taste, photosensitivity, lacrimation, leukocytosis, thrombocytopenia, eosinophilia.

Nursing considerations: For external use only; apply with care near the eyes, nose, and mouth. If applied with fingers, wash hands immediately after use. A caregiver applying the drug should be sure to wear gloves. Avoid prolonged exposure to ultraviolet rays while under treatment. Reaction to treatment may be unsightly during therapy and possibly for several weeks after. Use porous gauze if dressing is needed. Avoid occlusive dressing.

ANTIHYPERTENSIVE AGENT

Minoxidil (2% solution) (Rogaine)

Minoxidil topical solution stimulates hair growth in men with balding of the vertex of the scalp and in women with diffuse hair loss. It has no effect on frontal hair loss. Its mechanism of action is not known, but it is thought to be due to arterial dilation. Topical minoxidil is poorly absorbed.

Indications: Treatment of androgenic alopecia in men and of diffuse hair loss or thinning of the frontal parietal areas in women.

Administration: Apply 1 ml to total affected areas of the scalp twice daily (AM, PM). Hair and scalp should be dry before applying. Twice daily application for at least 4 months may be needed before evidence of hair growth is noted.

Precautions/contraindications: Contraindicated with hypersensitivity to any components of the product. Patient must have a normal, healthy scalp with no abrasions or dermatitis that may increase absorption. Greater absorption due to misuse may lead to systemic effects. Do not use in conjunction with other topical drugs such as corticosteroids, retinoids, or petrolatum, all of which may enhance absorption. Use with caution in patients with heart disease; monitor the patients for tachycardia and fluid retention. Do not use in pregnant or nursing women. Patient should have a physical examination before using minoxidil and should be monitored at least 1 month after starting and every 6 months thereafter.

Side effects/adverse reactions: Irritant dermatitis, allergic contact dermatitis, eczema, hypertrichosis, dry skin, scalp flaking, headache, tachycardia, blood pressure changes, dizziness, edema, chest pain.

Nursing considerations: For external use to the scalp only; avoid eyes and mucous membranes. Do not inhale spray mist. Do not use on broken or irritated skin or with other topical drugs because of potential for increased absorption. Evidence of hair growth takes at least 4 months. First hair will be soft and colorless but will fill in like new hair with further treatment. Twice a day dosage only. Do not make up for missed applications. More frequent applications will not speed up hair growth and may lead to an increased chance of side effects. The solution contains alcohol and can cause irritation or burning. Contact physician if irritation develops and persists. If fingers are used to apply, wash hands afterward. A caregiver applying the drug should be sure to wear gloves. New hair will probably be shed within a few months after treatment stops. If no response is noted after 4 months, reconsider therapy.

DRUGS FOR THE TREATMENT OF ACNE

Benzoyl Peroxide (2.5%, 5%, 10% lotion, cream, gel, bar, liquid) (Benzac, Desquam-X, Oxy-5, Oxy-10, Clearasil, Fostex)

Benzoyl peroxide is an antibacterial agent. The drying vehicle aids in removing excess sebum and shrinking the papules and pustules.

Indications: Treatment of mild to moderate acne.

Administration: *Cleansers:* Use once or twice daily to wet skin. Rinse and dry well. *Creams, lotions, gels:* Apply once daily initially. Gradually increase as needed and as tolerated to twice a day. Control side effects and excessive irritation with changes in percentage strength and frequency of application.

Precautions/contraindications: Contraindicated with hypersensitivity to any component of the product. Cross-sensitization between benzoic acid derivatives (cinnamon, certain topical anesthetics) may occur. May bleach hair and fabrics. Pregnancy category C; use only if clearly needed. Use with caution in nursing women. Concurrent use with tretinoin may cause serious skin irritation.

Side effects/adverse reactions: Dry skin, peeling, redness, sensation of warmth, edema, stinging.

Nursing considerations: For external use only. Avoid contact with eyes, mouth, mucous membranes, and inflamed skin. Dryness, redness, and peeling are expected. Severe redness, pruritus, blisters, burning, and edema require using a lower percentage formulation or discontinuing use temporarily. Do not use with other acne medications, and avoid excessive sunlight unless directed. May bleach hair and fabrics.

Isotretinoin (10 mg, 20 mg, 40 mg capsules) (Accutane)

Isotretinoin is an isomer of retinoic acid, which is a metabolite of vitamin A. Its exact mechanism of action is unknown, but it appears to reduce the secretion of sebum and the size of the sebaceous glands, as well as inhibit sebaceous gland differentiation. Isotretinoin also may prevent abnormal keratinization.

Indications: Treatment of severe, recalcitrant cystic acne in patients who are unresponsive to conventional therapy.

Administration: 0.5 to 2 mg/kg/day orally in two divided doses for 15 to 20 weeks. A second course, if warranted, may be started after patient has been off therapy for 2 months or longer.

Precautions/contraindications: Contraindicated with hypersensitivity to any component of the product and sensitivity to parabens. Use with caution in diabetics and patients with hepatic disease. Do not donate blood while taking this drug or for 30 days following treatment. May cause photosensitivity. Topical drugs used for acne should be discontinued before starting isotretinoin.

> **Pregnancy category X; do not give to pregnant women, or to women who may become pregnant while taking this drug or within 1 month after discontinuing the drug. Do not use in nursing mothers.**

Side effects/adverse reactions: Cheilitis, conjunctivitis, skin fragility, dry skin, pruritus, epistaxis, dry nose, dry mouth. Pseudotumor cerebri, corneal opacities, decreased night vision, contact lens intolerance, inflammatory bowel disease, hypertriglyceridemia, arthralgia, hepatotoxicity, initial exacerbation of acne, photosensitivity. Peeling of palms and soles, nausea, vomiting, abdominal pain. Fatigue, headache, hair problems, nail brittleness, increased liver enzymes, hematuria, proteinuria, thrombocytopenia, papilledema, elevation of sedimentation rates.

Pharmacokinetics: Peak plasma concentrations are at 2.9 to 3.2 hours. Half-life is 10 to 20 hours. Drug is metabolized in the liver and excreted in the urine and feces in approximately equal portions in patients with normal renal and hepatic function.

Interactions: Do not take vitamin A concomitantly with isotretinoin. Minocycline and tetracycline have been associated with pseudotumor cerebri or papilledema in patients taking isotretinoin.

Nursing considerations: Take whole—do not crush. Take with meals (absorption is increased when drug is taken with food or milk). Wait at least 2 months before starting second course of therapy. **Females must have a negative pregnancy test before treatment is initiated; they must use a reliable form of birth control during therapy, and for 1 month after completion of therapy.** Initially acne may worsen during therapy. Avoid prolonged exposure to sunlight due to photosensitivity. Minimize or avoid alcohol consumption. Monitor for triglyceride levels, liver enzymes, proteinuria, hematoma, diabetes. Monitor for symptoms of pseudotumor cerebri (headache, vomiting, nausea, visual disturbances); if present, discontinue drug.

Tretinoin (0.025%, 0.05%, 0.1% cream; 0.025%, 0.01% gel; 0.05% liquid) (Retin-A)

Tretinoin is used in the treatment of acne vulgaris. It is an irritant that stimulates epidermal cell turnover, causing skin peeling and extrusion of the comedones. It has no antibacterial activity.

Indications: Topical treatment of acne vulgaris.

Administration: Apply once a day at bedtime to clean, dry skin. Cover entire area lightly.

Precautions/contraindications: Contraindicated with hypersensitivity to any component of the product. May cause photosensitivity. Pregnancy category C; use only if clearly needed. Use with caution if breast-feeding. Excessive application will not improve effectiveness and may cause redness, peeling, and discomfort.

Side effects/adverse reactions: Erythema, edematous, blistered or crusted skin; temporary changes in pigmentation; photosensitivity, dry skin, peeling, stinging.

Interactions: Absorption of topical minoxidil is increased when that drug is taken with tretinoin. Significant skin irritation may result if used concomitantly with keratolytic medications such as sulfur and salicylic acid, resorcinol, or benzoyl peroxide.

Nursing considerations: For external use only. Keep away from eyes, mouth, angles of the nose, and mucous membranes. Avoid excessive exposure to sunlight and sunlamps. Wear a sunscreen and protective clothing. Redness and peeling may occur; if excessive, decrease dosage or discontinue temporarily. Avoid using or use cautiously with keratolytics, products with a high alcohol content, abrasive cleansers, astringents, and topical products containing spices or lime. Apply after carefully cleansing the face and allowing it to dry for at least 30 minutes for skin to dry thoroughly. Applying the drug to moist or wet skin increases irritation. Use topical moisturizer if skin becomes too dry. Cosmetics can be used. Therapeutic response may be seen after 2 to 3 weeks but may take up to 6 weeks for optimum response. Once response is satisfactory, less frequent application or a lower dosage can be used. Some patients respond to less frequent applications or a lower concentration; others may need a higher dosage.

CORTICOSTEROIDS

Topical corticosteroids are adrenocorticosteroid derivatives that have antiinflammatory, antipruritic, and vasoconstrictive effects. They are incorporated into various vehicles, depending on the condition being treated. Ointments are more occlusive and are used to treat dry, scaly, thickened, pruritic skin; ointments tend to be greasier than creams or gels. Creams are used for oozing lesions or in intertriginous areas; they have a more drying effect than ointments. Sprays, gels, and lotions are useful on hairy areas of the body. Sprays are also good for weeping lesions.

The vehicle used is a factor in the potency and effectiveness of the corticosteroid, because it affects the drug's ability to penetrate the skin. Ointments usually allow the greatest penetration, followed by gels, creams, then lotions. Corticosteroids can be chemically altered by hydroxylation, methylation, fluorination, or esterification, all of which increase the drug's potency and lipid solubility and decrease the mineralocorticoid effects. Systemic absorption of the drug is increased when applied to a large surface area; the condition of the skin may also affect drug absorption.

Topical corticosteroids are grouped by potency into four classes (Table 13-1), class I being the strongest. Class I drugs sometimes are used as an alternative to systemic corticosteroid therapy. The topical preparations are more likely to cause skin atrophy and should be used only for short periods on a small area. They should not be applied to the face, and occlusive dressings should not be used with these products.

Class I topical corticosteroids can induce adrenal suppression.

Class II preparations can be used for an intermediate period. They may be used on the face and in intertriginous areas for brief periods.

Class III corticosteroids can be used for chronic cases and for a limited time on the face and in intertriginous areas.

Class IV corticosteroids are safe for chronic cases. They can be used with occlusive dressings, in intertriginous areas, on the face and genital area, and for large areas of the body. They also can be used on children.

Aclometasone Dipropionate (0.05% cream, ointment) (Aclovate)

Aclometasone dipropionate is a low-potency (class IV) topical corticosteroid.

Indications: Relief of inflammatory and pruritic manifestations of corticosteroid-responsive dermatoses (e.g., contact dermatitis, eczema, psoriasis, insect bites, burns, and sunburn).

Administration: Apply a thin film to affected areas two or three times daily. Rub in until medication disappears.

Precautions/contraindications: Contraindicated with hypersensitivity to any components of the product. Use with caution in children and infants. Pregnancy category C; use only if benefits outweigh risks. Use with caution in nursing mothers. Use with caution with viral, bacterial, and fungal infections. Use an appropriate antiinfective agent for underlying infections. If a favorable response is not seen, stop corticosteroid therapy until infection is controlled. Use with caution on face,

Table 13-1

CLASSES OF TOPICAL CORTICOSTEROIDS

Generic name	Trade name	Strength
Class I (very high potency)		
Augmented betamethasone dipropionate	Diprolene, Diprolene AF ointment	0.05%
Clobetasol propionate	Temovate	0.05%
Diflorasone diacetate	Psorcon	0.05%
Halobetasol propionate	Ultravate	0.05%
Class II (high potency)		
Amcinonide	Cyclocort	0.1%
Augmented betamethasone dipropionate	Diprolene, Diprolene AF cream	0.05%
Betamethasone dipropionate	Diprosone, Maxivate cream, ointment	0.05%
Desoximetasone	Topicort, Topicort LP cream, ointment	0.25%
	gel	0.05%
Diflorasone diacetate	Florone, Maxiflor	0.05%
Fluocinolone acetonide	Synalar-HP cream	0.2%
Fluocinonide	Lidex, Lidex-E	0.05%
Halcinonide	Halog, Halog-E	0.1%
Triamcinolone acetonide	Aristocort, Kenalog	0.5%
Class III (medium potency)		
Betamethasone benzoate	Uticort	0.025%
Betamethasone dipropionate	Diprosone (lotion)	0.05%
Betamethasone valerate	Valisone (cream)	0.1%
Clocortolone pivalate	Cloderm	0.1%
Desoximetasone	Topicort (cream)	0.05%
Fluocinolone acetonide	Synalar cream, ointment	0.025%
Flurandrenolide	Cordran cream, ointment	0.025%
	cream, ointment, lotion	0.05%
	tape	4 μg/cm^2
Fluticasone propionate	Cutivate cream	0.05%
	ointment	0.005%
Hydrocortisone butyrate	Locoid	0.1%
Hydrocortisone valerate	Wescort	0.2%
Mometasone furoate	Elocon	0.1%
Triamcinolone acetonide	Kenalog, Aristocort	0.1%
Class IV (low potency)		
Aclometasone dipropionate	Aclovate	0.05%
Desonide	DesOwen, Tridesilon	0.05%
Dexamethasone sodium phosphate	Decadron	0.1%

Table 13-1

CLASSES OF TOPICAL CORTICOSTEROIDS—cont'd

Generic name	Trade name	Strength
Fluocinolone acetonide	Synalar	
	cream, solution	0.01%
Hydrocortisone	Hytone, Cortaid, others	
	lotion	0.25%
	cream, ointment, gel	0.5%
	cream, ointment, lotion, solution	1%
	lotion	2%
	cream, lotion	2.5%
Triamcinolone acetonide	Aristocort, Kenalog	0.025%

groin, axillae, and intertriginous areas because of resulting striae and atrophy. Systemic absorption may occur; monitor for symptoms (Cushing syndrome, HPA axis suppression, hyperglycemia, glycosuria), especially in children and infants and in patients with liver failure.

Side effects/adverse reactions: Burning, itching, dryness, irritation, stinging, soreness, acne, numbness of the fingers, folliculitis, hypertrichosis, hypopigmentation, atrophy, secondary infections.

Nursing considerations: For external use only. Avoid contact with eyes. Do not bandage, wrap, cover, or use occlusive dressing unless otherwise directed. Apply only to affected area. Apply sparingly and rub in well. Do not apply to weeping, denuded, or infected areas. If irritation develops, discontinue and notify physician. If treating a child or infant's diaper area, do not use tight-fitting diapers or plastic pants, which may act as an occlusive dressing. With long-term use, do not discontinue treatment abruptly.

Amcinonide (0.1% cream, lotion, ointment) (Cyclocort)

Amcinonide is a high-potency (class II) topical corticosteroid.

Indications: Relief of inflammatory and pruritic manifestations of corticosteroid-responsive dermatoses (e.g., contact dermatitis, eczema, psoriasis, insect bites, burns, and sunburn).

Administration: Apply a thin film two or three times daily. Rub in gently.

Precautions/contraindications: Contraindicated with hypersensitivity to any component of the product. Use with caution in children and infants. Pregnancy category C; use only if the benefits outweigh the risks. Use with caution in nursing mothers. Use with caution with viral, bacterial, and fungal infections. Use an ap-

propriate antiinfective agent for underlying bacterial or fungal infection; if a favorable response is not seen, stop corticosteroid therapy until infection is controlled. Do not use on the face or groin or in intertriginous areas because of resulting striae and atrophy. Systemic absorption may occur; side effects consistent with systemic absorption include Cushing syndrome, hypothalamo-pituitary-adrenocortical (HPA) axis suppression, hyperglycemia, and glycosuria, especially in children, infants, and patients with liver failure.

Side effects/adverse reactions: Burning, dryness, itching, irritation, stinging, soreness, acne, folliculitis, hypertrichosis, numbness of the fingers, hypopigmentation, atrophy, secondary infection.

Nursing considerations: For external use only to affected areas. Avoid contact with the eyes. Do not bandage, wrap, cover, or use occlusive dressing on affected area unless otherwise directed. Do not apply to weeping, denuded, or infected areas. If irritation develops, discontinue treatment and notify physician. If treating a child or infant in the diaper area, do not use tight-fitting diapers or plastic pants, which can act as an occlusive dressing. With long-term use, do not discontinue treatment abruptly.

Betamethasone Benzoate (0.025% cream, lotion, gel) (Uticort)

Betamethasone benzoate is a medium-potency (class III) topical corticosteroid.

Indications: Relief of inflammatory and pruritic manifestations of corticosteroid-responsive dermatoses (e.g., contact dermatitis, eczema, psoriasis, insect bites, burns, and sunburn).

Administration: Apply sparingly two or three times daily.

Precautions/contraindications: Contraindicated with

hypersensitivity to any components of the product. Use with caution in children and infants. Pregnancy category C; use only if benefits outweigh risks. Use with caution in nursing mothers. Use with caution with viral, bacterial, and fungal infections. Use an appropriate antiinfective agent for underlying infections. If a favorable response is not seen, stop corticosteroid therapy until infection is controlled. Use with caution on face, groin, axillae, and intertriginous areas because of resulting striae and atrophy. Systemic absorption may occur; monitor for symptoms (Cushing syndrome, HPA axis suppression, hyperglycemia, glycosuria) especially in children and infants and in patients with liver failure.

Side effects/adverse reactions: Burning, itching, dryness, irritation, stinging, soreness, acne, numbness of the fingers, folliculitis, hypertrichosis, hypopigmentation, atrophy, secondary infections.

Nursing considerations: For external use only. Avoid contact with eyes. Do not bandage, wrap, cover, or use occlusive dressing unless otherwise directed. Apply only to affected area. Apply sparingly and rub in well. Do not apply to weeping, denuded, or infected areas. If irritation develops, discontinue and notify physician. If treating a child's or infant's diaper area, do not use tight-fitting diapers or plastic pants, which may act as an occlusive dressing. With long-term use, do not discontinue treatment abruptly.

Betamethasone Dipropionate (0.05% ointment, cream, lotion) (Diprosone, Maxivate)

Betamethasone dipropionate ointment and cream are high-potency (class II) topical corticosteroids. Betamethasone dipropionate lotion is a medium-potency (class III) corticosteroid.

Augmented Betamethasone Dipropionate (0.05% cream, ointment, lotion, gel) (Diprolene, Diprolene AF)

Augmented betamethasone dipropionate is betamethasone dipropionate in a special vehicle that augments the penetration of the steroid. The ointment is a very-high-potency (class I) corticosteroid; the cream is a high-potency (class II) corticosteroid. The lotion is a medium-potency (class III) corticosteroid.

Indications: For the treatment of psoriasis, contact dermatitis, eczema, and pruritus.

Administration: Apply sparingly once or twice daily.

Precautions/contraindications: Contraindicated with hypersensitivity to any component of the product. Use with caution in children and infants. Pregnancy category C; use only if benefits outweigh risks. Use with caution in nursing mothers. Use with caution with viral, bacterial, and fungal infections. Use an appropriate antiinfective agent for underlying infections. If a favorable response is not seen, stop corticosteroid therapy until infection is controlled. Use with caution on face, groin, axillae, and intertriginous areas because of resulting striae and atrophy. Systemic absorption may occur; monitor for symptoms (Cushing syndrome, HPA axis suppression, hyperglycemia, glycosuria), especially in children and infants and in patients with liver failure. Do not use an occlusive dressing with this product.

Side effects/adverse reactions: Burning, itching, dryness, irritation, stinging, soreness, acne, numbness of the fingers, folliculitis, hypertrichosis, hypopigmentation, atrophy, secondary infections.

Nursing considerations: For external use only. Avoid contact with eyes. Do not bandage, wrap, cover, or use occlusive dressing unless otherwise directed. Apply only to affected area. Apply sparingly and rub in well. Do not apply to weeping, denuded, or infected areas. If irritation develops, discontinue and notify physician. If treating a child or infant's diaper area, do not use tight-fitting diapers or plastic pants, which may act as an occlusive dressing. With long-term use, do not discontinue treatment abruptly.

Clobetasol Propionate (0.05% ointment, cream) (Temovate)

Clobetasol propionate is a very-high-potency (class I) topical corticosteroid.

Indications: For the treatment of psoriasis, eczema, contact dermatitis, and pruritus.

Usual dosage: Apply a thin layer twice daily (AM, PM).

Precautions/contraindications: Contraindicated with hypersensitivity to any component of the product. Treatment must be limited to 2 consecutive weeks, and no more that 50 g/week should be used. Do not use in children under 12 years of age. Pregnancy category C; use only if benefits outweigh risks. Use with caution in nursing mothers. Use with caution with bacterial, fungal, or viral infections. Use an appropriate antiinfective agent for underlying infections; if a favorable response is not seen, stop corticosteroid therapy until infection is controlled. Do not use on the face, groin, or axillae, or in intertriginous areas because of resulting atrophy and striae. Systemic absorption may occur; symptoms consistent with systemic absorption include Cushing syndrome, HPA axis suppression, hyperglycemia, and glycosuria.

Side effects/adverse reactions: Same as for betamethasone benzoate.

Nursing considerations: For external use only. Avoid contact with the eyes. Do not use an occlusive dressing with this product. Apply only to affected areas; apply sparingly and rub in well. Do not apply to weeping, denuded, or infected areas. If irritation develops, discontinue treatment and notify physician.

Clocortolone Pivalate (0.1% cream) (Cloderm)

Clocortolone pivalate is a medium-potency (class III) topical corticosteroid.

Indications: For the treatment of psoriasis, eczema, contact dermatitis, and pruritus.

Administration: Apply a thin layer once or twice daily.

Precautions/contraindications: Contraindicated with hypersensitivity to any component of the product. Use with caution in children and infants. Pregnancy category C; use only if benefits outweigh risks. Use with caution in nursing mothers. Use with caution with viral, bacterial, and fungal infections. Use an appropriate antiinfective agent for underlying infections. If a favorable response is not seen, stop corticosteroid therapy until infection is controlled. Use with caution on face, groin, axillae, and intertriginous areas because of resulting striae and atrophy. Systemic absorption may occur; monitor for symptoms (Cushing syndrome, HPA axis suppression, hyperglycemia, glycosuria), especially in children and infants and in patients with liver failure.

Side effects/adverse reactions: Burning, itching, dryness, irritation, stinging, soreness, acne, numbness of the fingers, folliculitis, hypertrichosis, hypopigmentation, atrophy, secondary infections.

Nursing considerations: For external use only. Avoid contact with eyes. Do not bandage, wrap, cover, or use occlusive dressing unless otherwise directed. Apply only to affected area. Apply sparingly and rub in well. Do not apply to weeping, denuded, or infected areas. If irritation develops, discontinue and notify physician. If treating a child or infant's diaper area, do not use tight-fitting diapers or plastic pants, which may act as an occlusive dressing. With long-term use, do not discontinue treatment abruptly.

Desonide (0.05% ointment, cream, lotion) (DesOwen, Tridesilon)

Desonide is a low-potency (class IV) topical corticosteroid.

Indications: For the treatment of psoriasis, eczema, contact dermatitis, and pruritus.

Administration: Apply a thin layer two to four times daily. Rub in gently.

Precautions/contraindications: Contraindicated with hypersensitivity to any component of the product. Use with caution in children and infants. Pregnancy category C; use only if benefits outweigh risks. Use with caution in nursing mothers. Use with caution with viral, bacterial, and fungal infections. Use an appropriate antiinfective agent for underlying infections. If a favorable response is not seen, stop corticosteroid therapy until infection is controlled. Use with caution on face, groin, axillae, and intertriginous areas because of re-

sulting striae and atrophy. Systemic absorption may occur; monitor for symptoms (Cushing syndrome, HPA axis suppression, hyperglycemia, glycosuria), especially in children and infants and in patients with liver failure.

Side effects/adverse reactions: Burning, itching, dryness, irritation, stinging, soreness, acne, numbness of the fingers, folliculitis, hypertrichosis, hypopigmentation, atrophy, secondary infections.

Nursing considerations: For external use only. Avoid contact with eyes. Do not bandage, wrap, cover, or use occlusive dressing unless otherwise directed. Apply only to affected area. Apply sparingly and rub in well. Do not apply to weeping, denuded, or infected areas. If irritation develops, discontinue and notify physician. If treating a child or infant's diaper area, do not use tight-fitting diapers or plastic pants, which may act as an occlusive dressing. With long-term use, do not discontinue treatment abruptly.

Desoximetasone (0.05% cream; 0.25% cream, ointment; 0.05% gel) (Topicort, Topicort LP)

Desoximetasone 0.25% cream and ointment and 0.05% gel are high-potency (class II) topical corticosteroids. Desoximetasone 0.05% cream is a medium-potency (class III) corticosteroid.

Indications: Relief of inflammatory and pruritic manifestations of corticosteroid-responsive dermatoses (e.g., contact dermatitis, eczema, psoriasis, pruritus).

Administration: Apply a thin film twice daily. Rub in gently.

Precautions/contraindications: Contraindicated with hypersensitivity to any component of the product. Use with caution in children and infants. Pregnancy category C; use only if the benefits outweigh the risks. Use with caution in nursing mothers. Use with caution with viral, bacterial, and fungal infections. Use an appropriate antiinfective agent for underlying bacterial or fungal infection; if a favorable response is not seen, stop corticosteroid therapy until infection is controlled. Do not use on the face or groin or in intertriginous areas because of resulting striae and atrophy. Systemic absorption may occur; side effects consistent with systemic absorption include Cushing syndrome, hypothalmo-pituitary-adrenocortical (HPA) axis suppression, hyperglycemia, and glycosuria, especially in children, infants, and patients with liver failure.

Side effects/adverse reactions: Burning, dryness, itching, irritation, stinging, soreness, acne, folliculitis, hypertrichosis, numbness of the fingers, hypopigmentation, atrophy, secondary infection.

Nursing considerations: For external use only to affected areas. Avoid contact with the eyes. Do not bandage, wrap, cover, or use occlusive dressing on affected area unless otherwise directed. Do not apply to weeping, denuded, or infected areas. If irritation develops, discontinue treatment and notify physician. If treating a child or infant in the diaper area, do not use tight-fitting diapers or plastic pants, which can act as an occlusive dressing. With long-term use, do not discontinue treatment abruptly.

Diflorasone Diacetate (0.05% ointment, cream) (Psorcon, Florone, Maxiflor)

Diflorasone diacetate ointment (Psorcon) is a very-high-potency (class I) topical corticosteroid. The cream and emollient-based ointment are high-potency (class II) corticosteroids.

Indications: Relief of inflammatory and pruritic manifestations of corticosteroid-responsive dermatoses (e.g., contact dermatitis, eczema, psoriasis, pruritus).

Administration: Apply to affected areas twice daily. Rub in gently.

Precautions/contraindications: Contraindicated with hypersensitivity to any component of the product. Use with caution in children and infants. Pregnancy category C; use only if the benefits outweigh the risks. Use with caution in nursing mothers. Use with caution with viral, bacterial, and fungal infections. Use an appropriate antiinfective agent for underlying bacterial or fungal infection; if a favorable response is not seen, stop corticosteroid therapy until infection is controlled. Do not use on the face or groin or in intertriginous areas because of resulting striae and atrophy. Systemic absorption may occur; side effects consistent with systemic absorption include Cushing syndrome, hypo-thalamo-pituitary-adrenocortical (HPA) axis suppression, hyperglycemia, and glycosuria, especially in children, infants, and patients with liver failure.

Side effects/adverse reactions: Burning, dryness, itching, irritation, stinging, soreness, acne, folliculitis, hypertrichosis, numbness of the fingers, hypopigmentation, atrophy, secondary infection.

Nursing considerations: For external use only to affected areas. Avoid contact with the eyes. Do not bandage, wrap, cover, or use occlusive dressing on affected area unless otherwise directed. Do not apply to weeping, denuded, or infected areas. If irritation develops, discontinue treatment and notify physician. If treating a child or infant in the diaper area, do not use tight-fitting diapers or plastic pants, which can act as an occlusive dressing. With long-term use, do not discontinue treatment abruptly.

Halcinonide (0.1% cream, ointment) (Halog, Halog-E)

Halcinonide is a high-potency (class II) topical corticosteroid.

Indications: Relief of inflammatory and pruritic manifestations of corticosteroid-responsive dermatoses

(e.g., contact dermatitis, eczema, psoriasis, pruritus).

Administration: Apply a thin layer to affected area two to four times daily. Rub in gently.

Precautions/contraindications: Contraindicated with hypersensitivity to any component of the product. Use with caution in children and infants. Pregnancy category C; use only if the benefits outweigh the risks. Use with caution in nursing mothers. Use with caution with viral, bacterial, and fungal infections. Use an appropriate antiinfective agent for underlying bacterial or fungal infection; if a favorable response is not seen, stop corticosteroid therapy until infection is controlled. Do not use on the face or groin or in intertriginous areas because of resulting striae and atrophy. Systemic absorption may occur; side effects consistent with systemic absorption include Cushing syndrome, hypo-thalamo-pituitary-adrenocortical (HPA) axis suppression, hyperglycemia, and glycosuria, especially in children, infants, and patients with liver failure.

Side effects/adverse reactions: Burning, dryness, itching, irritation, stinging, soreness, acne, folliculitis, hypertrichosis, numbness of the fingers, hypopigmentation, atrophy, secondary infection.

Nursing considerations: For external use only to affected areas. Avoid contact with the eyes. Do not bandage, wrap, cover, or use occlusive dressing on affected area unless otherwise directed. Do not apply to weeping, denuded, or infected areas. If irritation develops, discontinue treatment and notify physician. If treating a child or infant in the diaper area, do not use tight-fitting diapers or plastic pants, which can act as an occlusive dressing. With long-term use, do not discontinue treatment abruptly.

Fluocinolone Acetonide (0.025% cream, ointment; 0.01% cream, solution; 0.2% cream) (Synalar, Synalar-HP)

Fluocinolone acetonide 0.2% cream is a high-potency (class II) topical corticosteroid. Fluocinolone acetonide 0.025% cream and ointment are medium-potency (class III) corticosteroids. Fluocinolone acetonide 0.01% cream and solution are low-potency (class IV) corticosteroids.

Indications: Relief of inflammatory and pruritic manifestations of corticosteroid-responsive dermatoses (e.g., contact dermatitis, eczema, psoriasis, pruritus).

Administration: Apply a thin film two to four times daily. Rub in gently.

Precautions/contraindications: Contraindicated with hypersensitivity to any component of the product. Use with caution in children and infants. Pregnancy category C; use only if the benefits outweigh the risks. Use with caution in nursing mothers. Use with caution with viral, bacterial, and fungal infections. Use an appropriate antiinfective agent for underlying bacterial or fungal infection; if a favorable response is not seen, stop corticosteroid therapy until infection is controlled. Do not use on the face or groin or in intertriginous areas because of resulting striae and atrophy. Systemic absorption may occur; side effects consistent with systemic absorption include Cushing syndrome, hypothalamo-pituitary-adrenocortical (HPA) axis suppression, hyperglycemia, and glycosuria, especially in children, infants, and patients with liver failure.

Side effects/adverse reactions: Burning, dryness, itching, irritation, stinging, soreness, acne, folliculitis, hypertrichosis, numbness of the fingers, hypopigmentation, atrophy, secondary infection.

Nursing considerations: For external use only to affected areas. Avoid contact with the eyes. Do not bandage, wrap, cover, or use occlusive dressing on affected area unless otherwise directed. Do not apply to weeping, denuded, or infected areas. If irritation develops, discontinue treatment and notify physician. If treating a child or infant in the diaper area, do not use tight-fitting diapers or plastic pants, which can act as an occlusive dressing. With long-term use, do not discontinue treatment abruptly.

Fluocinonide (0.05% cream, ointment, gel, solution) (Lidex, Lidex-E)

Fluocinonide is a high-potency (class II) topical corticosteroid.

Indications: Relief of inflammatory and pruritic manifestations of corticosteroid-responsive dermatoses (e.g., contact dermatitis, eczema, psoriasis, pruritus).

Administration: Apply a thin film to affected area two to four times daily. Rub in well.

Precautions/contraindications: Contraindicated with hypersensitivity to any component of the product. Use with caution in children and infants. Pregnancy category C; use only if the benefits outweigh the risks. Use with caution in nursing mothers. Use with caution with viral, bacterial, and fungal infections. Use an appropriate antiinfective agent for underlying bacterial or fungal infection; if a favorable response is not seen, stop corticosteroid therapy until infection is controlled. Do not use on the face or groin or in intertriginous areas because of resulting striae and atrophy. Systemic absorption may occur; side effects consistent with systemic absorption include Cushing syndrome, hypothalamo-pituitary-adrenocortical (HPA) axis suppression, hyperglycemia, and glycosuria, especially in children, infants, and patients with liver failure.

Side effects/adverse reactions: Burning, dryness, itching, irritation, stinging, soreness, acne, folliculitis, hypertrichosis, numbness of the fingers, hypopigmentation, atrophy, secondary infection.

Nursing considerations: For external use only to affected areas. Avoid contact with the eyes. Do not bandage, wrap, cover, or use occlusive dressing on affected area unless otherwise directed. Do not apply to weeping, denuded, or infected areas. If irritation develops, discontinue treatment and notify physician. If treating a child or infant in the diaper area, do not use tight-fitting diapers or plastic pants, which can act as an occlusive dressing. With long-term use, do not discontinue treatment abruptly.

Hydrocortisone (0.25% lotion; 0.5% cream, ointment, gel; 1% cream, ointment, lotion, solution; 2% lotion; 2.5% cream, lotion) (Hytone, Cort-Dome, Cetacort, Cortaid)

Hydrocortisone is a low-potency (class IV) topical corticosteroid.

Indications: For the treatment of psoriasis, eczema, contact dermatitis, pruritus.

Administration: Apply a thin film two to four times daily. Rub in gently.

Precautions/contraindications: Contraindicated with hypersensitivity to any components of the product. Use with caution in children and infants. Pregnancy category C; use only if benefits outweigh risks. Use with caution in nursing mothers. Use with caution with viral, bacterial, and fungal infections. Use an appropriate antiinfective agent for underlying infections. If a favorable response is not seen, stop corticosteroid therapy until infection is controlled. Use with caution on face, groin, axillae, and intertriginous areas because of resulting striae and atrophy. Systemic absorption may occur; monitor for symptoms (Cushing syndrome, HPA axis suppression, hyperglycemia, glycosuria), especially in children and infants and in patients with liver failure.

Side effects/adverse reactions: Burning, itching, dryness, irritation, stinging, soreness, acne, numbness of the fingers, folliculitis, hypertrichosis, hypopigmentation, atrophy, secondary infections.

Nursing considerations: For external use only. Avoid contact with eyes. Do not bandage, wrap, cover, or use occlusive dressing unless otherwise directed. Apply only to affected area. Apply sparingly and rub in well. Do not apply to weeping, denuded, or infected areas. If irritation develops, discontinue and notify physician. If treating a child's or infant's diaper area, do not use tight-fitting diapers or plastic pants, which may act as an occlusive dressing. With long-term use, do not discontinue treatment abruptly.

Mometasone Furoate (0.1% cream, ointment, lotion) (Elocon)

Mometasone furoate is a medium-potency (class III) topical corticosteroid.

Indications: For the treatment of psoriasis, eczema, contact dermatitis, pruritus.

Administration: Apply a thin film to affected areas once daily. Rub in gently.

Precautions/contraindications: Contraindicated with hypersensitivity to any components of the product. Use with caution in children and infants. Pregnancy category C; use only if benefits outweigh risks. Use with caution in nursing mothers. Use with caution with viral, bacterial, and fungal infections. Use an appropriate antiinfective agent for underlying infections. If a favorable response is not seen, stop corticosteroid therapy until infection is controlled. Use with caution on face, groin, axillae, and intertriginous areas because of resulting striae and atrophy. Systemic absorption may occur; monitor for symptoms (Cushing syndrome, HPA axis suppression, hyperglycemia, glycosuria), especially in children and infants and in patients with liver failure. Do not use an occlusive dressing with this product.

Side effects/adverse reactions: Burning, itching, dryness, irritation, stinging, soreness, acne, numbness of the fingers, folliculitis, hypertrichosis, hypopigmentation, atrophy, secondary infections.

Nursing considerations: For external use only. Avoid contact with eyes. Do not bandage, wrap, cover, or use occlusive dressing unless otherwise directed. Apply only to affected area. Apply sparingly and rub in well. Do not apply to weeping, denuded, or infected areas. If irritation develops, discontinue and notify physician. If treating a child's or infant's diaper area, do not use tight-fitting diapers or plastic pants, which may act as an occlusive dressing. With long-term use, do not discontinue treatment abruptly.

Triamcinolone Acetonide (0.025% cream, ointment, lotion; 0.1% cream, ointment, lotion; 0.5% cream, ointment) (Aristocort, Kenalog)

Triamcinolone acetonide 0.5% is a high-potency (class II) topical corticosteroid. The 0.1% strength is a medium-potency (class III) corticosteroid. The 0.025% formulation is a low-potency (class IV) corticosteroid.

Indications: For the treatment of psoriasis, eczema, contact dermatitis, and pruritus.

Administration: Apply to affected area two to four times daily. Rub in gently.

Precautions/contraindications: Contraindicated with hypersensitivity to any components of the product. Use with caution in children and infants. Pregnancy category C; use only if benefits outweigh risks. Use with caution in nursing mothers. Use with caution with viral, bacterial, and fungal infections. Use an appropriate antiinfective agent for underlying infections. If a favorable response is not seen, stop corticosteroid therapy until infection is controlled. Use with caution on face, groin, axillae, and intertriginous areas because of resulting striae and atrophy. Systemic absorption may oc-

cur; monitor for symptoms (Cushing syndrome, HPA axis suppression, hyperglycemia, glycosuria), especially in children and infants and in patients with liver failure.

Side effects/adverse reactions: Burning, itching, dryness, irritation, stinging, soreness, acne, numbness of the fingers, folliculitis, hypertrichosis, hypopigmentation, atrophy, secondary infections.

Nursing considerations: For external use only. Avoid contact with eyes. Do not bandage, wrap, cover, or use occlusive dressing unless otherwise directed. Apply only to affected area. Apply sparingly and rub in well. Do not apply to weeping, denuded, or infected areas. If irritation develops, discontinue and notify physician. If treating a child or infant's diaper area, do not use tight-fitting diapers or plastic pants, which may act as an occlusive dressing. With long-term use, do not discontinue treatment abruptly.

PHOTOSENSITIZERS

Methoxsalen (10 mg capsules; 1% lotion) (Oxsoralen, Oxsoralen-Ultra, 8-Mop)

Methoxsalen is a psoralen derivative that is used as a pigmentating agent. It increases melanization of the epidermis and thickening of the stratum corneum. It also acts as a photosensitizer, bonding with cellular DNA and causing cell damage when exposed to UVA, with a resultant decrease in cell turnover.

Indications: Treatment of severe psoriasis and vitiligo.

Usual dosage: *Psoriasis:* Individualized according to weight. Take dose 2 hours before UVA exposure. Take with food or milk. (Oxsoralen-Ultra has greater bioavailability and an earlier photosensitization onset time of 1.5 to 2 hours. It is *not* interchangeable with Oxsoralen.)

Vitiligo: 20 mg once a day with food or milk 2 to 4 hours before UVA exposure. Administer on alternate days only. *Lotion:* Apply to a small, well-defined area 1 to 2 hours before exposure to UVA light. Treatment intervals are regulated by erythematous response, but are usually once a week or less frequent.

Precautions/contraindications: Contraindicated with hypersensitivity, increased risk for the development of melanoma, squamous cell carcinoma, aphakia, diseases associated with photosensitivity, albinism, and cataracts. Do not give to children 12 years of age or younger. Pregnancy category C; use only if clearly needed. Use with caution in nursing mothers. Methoxsalen accumulates in the lens of the eye and can cause cataracts if exposed to UVA. Have patient wear UVA-absorbing wraparound sunglasses for 24 hours after taking methoxsalen. Use with caution in patients with hepatic or cardiac disease, in individuals with tartrazine sensitivity, and in those taking photosensitizing drugs. Eating foods containing furocoumarin (limes, figs, parsley, parsnips, mustard, carrots, and celery) may be harmful. Do not dispense lotion to patient.

Side effects/adverse reactions: Severe burns when exposure to UV light is severe, rash, pruritus, peeling, erythema, nausea, nervousness, insomnia, dizziness, headache, depression, malaise, hypopigmentation, leg cramps, herpes simplex, hypotension.

Pharmacokinetics: 95% absorbed from the GI tract. Food increases peak serum concentrations. Oxsoralen-Ultra reaches peak levels in 30 minutes to 1 hour. Regular Oxsoralen reaches peak levels in 1½ to 6 hours. Half-life is 2 hours. Methoxsalen is rapidly metabolized in the liver, and primarily excreted in the urine.

Interactions: Photosensitizing drugs (phenothiazines, thiazides, sulfonamides, tetracyclines, griseofulvin, coal tar derivatives, nalidixic acid, and halogenated salicylamides) can increase the effects of methoxsalen.

Nursing considerations: Take with food or milk to prevent GI upset. Give on alternate days, not consecutive days. Use lotion for small areas. Treat systemically for large areas. Protect eyes with UVA-absorbing wraparound sunglasses for at least 24 hours. Protect lips and skin from UVA exposure for at least 8 hours after oral treatment. Protect eyes for 24 hours after ingestion of the drug. With use of lotion, treated skin may be highly photosensitive for several days. Avoid direct or indirect sunlight. Use sunscreen or protective clothing. Pruritus can be treated with bland emollients. Repigmentation in vitiligo may take 6 to 9 months.

TOPICAL ANESTHETIC

Pramoxine Hydrochloride (0.5% cream; 1% cream, liquid, lotion, gel, ointment) (Pramegel, Tronothane, Procto Foam)

Pramoxine is a topical anesthetic that inhibits impulses from sensory nerves.

Indications: Treatment of pruritus, sunburn, minor burns, and rectal pain and irritation.

Usual dosage: Apply to affected areas as needed, usually every 3 to 4 hours. Use rectally up to five times daily or after each bowel movement.

Precautions/contraindications: Contraindicated with hypersensitivity to any components of the products. Not for ophthalmic use. For external use only. Use the lowest amount effective, and do not apply to large areas of the body. Pregnancy category C; use only if clearly

needed. Use with caution in children under 12 years of age.

Side effects/adverse reactions: Rash, irritation, burning, stinging, urticaria, eczema, sensitization.

Nursing considerations: Apply to clean, dry affected area. Monitor for allergic reactions, rash, erythema, swelling. Do not apply to infected or denuded skin. When using rectally, use applicator. Can be applied to gauze or bandage before applying to the skin.

ANTIHISTAMINES

Astemizole (10 mg tablets) (Hismanal)

Astemizole is a histamine H_1-receptor antagonist that is chemically distinct from other antihistamines. It affects peripheral H_1-receptors and does not reach central receptors in the brain; as a result, astemizole has fewer side effects than most antihistamines.

Indications: Relief of allergic rhinitis and chronic idiopathic urticaria.

Usual dosage: One table daily, taken on an empty stomach at least 1 hour before eating or 2 hours after.

Precautions/contraindications: Contraindicated with hypersensitivity to any component of the product. Pregnancy category C; use only if benefits justify risks. Use with caution in nursing mothers. Do not give concomitantly with macrolide antibiotics (erythromycin, azithromycin, clarithromycin, troleandomycin) or with ketoconazole, itraconazole, or other azole-type antifungal agents (fluconazole, miconazole). These drugs inhibit astemizole metabolism via the cytochrome P-450 pathway, resulting in elevated plasma levels of astemizole, which can lead to prolonged QT intervals and serious cardiac effects (death, cardiac arrest, and ventricular arrhythmia, including torsades de pointes). Do not use in patients with conditions that may lead to prolongation of QT intervals, or in those taking antiarrhythmic drugs, bepridil, or certain psychotropic drugs. Do not use in patients with electrolyte abnormalities or significant hepatic dysfunction.

Use with caution in patients with impaired renal function, and in those with lower respiratory disease caused by anticholinergic (drying effect) action.

Side effects/adverse reactions: Adverse cardiovascular effects: Ventricular tachyrhythmias (torsades de pointes, ventricular fibrillation, and cardiac arrest). Hypotension, palpitations, syncope, and dizziness are also possible and may reflect undetected ventricular arrhythmias. Other side effects may include headache, increased appetite, weight gain, nausea, nervousness, dizziness, dry mouth, elevated liver enzymes, bronchospasm, depression, photosensitivity, and rash.

Pharmacokinetics: Peak plasma concentrations are reached within 1 hour. The half-life is biphasic: distribution phase, 20 hours; elimination phase, 7 to 11 days. Astemizole is almost completely metabolized by the liver and is excreted primarily in the feces (50% to 70%).

Nursing considerations: Do not exceed dosage of 10 mg daily. Absorption is reduced by 60% when drug is taken with food. Because the onset of action is slow, astemizole should not be given for acute relief of symptoms. Monitor for symptoms of underlying ventricular arrhythmias (hypotension, palpitations, syncope). Store in a tightly closed container in a cool, dry place, away from heat or direct sunlight.

Clemastine Fumarate (1.34 mg; 2.68 mg tablet; 0.67 mg/5 ml syrup) (Tavist, Tavist-1)

Clemastine fumarate is an antihistamine belonging to the ethanolamine class. It acts by competitively antagonizing histamine at the H_1-receptor site.

Indications: For relief of symptoms associated with allergic rhinitis and for mild uncomplicated allergic skin manifestations of urticaria and angioedema. Clemastine fumarate is indicated for dermatologic conditions at the 2.68 mg dosage only.

Usual dosage: 1.34 mg twice daily, or up to 6 tablets/day; 2.68 mg once daily, or up to three times daily.

Precautions/contraindications: Contraindicated with hypersensitivity to any component of the product. Pregnancy category B; use only if clearly needed. Do not use in nursing mothers. Do not use to treat lower respiratory tract symptoms, including asthma. Do not give concomitantly with monoamine oxidase (MAO) inhibitors. Use with caution in patients who have narrow-angle glaucoma, stenosing peptic ulcer, pyloroduodenal obstruction, prostatic hypertrophy, bladder neck obstruction, bronchial asthma, glaucoma, hyperthyroidism, cardiovascular disease, or hypertension. Use with caution in conjunction with other CNS depressants and alcohol.

Side effects/adverse reactions: Drowsiness is the most common side effect. Dizziness, sedation, and hypotension also may occur and are seen more often in the elderly. Epigastric distress is another common side effect. Other side effects include urticaria, rash, photosensitivity, dry mouth, headache, palpitations, hemolytic anemia, thrombocytopenia, agranulocytosis, urinary frequency, difficulty urinating, thickening of bronchial secretions, tightness of the chest, wheezing, and nasal congestion.

Pharmacokinetics: Peak plasma levels occur in 2 to 4 hours. Drug is excreted primarily in the urine.

Interactions: MAO inhibitors prolong and intensify the anticholinergic effects of clemastine fumarate. CNS depression is increased by interaction with barbiturates, narcotics, hypnotics, alcohol, and tricyclic antidepressants.

Nursing considerations: Caution patients about drowsiness and use of the drug while driving or performing hazardous activities. If GI upset occurs, take drug with food. Watch for urinary retention, frequency, or dysuria. Monitor respiratory status for thickening of bronchial secretions, wheezing.

Cyproheptadine Hydrochloride (4 mg tablets; 2 mg/5 ml syrup) (Periactin)

Cyproheptadine hydrochloride is an antihistamine belonging to the piperidine class. It has both antiserotonin and antihistamine actions. It acts by competing with serotonin and histamine at their respective receptor sites.

Indications: Treatment of allergic rhinitis, allergic conjunctivitis, and allergic skin manifestations of urticaria, cold urticaria, and angioedema.

Usual dosage: *Adults:* 4 mg three times daily, or up to 0.5 mg/kg/day.

Children 7 to 14 years: 4 mg two or three times daily, not to exceed 16 mg/day.

Children 2 to 6 years: 2 mg two or three times daily, not to exceed 12 mg/day.

Precautions/contraindications: Contraindicated with hypersensitivity to any component of the product. Pregnancy category B; use only if clearly needed. Do not give to nursing mothers (drug is excreted in breast milk). Do not give to newborns or premature infants. Do not give with MAO inhibitors. Use with considerable caution in elderly or debilitated patients (side effects are more pronounced in the elderly), and in patients with angle-closure glaucoma, stenosing peptic ulcer, prostatic hypertrophy, bladder neck obstruction, or pyloroduodenal obstruction. Use with caution in children (safety for use in children under 2 years of age has not been established) and in patients with lower respiratory disease, glaucoma, hyperthyroidism, hypertension, or cardiovascular disease. Use with caution when taking other CNS depressants or alcohol, and when driving or performing hazardous activities.

Side effects/adverse reactions: Drowsiness; dizziness; poor coordination; confusion; restlessness; rash; photosensitivity; blurred vision; tinnitus; hypotension; palpitations; tachycardia; mouth, nose, and throat dryness; GI upset; urinary retention or frequency; thickening of respiratory secretions; chest tightness; wheezing; increased appetite.

Interactions: MAO inhibitors prolong and intensify the anticholinergic effects of cyproheptadine. Alcohol and other depressants increase cyproheptadine's CNS depressant effects.

Pharmacokinetics: The duration of action of cyproheptadine is 4 to 6 hours. The drug is metabolized in the liver, excreted by the kidneys, and excreted in breast milk.

Nursing considerations: Caution patient about use while driving or performing hazardous activities. Urge patient to try to avoid use with alcohol and other CNS depressant drugs. Watch for urinary retention, urinary frequency, or dysuria. Monitor respiratory status: thickening of bronchial secretions, wheezing. Give with food if GI upset occurs.

Diphenhydramine Hydrochloride (25 mg-50 mg capsule; 12.5 mg/5 ml elixir; 10 mg/ml and 50 mg/ml injection) (Benadryl, Nytol, Sominex)

Diphenhydramine hydrochloride is an antihistamine in the ethanolamine class. It acts by competing with histamine at the H_1-receptor sites.

Indications: Treatment of allergy symptoms, rhinitis, urticaria, motion sickness, and parkinsonism; insomnia, and as a cough suppressant.

Usual dosage: *Adults:* 25 to 50 mg three or four times daily, not to exceed 400 mg/day. For nighttime sleep, 50 mg hs. IM/IV: 10 to 50 mg, not to exceed 400 mg/day.

Children (over 20 pounds): 12.5 to 25 mg three or four times daily, not to exceed 300 mg/day. PO/IM/IV: 5 mg/kg/day.

Precautions/contraindications: Contraindicated with hypersensitivity to any component of the product. Pregnancy category B; use only if clearly needed. Do not give to nursing mothers (drug is excreted in breast milk). Do not give to newborns or premature infants. Use with considerable caution in patients with angle-closure glaucoma, stenosing peptic ulcer, prostatic hypertrophy, bladder neck obstruction, or pyloroduodenal obstruction. Use with caution in children or the elderly or debilitated (side effects are more pronounced in the elderly), and in patients with lower respiratory disease, glaucoma, hyperthyroidism, hypertension, or cardiovascular disease. Use with caution when taking other CNS depressants or alcohol, and when driving or performing hazardous activities.

Side effects/adverse reactions: Sedation, sleepiness, dizziness, disturbed coordination, stomach upset, and thickening of bronchial secretions are the most common side effects. Restlessness; irritability; rash; photosensitivity; blurred vision; tinnitus; hypotension; palpitations; tachycardia; dry mouth, nose, and throat; urinary retention; urinary frequency; dysuria; wheezing; chest tightness; hemolytic anemia; thrombocytopenia; and agranulocytosis also may occur.

Pharmacokinetics: *PO:* Peak levels in 1 to 3 hours; duration, 4 to 6 hours. *IM:* Onset, ½ hour; peak in 1 to 4 hours; duration, 4 to 6 hours. *IV:* Onset, immediate; duration, 4 to 6 hours. Half-life is 2 to 7 hours. The drug is metabolized in the liver and excreted in the urine.

Interactions: MAO inhibitors prolong and intensify the anticholinergic effects of diphenhydramine. Alcohol and other CNS depressants increase the CNS depressant effects of the drug.

Nursing considerations: Caution patient about use when driving or performing hazardous activities. Urge patient to try to avoid use with alcohol and other CNS depressants. Watch for urinary retention, urinary frequency, dysuria. Monitor respiratory status: thickening of bronchial secretions, wheezing. Give with food if GI upset occurs.

Methdilazine Hydrochloride (3.6 mg chewable tablet; 8 mg tablet; 4 mg/5 ml syrup) (Tacaryl)

Tacaryl is an antihistamine. It is a phenothiazine derivative.

Indications: Treatment of pruritic symptoms in urticaria, nasal allergies, and dermatitis.

Usual dosage: *Adults:* 7.2 to 8 mg two to four times daily.

Children over 3 years: 3.6 to 4 mg two to four times a day.

Precautions/contraindications: Contraindicated in comatose patients or patients taking large amounts of CNS depressants, and patients with bone marrow depression, jaundice, or hypersensitivity to any component of the product or to other phenothiazines. Contraindicated during pregnancy and in newborns, premature infants, and nursing mothers. Do not use with alcohol.

Use with caution in (1) the elderly; (2) patients with underlying diseases that are adversely affected by anticholinergics (e.g., asthma, narrow-angle glaucoma, prostatic hypertrophy, stenosing peptic ulcer, pyloroduodenal obstruction, and bladder neck obstruction); (3) patients taking monoamine oxidase inhibitors; (4) children with sleep apnea or a family history of sudden infant death syndrome (SIDS); and (5) patients with cardiovascular disease, impaired liver function, or a history of ulcers.

Side effects/adverse reactions: Drowsiness is the most common side effect. Extrapyramidal reactions may occur, especially with high doses. Dizziness, headache, tinnitus, blurred vision, postural hypotension, anorexia, nausea, urinary frequency, urinary retention, and thickening of bronchial secretions may also occur. Allergic reactions, including urticaria, dermatitis, asthma, and laryngeal edema, have been reported. Other reactions reported include leukopenia, agranulocytosis, pancytopenia, elevated cholesterol levels, jaundice, and increased prolactin levels.

Interactions: Monoamine oxidase inhibitors used in combination with trimeprazine may cause hypertension and extrapyramidal reactions. The CNS depressant effects of narcotics are potentiated by trimeprazine. Oral contraceptives, reserpine, nylidrin, and thiazides may potentiate the side effects of trimeprazine.

Nursing considerations: Do not crush or chew time-release formulation. May cause drowsiness; warn patient about driving or operating heavy machinery. Watch for urinary retention, dysuria, urinary frequency, extrapyramidal symptoms, and hypotension. In patients with respiratory impairment, watch for thickening of bronchial secretions, wheezing, and chest tightness.

Terfenadine (60 mg tablets) (Seldane)

Terfenadine is a histamine-1 receptor antagonist that is chemically distinct from other antihistamines. It is classified as a butyrophenone derivative. It acts on peripheral H_1-receptors and not central H_1-receptors in the brain; as a result, it causes fewer side effects than are normally associated with antihistamines.

Indications: Relief of allergic rhinitis and associated symptoms (sneezing, rhinorrhea, pruritus, lacrimation).

Usual dosage: *Adults, children 12 years or older:* One tablet (60 mg) twice daily. *Children 6 to 12 years:* 30 to 60 mg twice daily. *Children 3 to 6 years:* 15 mg twice daily.

Precautions/contraindications: Contraindicated with hypersensitivity to any component of the product. Pregnancy category C; use only if benefits justify risks. Not recommended for nursing mothers. Do not give concomitantly with macrolides (erythromycin, azithromycin, clarithromycin, troleandomycin) or with ketoconazole, itraconazole, or other azole-type antifungal agents (fluconazole, miconazole); these drugs inhibit terfenadine metabolism via a cytochrome P-450 pathway. This inhibition results in elevated plasma levels of terfenadine, which can lead to prolonged QT intervals and serious ventricular arrhythmias, including torsades de pointes. This reaction can be fatal. Do not use in patients with conditions that may lead to prolongation of QT intervals, or in patients taking antiarrhythmic drugs, bepridil, or certain psychotropic drugs. Do not use in patients with electrolyte abnormalities or significant hepatic dysfunction.

Side effects/adverse reactions: Adverse cardiovascular effects: Ventricular tachyrhythmias (torsades de pointes, ventricular fibrillation) and cardiac arrest. Hypotension, palpitations, syncope, and dizziness are also possible and may reflect undetected ventricular arrhythmias. Other side effects may include alopecia, visual disturbances, skin eruption, itching, bronchospasm, cough, depression, dry mouth, change in bowel habits, and elevated liver enzymes. Terfenadine causes less drowsiness than most other antihistamines, because it does not cross the blood-brain barrier.

Pharmacokinetics: Peak plasma levels are reached in 2 hours. Terfenadine is 99% metabolized in the liver by a cytochrome P-450 isoenzyme. The half-life is biphasic: distribution phase, 3½ hours; elimination phase, 20 hours. The drug is 97% protein bound; 40% is excreted in the urine, 60% in the feces.

Nursing considerations: Do not exceed dosage of 60 mg twice a day. Monitor for symptoms of underlying arrhythmias (hypotension, palpitations, syncope). Store in a tightly closed container in a cool place, away from heat or direct sunlight.

Trimeprazine Tartrate (2.5 mg tablets; 5 mg sustained-release capsule; 2.5 mg/5 ml syrup) (Temaril)

Trimeprazine tartrate is a phenothiazine derivative that has antipruritic and antihistaminic properties.

Indications: Treatment of allergic and nonallergic pruritic symptoms, urticaria, and dermatitis.

Usual dosage: *Adults:* 2.5 mg four times a day.

Children over 3 years: 2.5 mg at bedtime or three times a day if needed.

Children 6 months to 3 years: 1.25 mg (½ teaspoon) at bedtime or three times a day if needed.

Precautions/contraindications: Contraindicated in comatose patients or patients taking large amounts of CNS depressants, and patients with bone marrow depression, jaundice, or hypersensitivity to any component of the product or to other phenothiazines. Contraindicated during pregnancy and in newborns, premature infants, and nursing mothers. Do not use with alcohol. Use with caution in (1) the elderly; (2) patients with underlying diseases that are adversely affected by anticholinergics (e.g., asthma, narrow-angle glaucoma, prostatic hypertrophy, stenosing peptic ulcer, pyloroduodenal obstruction, and bladder neck obstruction); (3) patients taking monoamine oxidase inhibitors; (4) children with sleep apnea or a family history of sudden infant death syndrome (SIDS); and (5) patients with cardiovascular disease, impaired liver function, or a history of ulcers.

Side effects/adverse reactions: Drowsiness is the most common side effect. Extrapyramidal reactions may occur, especially with high doses. Dizziness, headache, tinnitus, blurred vision, postural hypotension, anorexia, nausea, urinary frequency, urinary retention, and thickening of bronchial secretions may also occur. Allergic reactions, including urticaria, dermatitis, asthma, and laryngeal edema, have been reported. Other reactions reported include leukopenia, agranulocytosis, pancytopenia, elevated cholesterol levels, jaundice, and increased prolactin levels.

Interactions: Monoamine oxidase inhibitors used in combination with trimeprazine may cause hypertension and extrapyramidal reactions. The CNS depressant effects of narcotics are potentiated by trimeprazine. Oral contraceptives, reserpine, nylidrin, and thiazides may potentiate the side effects of trimeprazine.

Nursing considerations: Do not crush or chew time-release formulation. May cause drowsiness; warn patient about driving or operating heavy machinery. Watch for urinary retention, dysuria, urinary frequency, extrapyramidal symptoms, and hypotension. In patients with respiratory impairment, watch for thickening of bronchial secretions, wheezing, and chest tightness.

A STRINGENTS

Burow's Solution (tablets, packets) (Domeburo, Boropak, Bluboro)

Burow's solution is an astringent wet dressing used to relieve minor skin irritations.

Indications: Treatment of poison ivy, insect bites, athlete's foot, rashes, allergies.

Usual dosage: Dissolve one or two tablets or packets in 16 ounces of water. Do not strain or filter solution. One packet in 16 ounces of water yields a 1:40 dilution; two packets, a 1:20 dilution.

Precautions/contraindications: For external use only; avoid contact with the eyes. Do not use with an occlusive dressing.

Nursing considerations: Can be used as a compress, wet dressing, or soak. When used as a soak, soak affected area for 15 to 30 minutes three times a day. Do not reuse solution. Discard after use. When used as a wet dressing or compress, saturate a clean white cloth or gauze and apply to area. Rewet every 15 to 30 minutes. Repeat as needed. If condition worsens or does not respond after 7 days, discontinue and contact physician.

E MOLLIENTS

Emollients are used to moisturize, lubricate, and soothe dry, irritated skin. Emollients are divided into several types: lanolin; petrolatum; mineral oil; glycerin; vitamins A, D, and E oils; and parabens. The following emollients are commercially available over-the-counter:

Aquaphor
Complex-15
Curel
Eucerin
Keri creme/lotion
Lubriderm
Moisturel
Nivea cream/lotion
Nutraderm
Vaseline

Aveeno Bath (Regular: 100% colloidal oatmeal; oilated: 43% colloidal oatmeal, mineral oil)

Aveeno contains colloidal oatmeal, which acts as an emollient and a natural moisturizer. Oilated Aveeno, which contains mineral oil as well, also acts as an adsorbent skin cleanser.

Indications: Temporary relief of itching and irritation of the skin caused by rashes, eczema, chickenpox, hives, poison ivy, and dry skin. Also used as a skin cleanser.

Usual dosage: Sprinkle contents of one packet into tube under warm running water. Stir to prevent clumping. Bathe once or twice daily for 15 to 20 minutes.

Precautions/contraindications: For external use only; avoid contact with the eyes. Do not use on acutely inflamed areas. Use with caution in tub to avoid slipping.

Nursing considerations: Aveeno is also available as a lotion to be applied topically and as a shower and bath oil, which is used as a skin cleanser and moisturizer.

Lac-Hydrin (12% lactic acid lotion)

Lac-Hydrin is a lotion containing 12% lactic acid that is used to treat dry, rough, scaling skin. Lactic acid is an alpha-hydroxy acid, a naturally occurring humectant. Lac-Hydrin also acts to reduce excessive epidermal keratinization in patients with hyperkeratotic conditions.

Indications: Treatment of dry, scaly skin and ichthyosis vulgaris, and relief of itching caused by these conditions.

Usual dosage: Shake well. Apply twice daily to affected area. Rub in well.

Precautions/contraindications: Contraindicated with hypersensitivity to any components of the product. Use with caution on the face. Mild stinging may occur with use on irritated, inflamed, or sensitive skin. Pregnancy category C; use only when clearly necessary. Use with caution in nursing mothers.

Side effects/adverse reactions: Transient stinging, burning, erythema, peeling, eczema, dryness, hyperpigmentation.

Nursing considerations: For external use only; avoid use in eyes or on lips or mucous membranes. Side effects are more numerous in people with sensitive skin or with ichthyosis vulgaris. Shake bottle well before using.

References

1. Abel EA et al: Drugs in exacerbation of psoriasis, *J Am Acad Dermatol* 15:1007-1022, 1986.
2. American Cancer Society: *Cancer facts and figures—1991*, Atlanta, 1991 The Society.
3. Beare PG, Myers JL: *Principles and practice of adult health nursing*, St Louis, 1990, Mosby.
4. Becker LE, Jraus EW, Tschen E: In Demis D, ed: *Clinical Dermatology*, ed 19, Philadelphia, 1992, JB Lippincott.
5. Belcher A: *Cancer nursing*, St Louis, 1994, Mosby.
6. Bryant RA: *Acute and chronic wounds: nursing management*, St Louis, 1992, Mosby.
7. Burton CS: Stasis dermatitis. In Demis D, ed: *Clinical dematology*, ed 19, Philadelphia, 1992, JB Lippincott.
8. Chapman-Winokur RL, Krull, EA: Senile purpura. In Demis D, ed: *Clinical dermatology*, ed 19, Philadelphia 1992, JB Lippincott.
9. Clark RAF, Adinoff AD: Aeroallergen contact can exacerbate atopic dermatitis: patch tests as a diagnostic tool, *J Am Acad Dermatol* 21(4):863-869, 1989.
10. Clark RAF, Nicol N, Adinoff A: Current concepts in the management of the patient with atopic dermatitis, *Modern Medicine*, 58(3): 78-94, 1990.
11. Clark RAF, Nicol NH, Adinoff AD: Atopic dermatitis. In Sams M, Lynch P, eds: *Principles and practice of dermatology*, Philadelphia, 1990, WB Saunders, pp 365-380.
12. Demis D, ed: *Clinical dermatology*, ed 19, Philadelphia, 1992, JB Lippincott.
13. Diette KM et al: Psoralens and UV-A and UV-B twice weekly for the treatment of psoriasis, *Arch Dermatol* 120:1169-1173, 1984.
14. Driscoll M, Rothi M, Abrahamian L, Grant-Kels J: *J Am Acad Dermatol*, April 1993, pp 595-601.
15. Dunn ML et al: Treatment options for psoriasis, *Am J Nurs*, 88(8):1082-1087, 1988.
16. Ellis CN, Voorhees JJ: Etretinate theraphy, *J Am Acad Dermatol* 1:267-291, 1987.
17. Epstein E: *Common skin disorders*, ed 3, Oradell, NJ, 1988, Medical Economics.
18. Farber EM, Abel EA, Charuworn A: Recent advances in the treatment of psoriasis, *J Am Acad Dermatol* 8:311-321, 1983.
19. Farber EM, Abel EA, Cox AJ: Long-term risks of psoralen and UV-A therapy for psoriasis, *Arch Dermatol* 119:426-431, 1983.
20. Farber EM, Nall L: An appraisal of measures to prevent and control psoriasis, *J Am Acad Dermatol* 10:511-517, 1984.
21. Fekety FR: Erysipelas. In Demis D, ed: *Clinical dermatology*, ed 19, Philadelphia, 1992, JB Lippincott.
22. Fitzpatrick TB: Fundamentals of dermatologic diagnosis. In Fitzpatrick TB, Eisen AZ, Wolff K, Freedberg IM, Austen KF, ed: *Dermatology in general medicine*, New York, 1971, McGraw-Hill.
23. Flory C: Skin assessment, *RN*, June 1992, pp 22-26.
24. Garver J, Wilkin J: Flushing and rosacea: overview and nursing interventions, *Dermatology Nursing*, August 1992, pp 271-277.

25. Habif T: *Clinical dermatology: a color guide to diagnosis and therapy*, ed 2, St Louis, 1990, Mosby.

26. Hill M: Nursing management of adults with skin disorders. In Beare PG, Myers JL, eds: *Principles and practice of adult health nursing*, St Louis, 1994, Mosby.

27. Hill M: The skin: anatomy and physiology, *Dermatology Nursing* 2(1): 13-17, 1990.

28. Huff JC: Erythema multiforme. In Demis D, ed: *Clinical dermatology*, ed 19, Philadelphia, 1992, JB Lippincott.

29. Jablonska S: Warts. In Demis D, ed: *Clinical dermatology*, ed 19, Piladelphia, 1992, JB Lippincott.

30. Kaplan RP, Ahmed AR: Behçet's syndrome. In Demis D, ed: *Clinical dermatology*, ed 19, Philadelphia, 1992, JB Lippincott.

31. Kozinn PJ, Taschdjian CL: Candidosis. In Demis D, ed: *Clinical dermatology*, ed 19, Philadelphia, 1992, JB Lippincott.

32. Lash AA: Systemic lupus erythematosus. II. Diagnosis, treatment modalities, and nursing management, *Medsurg Nursing*, October 1993, pp 375-385.

33. Lash AA: Why so many women? I. Systemic lupus erythematosus, *Medsurg Nursing*, August 1993, pp 259-264.

34. Laudano J, Leach E, Armstrong, R: Acne: therapeutic perspectives with an emphasis on the role of isotretinoin, *Dermatology Nursing*, December 1990, pp 328-336.

35. LeVine MJ, Parrish JA: Outpatient phototherapy of psoriasis, *Arch Dermatol* 116:552-554, 1980.

36. Levy ML: Rubeola (typical and atypical measles). In Demis D, ed: *Clinical dermatology*, ed 19, Philadelphia, 1992, JB Lippincott.

37. Leyden JE, Marples RR, Kligman AM: *Staphylococcus aureus* in the lesions of atopic dermatitis, *Br J Dermatol* 90:525-530, 1974.

38. Lookingbill D, Marks J: *Principles of dermatology*, Philadelphia, 1986, WB Saunders.

39. Menkes A, Stern RS, Arndt KA: Psoriasis treatment with suberythemogenic ultraviolet B radiation and a coal tar extract, *J Am Acad Dermatol* 12:21-25, 1985.

40. Morton P: *Health assessment in nursing*, ed 2, Springhouse PA, 1993, Springhouse Corp.

41. Mudge-Grout C: *Immunologic Disorders*, St Louis, 1993, Mosby.

42. National Center for Health Statistics: Prevalence of dermatologic disease among persons 1-74 years of age: United States advance data from Vital and Health Statistics 572(4), Public Health Service, Washington, DC, Jan 26, 1977, US Government Printing Office.

43. Nicol NH: Atopic dermatitis: the (wet) wrap-up, *Am J Nursing*, 87(12):1560-1564, 1987.

44. Nicol NH: Current considerations and management of atopic dematitis, *Dermatology Nursing* 2:129-138, 1990.

45. Nicol NH: Clark RAF: Therapy of atopic dermatitis. In Farmer E, Provost T, eds: *Current therapy in dermatology—2*, Philadelphia, 1988, BC Decker.

46. Orkin M, Maibach H, Dahl M: *Dermatology*, East Norwalk, Conn, 1991, Appleton & Lange.

47. Pagan K, Pagan T: *Pocket Guide to Laboratory and Diagnostic Tests*, St Louis, 1986, Mosby.

48. Parrish J: *Dermatology and Skin Care*, New York, 1975, McGraw-Hill.

49. Patterson JB: Kaposi's sarcoma. In Demis D, ed: *Clinical dermatology*, ed 19, Philadelphia, 1992, JB Lippincott.

50. *Physicians' Desk Reference*, ed 46, Montvale, NJ, 1992, Medical Economics.

51. Ramier SS: Toxic shock syndrome. In Demis D, ed, *Clinical Dermatology*, ed 19, Philadelphia, 1992, JB Lippincott.

52. Raimer SS, Raimer BG: Rubella (German measles). In Demis D, ed: *Clinical dermatology*, ed 19, Philadelphia, 1992, JB Lippincott.

53. Rajka G: *Atopic dermatitis*, London, 1975, WB Saunders Co Ltd.

54. Reeves J, Maibach H: *Clinical dermatology illustrated: a regional approach*, Artarmon, Australia, 1986, Williams & Wilkins & Associates Pty Limited.

55. Ritchie SR, Thompson PJ: Primary bacterial skin infections, *Dermatology Nursing*, August 1992, pp 261-267.

56. Rosen T, Lanning M, Hill M: *The nurse's atlas of dermatology*, Boston, 1983, Little, Brown & Company.

57. Sampson HA: The role of food allergy and mediator release in atopic dermatitis. *J Allergy Clin Immunol* 81:635, 1988.

58. Sauer G: *Manual of skin diseases*, ed 6, Philadelphia, 1991, JB Lippincott.

59. Seidel H et al: *Mosby's guide to physical examination*, ed 2, St Louis, 1991, Mosby.

60. Sober A: Management of rosacea, *Dermatology Nursing*, December 1992, pp 454-456.

61. Thompson J et al: *Mosby's manual of clinical nursing*, ed 2, St Louis, 1989, Mosby.

62. Thibodeau G, Patton K: *Anatomy and physiology*, ed 2, St Louis, 1993, Mosby.

63. Tyring SK: Herpes simplex. In Demis D, ed, *Clinical dermatology*, ed 19, Philadelphia, 1992, JB Lippincott.

64. Tyring SK: Introduction to virus infections. In Demis S ed: *Clinical dermatology*, ed 19, Philadelphia, 1992, JB Lippincott.

65. Vasarinsh P: *Clinical dermatology*, Boston, 1982, Butterworth.

66. Werner Y: The water content of the stratum corneum in patients with atopic dermatitis, *Acta Derm Venereol* [Stockh] 66:281-284, 1986.

67. Wilkin JK: Erythema. In Demis D., ed, *Clinical dermatology*, ed 19, Philadelphia, 1992, JB Lippincott.

68. Wilkin JK: Introduction: diseases of the blood vessels. In Demis D, ed: *Clinical dermatology*, ed 19, Philadelphia, 1992, JB Lippincott.

Index

RESOURCES FOR PATIENTS AND NURSES

American Academy of Dermatology
Pkgs: 930 North Meacham Road
Schaumberg, IL 60173-4965
Corresp: P.O. Box 4014
Schaumberg, IL 60168-4014
(708)330-0230

American Cancer Society
National Headquarters
1599 Clifton Road, NE
Atlanta, GA 30329
(404)320-3333

The American Lupus Society
3914 Del Amo Blvd
Suite 922
Torrance, CA 90503
(310)542-8891 (800)331-1802

Arthritis Foundation
1314 Spring Street, NW
Atlanta, GA 30309
(800)283-7800 (general information)
(404)872-7100

Dermatology Nurses Association
East Holly Avenue
Box 56
Pitman, NJ 08071-0056
(609)256-2300

Dystrophic Epidermolysis Bullosa Research Association (DEBRA)
141 Fifth Avenue
Suite 7-South
New York, NY 10010
(212)995-2220

Ehlers-Danlos National Foundation
P.O. Box 1212
Southgate, MI 48195
(313)282-0180

Foundation for Ichthyosis and Related Skin Types (F.I.R.S.T.)
P.O. Box 20921
Raleigh, NC 27619-0921
(919)782-5728

Lupus Foundation of America
4 Research Place, Suite 180
Rockville, MD 20850-3226
(301)670-9292

National Arthritis and Musculoskeletal and Skin Disease Information Clearing House
Box AMS
National Institutes of Health
Bethesda, MD 20892
(301)496-8188

National Cancer Institute
Office of Cancer Communications
9000 Rockville Pike
Bethesda, MD 20892
(301)496-5583

National Organization for Rare Disorders (NORD)
P.O. Box 8923
New Fairfield, CT 06812
(203)746-6518

National Psoriasis Foundation
6600 SW 92nd Ave.
Suite 300
Portland, OR 97223
(503)244-7404

The Skin Cancer Foundation
245 Fifth Avenue
Suite 2402
New York, NY 10016
(212)725-5176